# Pervasive and Smart Technologies for Healthcare:
## Ubiquitous Methodologies and Tools

Antonio Coronato
*CNR, Italy*

Giuseppe De Pietro
*CNR, Italy*

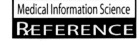

Medical Information Science
REFERENCE

**MEDICAL INFORMATION SCIENCE REFERENCE**

Hershey · New York

| Director of Editorial Content: | Kristin Klinger |
| Director of Book Publications: | Julia Mosemann |
| Acquisitions Editor: | Lindsay Johnston |
| Development Editor: | Christine Bufton |
| Publishing Assistant: | Devvin Earnest |
| Typesetter: | Michael Brehm |
| Production Editor: | Jamie Snavely |
| Cover Design: | Lisa Tosheff |
| Printed at: | Yurchak Printing Inc. |

Published in the United States of America by
Medical Information Science Reference (an imprint of IGI Global)
701 E. Chocolate Avenue
Hershey PA 17033
Tel: 717-533-8845
Fax: 717-533-8661
E-mail: cust@igi-global.com
Web site: http://www.igi-global.com/reference

Library of Congress Cataloging-in-Publication Data

Pervasive and smart technologies for healthcare : ubiquitous methodologies and tools / Antonio Coronato and Giuseppe De Pietro, editors.    p. ; cm.
  Includes bibliographical references and index.
  Summary: "This book reports several experiences concerning the application of pervasive computing technologies, methodologies and tools in healthcare"-- Provided by publisher.  ISBN 978-1-61520-765-7 (h/c)
  1. Ubiquitous computing. 2. Medical informatics. I. Coronato, Antonio, 1972- II. De Pietro, Giuseppe, 1962-
  [DNLM: 1. Biomedical Technology. 2. Delivery of Health Care--methods. 3. Computing Methodologies. 4. Medical Informatics Applications. W 82 P471 2010]
  R859.7.U27P46 2010
  610.285--dc22
                              2009036320

British Cataloguing in Publication Data
A Cataloguing in Publication record for this book is available from the British Library.

# Table of Contents

### Section 1
### Technologies and Applications

*Leroy Lai Yu Chan, The University of New South Wales, Australia*
*Branko George Celler, The University of New South Wales, Australia*
*James Zhaonan Zhang, The University of New South Wales, Australia*
*Nigel Hamilton Lovell, The University of New South Wales, Australia*

*Arianna D'Ulizia, CNR - Istituto di Ricerche sulla Popolazione e le Politiche Sociali, Italy*
*Fernando Ferri, CNR - Istituto di Ricerche sulla Popolazione e le Politiche Sociali, Italy*
*Patrizia Grifoni, CNR - Istituto di Ricerche sulla Popolazione e le Politiche Sociali, Italy*
*Tiziana Guzzo, CNR - Istituto di Ricerche sulla Popolazione e le Politiche Sociali, Italy*

*Shuyan Xie, The University of Alabama, USA*
*Yang Xiao, The University of Alabama, USA*
*Hsiao-Hwa Chen, National Cheng Kung University, Taiwan*

*Matti Linnavuo, Aalto University, Finland*
*Henry Rimminen, Aalto University, Finland*

**Section 3**
**Methodologies and Frameworks**

# Detailed Table of Contents

## Section 1
## Technologies and Applications

**Chapter 1**

*Leroy Lai Yu Chan, The University of New South Wales, Australia*
*Branko George Celler, The University of New South Wales, Australia*
*James Zhaonan Zhang, The University of New South Wales, Australia*
*Nigel Hamilton Lovell, The University of New South Wales, Australia*

It is becoming more critical for developed countries to deliver long-term and financially sustainable healthcare services to an expanding ageing population, especially in the area of residential aged care. There is a general consensus that innovations in the area of Wireless Sensor Networks (WSNs) are key enabling technologies for reaching this goal. The major focus of this chapter is on WSN design considerations for ubiquitous wellness monitoring systems in residential aged care facilities. The major enabling technologies for building a pervasive WSN will be explored, including details on sensor design, wireless communication protocols and network topologies. Also examined are various data processing methods and knowledge management tools to support the collection of sensor data and their subsequent analysis for health assessment. Future systems that incorporate the two aspects of wellness monitoring, vital signs and activities of daily living (ADL) monitoring, will also be introduced.

**Chapter 2**

*Arianna D'Ulizia, CNR - Istituto di Ricerche sulla Popolazione e le Politiche Sociali, Italy*
*Fernando Ferri, CNR - Istituto di Ricerche sulla Popolazione e le Politiche Sociali, Italy*
*Patrizia Grifoni, CNR - Istituto di Ricerche sulla Popolazione e le Politiche Sociali, Italy*
*Tiziana Guzzo, CNR - Istituto di Ricerche sulla Popolazione e le Politiche Sociali, Italy*

Today the biggest challenge of our aging society is to enable people with impairments to have a better quality of life maintaining their independence. The chapter explores how technology can support elderly and disabled people in their home. Firstly, a classification of Smart Home Systems in Safety systems, Environmental control systems, Energy-control-systems, Reminder systems, Medication Dispensing systems, Communication and Entertainment systems is presented. For each of these systems some examples of different technological solutions presented in the literature are described. Moreover, an analysis of social and economic impacts of the use of these technologies on the society is presented. Finally, some studies about the perception and acceptance of these technologies by user are given.

A nursing home is an entity that provides skilled nursing care and rehabilitation services to people with illnesses, injuries or functional disabilities, but most facilities serve the elderly. There are various services that nursing homes provide for different residents' needs, including daily necessity care, mentally disabled, and drug rehabilitation. The levels of care and the care quality provided by nursing homes have increased significantly over the past decade. The trend nowadays is the continuous quality development towards to residents' satisfaction; therefore healthcare technology plays a significant role in nursing home operations. This chapter points out the general information about current nursing home conditions and functioning systems in the United States, which indicates the way that technology and e-health help improve the nursing home development based on the present needs and demanding trends. We also provide a visiting report about Thomasville Nursing Home with the depth of the consideration to how to catch the trends by implementing the technologies.

The chapter describes the state of the art and potentialities of near-field imaging (NFI) technology, applications, and nursing tools in health care. First, principles of NFI are discussed. Various uses of NFI sensor data are presented. The data can be used for indoor tracking, automatic fall detection, activity monitoring, bed exit detection, passage control, vital functions monitoring, household automation and other applications. Special attention is given to the techniques and problems in localization, posture recognition, vital functions recording and additional functions for people identification. Examples of statistical analysis of person behavior are given. Three cases of realized applications of NFI technique are discussed.

    *Esteban Pino, Universidad de Concepción, Concepción, Chile*
    *Dorothy Curtis, Massachusetts Institute of Technology, USA*
    *Thomas Stair, Harvard Medical School, USA*
    *Lucila Ohno-Machado, University of California San Diego, USA*

Patient monitoring is important in many contexts: at mass-casualty disaster sites, in improvised emergency wards, and in emergency room waiting areas. Given the positive history of use of monitoring systems in the hospital during surgery, in the recovery room, or in an intensive care unit, we sought to use recent technological advances to enable patient monitoring in more diverse circumstances: at home, while traveling, and in some less well-monitored areas of a hospital. This chapter presents the authors' experiences in designing, implementing and deploying a wireless disaster management system prototype in a real hospital environment. In addition to a review of related systems, the sensors, algorithms and infrastructure used in our implementation are presented. Finally, general guidelines for ubiquitous methodologies and tools are shared based on the lessons learned from the actual implementation.

    *Nilmini Wickramasinghe, RMIT University, Australia*
    *Indrit Troshani, University of Adelaide Business School, Australia*
    *Steve Goldberg, INET International Inc., Canada*

Diabetes is one of the leading chronic diseases affecting Australians and its prevalence continues to rise. The goal of this study is to investigate the application of a pervasive technology solution developed by INET in the form of a wireless enabled mobile phone to facilitate superior diabetes self-care.

    *Vassiliki Koufi, University of Piraeus, Greece*
    *Flora Malamateniou, University of Piraeus, Greece*
    *George Vassilacopoulos, University of Piraeus, Greece*

Healthcare is an increasingly collaborative enterprise involving many individuals and organizations that coordinate their efforts toward promoting quality and efficient delivery of healthcare through the use of pervasive healthcare information systems. The latter can provide seamless access to well-informed, high-quality healthcare services anywhere, anytime by removing temporal, spatial and other constraints imposed by the technological heterogeneity of existing healthcare information systems. In such environments, concerns over the privacy and security of health information arise. Hence, it is essential to provide an effective access control mechanism that meets the requirements imposed by the least privilege principle by adjusting user permissions continuously in order to adapt to the current situation.

This chapter presents a pervasive grid-based healthcare information system architecture that facilitates authorized access to healthcare processes via wireless devices. Context-aware technologies are used to both automate healthcare processes and regulate access to services and data via a fine-grained access control mechanism.

## Section 2
### Security, Dependability, and Performability

**Chapter 8**

*Ioannis Krontiris, University of Mannheim, Germany*

Body-worn sensors and wireless interconnection of distributed embedded devices facilitate the use of lightweight systems for monitoring vital health parameters like heart rate, respiration rate and blood pressure. Patients can simply wear monitoring systems without restricting their mobility and everyday life. This is particularly beneficial in the context of world's ageing society with many people suffering chronic ailments. However, wireless transmission of sensitive patient data through distributed embedded devices presents several privacy and security implications. In this book chapter we first highlight the security threats in a biomedical sensor networks and identify the requirements that a security solution has to offer. Then we review some popular architectures proposed in the bibliography over the last few years and we discuss the methods that they employ in order to offer security. Finally we discuss some open research questions that have not been addressed so far and which we believe offer promising directions towards making these kinds of networks more secure.

**Chapter 9**

*Tristan Allard, University of Versailles, France*
*Nicolas Anciaux, INRIA Rocquencourt, France*
*Luc Bouganim, INRIA Rocquencourt, France*
*Philippe Pucheral, University of Versailles & INRIA Rocquencourt, France*
*Romuald Thion, INRIA Grenoble, France*

During the last decade, many countries launched ambitious Electronic Health Record (EHR) programs with the objective to increase the quality of care while decreasing its cost. Pervasive healthcare aims itself at making healthcare information securely available anywhere and anytime, even in disconnected environments (e.g., at patient home). Current server-based EHR solutions badly tackle disconnected situations and fail in providing ultimate security guarantees for the patients. The solution proposed in this chapter capitalizes on a new hardware device combining a secure microcontroller (similar to a smart card chip) with a large external Flash memory on a USB key form factor. Embedding the patient folder as well as a database system and a web server in such a device gives the opportunity to manage securely a healthcare folder in complete autonomy. This chapter proposes also a new way of personalizing access control policies to meet patient's privacy concerns with minimal assistance of practitioners. While both proposals are orthogonal, their integration in the same infrastructure allows building trustworthy pervasive healthcare folders.

# Chapter 10

This book chapter provides a systematic analysis of the communication technologies used in healthcare and homecare, their applications and the utilization of the mobile technologies in the healthcare sector by using in addition case studies to highlight the successes and concerns of homecare projects. There are several software applications, appliances, and communication technologies emerging in the homecare arena, which can be combined in order to create a pervasive mobile health system. This study highlights the key areas of concern and describes various types of applications in terms of communications' performance. A comprehensive overview of some of these homecare, healthcare applications and research are presented. The technologies regarding the provision of these systems are described and categorised in two main groups: synchronous and asynchronous communications' systems and technologies. The recent advances in homecare using wireless body sensors and on/off-body networks technologies are discussed along with the provision of future trends for pervasive healthcare delivery. Finally, this book chapter ends with a brief discussion and concluding remarks in succession to the future trends.

# Chapter 11

The evaluation of ubiquitous computing (Ubicomp) applications presents a number of challenges ranging from the optimal recreation of the contextual conditions where technologies will be implemented, to the definition of tasks which often go well beyond the model of human-computer interaction that people are used to interact with. Many contexts, such as hospitals and healthcare which are frequently explored for the deployment of Ubicomp raise additional challenges as a result of the nature of the work where human life can be in risk, privacy of personal records is paramount, and labor is highly distributed across space and time. For the last six years we have been creating and pilot-testing numerous Ubicomp applications in support of hospital work and healthcare (Ubihealth). In this chapter, we discuss the lessons learned from evaluating these applications and organize them as a frame of techniques that assists researchers in selecting the proper method and type of evaluation to be conducted. Based on that frame we discuss a set of principles that designers must consider during evaluation. These principles include maintaining consistency of the activities and techniques used during the evaluation, give proper credit of individual benefits, promote replication of the environment, balance constraints and consider the level of pervasiveness and complexity.

## Section 3
## Methodologies and Frameworks

### Chapter 12

*Werner Kurschl, Upper Austria University of Applied Sciences, Austria*
*Stefan Mitsch, Johannes Kepler University, Austria*
*Johannes Schoenboeck, Vienna University of Technology, Austria*

Pervasive healthcare applications aim at improving habitability by assisting individuals in living autonomously. To achieve this goal, data on an individual's behavior and his or her environment (often collected with wireless sensors) is interpreted by machine learning algorithms; their decision finally leads to the initiation of appropriate actions, e.g., turning on the light. Developers of pervasive healthcare applications therefore face complexity stemming, amongst others, from different types of environmental and vital parameters, heterogeneous sensor platforms, unreliable network connections, as well as from different programming languages. Moreover, developing such applications often includes extensive prototyping work to collect large amounts of training data to optimize the machine learning algorithms. In this chapter we present a model-driven prototyping approach for the development of pervasive healthcare applications to leverage the complexity incurred in developing prototypes and applications. We support the approach with a development environment that simplifies application development with graphical editors, code generators, and pre-defined components.

### Chapter 13

*Toshiyo Tamura, Chiba University, Japan*
*Isao Mizukura, Chiba University, Japan*
*Yutaka Kimura, Kansai Medical Univeristy, Japan*
*Haruyuki Tatsumi, Sapporo Medical University, Japan*

We propose a new home health care system for the acquisition and transmission of data from ordinary home health care appliances, such as blood pressure monitors and weight balances. In this chapter, we briefly explain a standard protocol for data collection and a simple interface to accommodate different monitoring systems that make use of different data protocols. The system provides for one-way data transmission, thus saving power and extending to CCITT. Our standardized protocol was verified during a 1-year field test involving 20 households in Japan. Data transmission errors between home health care devices and the home gateway were 4.21/day with our newly developed standard protocol. Over a 1 year period, we collected and analyzed data from 241,000 separate sources associated with both healthy, home-based patients and chronically ill, clinic-based patients, the latter with physician intervention. We evaluated some possible applications for collecting daily health care data and introduce some of our findings, relating primarily to body weight and blood pressure monitoring for elderly subjects in their own homes.

In this chapter, the program of the Technical University Munich regarding implementation of technologies for an aging society is introduced. Various departments from the faculties of both technology and medicine are working jointly to actualize a technological basis for the development of assistance devices. Industrialized countries such as Japan and Germany will be facing an extreme demographic shift over the next 15 years. More than half of the population will be over 50 years of age. Belief in technological progress – initiated by the innovations of computer and the Internet – harbors the risk that the time required for necessary technological advancements is being significantly underestimated. This article describes the motivation and the concept of hardware architecture for implementation of assistance devices and for integration of pre-existing (or concurrently developed) sensors and concepts.

# Chapter 15

The chapter reviews the state of the art of telemedicine and remote care in the home and the economic and organizational factors that impinge on its future success. Because of the constraints of distance, costs, and availability of providers (doctors and nurses) in specific areas of medical specialties, the model of treating patients in the general hospital is losing its luster in favor of dedicated clinics dispersed in the community and remote care in the home. Such a trend of decentralization of medical services has been in existence for some time. Yet, although technologies are quickly evolving and the need for telemedicine and home care is increasing, the progress of this mode of delivery of medical services has not kept up with the demand. The chapter attempts to review the economic and organizational factors which act as facilitators and barriers to the rapid diffusion of telemedicine and home care. In particular, the chapter explores the case of chronic diseases, and also offers a valuable comparison between two systems of national healthcare: the Italian and the American.

# Preface

The increasing aging of population and the growing number of chronically ill people require that national healthcare systems be prepared, in the next future, and equipped to face such issues and avoid collapses.

The shift to a more consumer driven healthcare market is impacting consumer expectations regarding the quality and consistency of the care they seek. Moreover, patients facing a potentially life threatening disease are seeking the rapid responses from healthcare systems and operators and, possibly, better plans for treatments. On the other hand, the wide diffusion of wireless technologies along with the emerging of new devices and sensors are opening a new market of better and cheaper healthcare applications.

Pervasive healthcare is the emerging discipline about the application of wireless, mobile and intelligent technologies to healthcare. It is related to the development and application of pervasive computing technologies -ubiquitous computing, context-aware computing, ambient intelligence, etc- for healthcare, health and wellness management.

It definitively aims at making healthcare available to anyone, anytime, and anywhere according to the original vision of the pervasive computing paradigm.

Pervasive healthcare, thus, seeks to respond to a variety of pressures on healthcare systems, including the increased incidence of life-style related and chronic diseases, emerging consumerism in healthcare, need for empowering patients and relatives for self-care and management of their own health, and need to provide seamless access to health care services, independent of time and place.

Pervasive healthcare s opening a wide range of innovative applications, from remote monitoring of elder people or ill patients, to new environments like advanced surgery rooms, smart spaces for doctor consulting, assisted living homes, smart hospitals, etc.

Research Community has been producing a remarkable effort with the aim of developing methodologies, techniques, technologies, tools, and applications of pervasive healthcare. Such an effort has been principally pushed by national governs and international organizations (e.g. European Commission) that have studied the benefits of adopting such technologies in healthcare and then funded myriad of projects.

This book reports several experiences concerning the application of pervasive computing technologies, methodologies and tools in healthcare.

It has received the contribution of members of prestigious universities, research institutes and industries, all working, day by day, for identifying solutions to decentralize patient care from hospital to home, to improve disease prevention and self-care, to provide seamless and pervasive access to health care services, etc.

This book is oriented both at ICT community members, who are willing to design and develop advanced pervasive healthcare application, and at healthcare managers and operators, who want to reorganize business processes into hospitals and in the healthcare system in general, as well as procedures for treating ill and/or old people.

The reader can easily figure out the potentialities of pervasive computing in healthcare. In particular, by means of the set of new applications described, as well as the methodologies, technologies and tools presented, the reader can catch the state of the art and future trends.

The book is organized in three main sections: "Technologies and Applications," "Security, Dependability, and Performability," and "Methodologies and Frameworks."

*Technologies and Applications* consists of seven chapters, which present different technologies, like body sensor networks, and relevant applications. *Security, Dependability, and Performability* is focused on critical issues like the reliability of pervasive healthcare solutions, the privacy of clinic information, the ability of remote monitoring services to perform correctly in real environments, etc. *Methodologies and Frameworks* presents methodological approaches to the design, implementation and business management of pervasive healthcare systems along with some enabling frameworks.

To conclude, we sincerely hope that you enjoy the experience of this state of the art book, and get excited by potentialities of new technologies in a crucial field of application like healthcare.

# Acknowledgment

Aside from our authors, to whom we are very grateful, many people contributed in different ways to this book. Obviously, we are very grateful to all reviewers and members of the editorial board who supported us during different steps of the development process. By the way, other people have contributed *in background*, to them our special thanks.

*Antonio Coronato*
*CNR, Italy*

*Giuseppe De Pietro*
*CNR, Italy*

# Section 1
# Technologies and Applications

# Chapter 1
# Pervasive Networks and Ubiquitous Monitoring for Wellness Monitoring in Residential Aged Care

**Leroy Lai Yu Chan**
*The University of New South Wales, Australia*

**Branko George Celler**
*The University of New South Wales, Australia*

**James Zhaonan Zhang**
*The University of New South Wales, Australia*

**Nigel Hamilton Lovell**
*The University of New South Wales, Australia*

## ABSTRACT

*It is becoming more critical for developed countries to deliver long-term and financially sustainable healthcare services to an expanding aging population, especially in the area of residential aged care. There is a general consensus that innovations in the area of Wireless Sensor Networks (WSNs) are key enabling technologies for reaching this goal. The major focus of this chapter is on WSN design considerations for ubiquitous wellness monitoring systems in residential aged care facilities. The major enabling technologies for building a pervasive WSN will be explored, including details on sensor design, wireless communication protocols and network topologies. Also examined are various data processing methods and knowledge management tools to support the collection of sensor data and their subsequent analysis for health assessment. Future systems that incorporate the two aspects of wellness monitoring, vital signs and activities of daily living (ADL) monitoring, will also be introduced.*

DOI: 10.4018/978-1-61520-765-7.ch001

## INTRODUCTION

In developed countries the lifespan of the population is lengthening and the elderly group constitutes an increasingly significant portion of the world population. In 2007, statistics from Australia, the European Union, Japan and the United States showed that people aged 65 years and above made up from 13% to 21% of the population in these areas (Australian Bureau of Statistics, 2008; Eurostat/US Bureau of the Census, 2008; Japan Statistics Bureau & Statistics Center, 2008; US Census Bureau, 2008). Assuming the current trends of fertility and mortality rates, the population in this age bracket is expected to grow to between 20% and 36% by 2050. Taking Australia as an example, the number of people aged 65 and over totals 2.75 million (or 13%). However, the more alarming statistic is that more than half the people in this group suffer from at least one chronic disease (Australian Bureau of Statistics, 2006) and as a result about one quarter of the annual government spending on healthcare services are used to provide corresponding treatment. Over the next 30 years, the estimated government healthcare expenditure will increase by 127%, amongst which spending on residential aged care is expected to experience the strongest growth (Australian Institute of Health and Welfare, 2008). This prediction coincides with Golant's (2008) view that "a large increase in the numbers of older persons at risk of needing the supportive services offered in assisted living residences is relatively certain" (p.12) as he assessed the growth demographic factors affecting the future of residential aged care in the United States (Golant, 2008). All these statistics and trends lead to the conclusion that provision of long-term support for the healthcare needs of the elderly, especially in terms of residential aged care services, is needed but burgeoning costs also mean that such services must be provided in a more financially sustainable way.

Recent innovations in the areas of sensor devices, wireless communication protocols and knowledge management are potential enabling information technologies for delivering future residential aged care services in an economic way. In fact the Commonwealth Government of Australia has recognized the promising benefits of these rising information technologies by piloting several key trial projects related to telehealth. These projects targeted the application areas of medication management (Australian Government, 2007a) and clinical well-being monitoring (Australian Government, 2007b; Branko G. Celler, Basilakis, Budge, & Lovell, 2006).

In simple terms, telehealth refers to the delivery of healthcare over distance. It covers a wide range of medical applications from remote surgery in a hospital to chronic disease management that takes place in a residential setting. This chapter, is centered on a discussion of how wireless sensor networks (WSNs) can be deployed pervasively in a residential aged care facility to achieve ubiquitous monitoring so that the functional health status of the residents can be assessed. It is organized into several inter-related sections. In the background section, existing models of residential aged care are presented, as well as how the research effort in wellness monitoring can potentially revolutionize care approaches. This is followed by a systems architecture description of WSN technologies and a discussion on how these technologies can change the way residential aged care is delivered. Future trends in this area will then be illustrated through analysis of data taken from a simulated residential aged care environment conducted within the authors' laboratories.

## BACKGROUND

In the past, healthcare systems were dominated by the so called "medical" model. In this model, the healthcare providers took the primary role in deciding what the patients' needs were and what clinical interventions would be undertaken. Elderly people with chronic conditions were either looked after by their families and carers in their own homes or in nursing homes. In the latter case there have been many reported incidents in which patients were deprived of choice, autonomy and even dignity.

More recently a "social healthcare" model has emerged as a result of changes in societal values, increased demand in the quality and choice of aged care services and a generally more educated public. In contrast to the medical model, the social healthcare model places its emphasis on the person receiving healthcare services, incorporating the "person's medical, psychological, social, and personal needs, as well as strengths, abilities, interests, and preferences – thereby recognizing a person's distinctive life history and set of experiences" (Hyde, Perez, & Reed, 2008)(p.48). In the context of residential aged care, the social healthcare model encourages the patients, if still capable, to make appropriate choices about how they live and the type of services they require. It also fosters an environment in which social interactions with other patients, visiting families and friends are seen to have positive therapeutic values.

As a result, modern residential aged care facilities need to change, both in terms of their environment and the services they provide, to cope with these new demands. The rate by which the residential aged care facilities can respond is largely dependent on overcoming some of the existing challenges. These include current, possibly out-of-date, government regulations and policies that restrict the growth of facilities such as those leading to funding deficiencies outlined in a report assessing the Australian market (Hogan, 2007). Staffing issues also contribute to the delivery of modern residential aged care services. For instance, the shortage of nursing staff is a major issue faced by the American healthcare system and the contributing factors are increased demand, retiring work force, inadequate trainers and alternative career options. Another major concern of the work force is the lack of appropriate training that empowers staff to respond to changing care demands (Hyde et al., 2008)(p.71, p.74). Another important challenge to be resolved is the reluctance of the elderly and nursing staff in adopting and using new technologies in the healthcare delivery process, largely due to fear and misunderstanding that machines will gradually outcast human interactions.

"Technologies are likely to help enhance the quality of the living environment and improve service delivery in the coming years" (Wylde, 2008)(p.179). Technology adoption in residential aged care must proceed with caution. The aim of implementing new technologies in aged care facilities should focus on how to assist staff to provide better and more cost-effective care instead of replacing personal relationships with robotic tools that simply perform a set task faster and cheaper. Assistive technologies showcase a diverse spectrum of devices ranging from low-end items such as wheelchairs and walking-aids, to high-end sophisticated electro-mechanical devices such as robotic bathtubs (Popular Mechanics, 2004). New types of devices – for example, sensors that detect falls, or computers that monitor adherence to medication regimens – are continually being introduced (Wolf & Jenkins, 2008)(p.207).

Broadly speaking, assistive technologies can be divided into categories according to their functional applications: (1) computer-based rehabilitation, cognitive stimulation, entertainment, and interpersonal communication systems; (2) resident assessment, data, and medical record software; (3) traditional emergency call systems; (4) passively-activated call systems; (5) wandering prevention and tracking systems; (6) vital signs monitoring; (7) fall detectors; and (8) more comprehensive activity monitoring systems (Kutzik, Glascock, Lundberg, & York, 2008)(p.224). In this chapter, the specific research area of wellness monitoring as a tool for functional health assessment in residential aged care settings using assisted technologies will be examined. Essentially, wellness monitoring draws on the collaboration of two of the aforementioned assistive technology categories, namely vital signs monitoring and comprehensive activity monitoring.

The objectives of wellness monitoring is three-fold; to discover the onset of certain conditions before obvious symptoms develop in an otherwise reasonably healthy person (Srovnal & Penhaker, 2007); to provide the tools and training to promote self care; and to ensure early hospital admission of chronically ill patients when the condition requires immediate treatment. The first two objectives focus on the growing importance of prevention or early detection of a medical condition while the latter focuses on the urgency in providing necessary therapies to minimize patient morbidity crises and medical costs.

Vital signs monitoring, whether real time or periodic, provide an insight into essential statistics about the patient including heart rate and rhythm disturbances, blood oxygen content, respiratory rate, blood pressure, body temperature, etc.. Taken collectively these clinical measurements can be skillfully combined by an experienced caregiver to infer the well-being of the patient. An elevated body temperature in a normally healthy subject may signal the onset of influenza or gradual weight gain in a congestive heart failure patient may indicate edema related to a failing heart. For a diabetic patient, a steady and uncontrollable increase in blood glucose level above the target range warrants immediate treatment. A conventional vital signs recording session involves the health worker who manually measures a patient's body temperature, records the result and enters the data into the patient health record database. Drawbacks of this approach are numerous and include errors and delays in data entry, lost data records, and clinicians being unable to concurrently access the latest patient health data.

Due to the importance of physiological measurements, vital signs monitoring technology research has proliferated over the past decade. One approach for collecting a patient's physiological data is by means of a home clinical workstation located in a common area, such as the lounge, within an aged care facility. Residents can, and are encouraged to, visit the workstation periodically to have their vital signs checked. Collected data can be stored locally, transferred to an on-site database to be reviewed by staff later, or even transmitted to a remote clinician's site for assessment. The communication protocols that can be used vary from wired platforms such as Ethernet, traditional phone line or Asymmetric Digital Subscriber Line (ADSL) to wireless technologies that are becoming more commonplace such as Wireless Local Area Network (WLAN), Bluetooth, Zig-Bee, Global System for Mobile communications (GSM), General Packet Radio Service (GPRS) or Universal Mobile Telecommunications System (UMTS). The major advantage of using such a shared system is the reduction in cost since there is no need for an individual monitoring system for each patient. However, as with all other types of shared computers, data security and privacy is an issue not to be overlooked.

One successful example of such a system is the TeleMedCare Home Monitoring System (TeleMedCare, Sydney, Australia) (Figure 1) developed at the University of New South Wales, Sydney Australia (Branko G. Celler et al., 2006; Lovell et al., 2002). The system has features to measure a single lead electrocardiogram (ECG), arterial blood oxygen saturation, body temperature, body weight and spirometry. It also provides an interface for medication management, patient education and secure staff access for patient medical records and service provision history. Other systems that have been in clinical use throughout the world include the HomMed system (Honeywell, Milwaukee, USA) and doc@Home (Docobo Ltd., Bookham, UK).

Unfortunately in a residential aged care setting, it is often infeasible for the elderly to self-perform routine vital signs monitoring due to their immobility and the lack of necessary motor and cognitive skills to interact with the devices. Therefore, in contrast with the shared workstation method for

*Figure 1. The TeleMedCare Home Monitoring System is capable of recording multiple clinical measurements, including single lead ECG, blood pressure, spirometry and pulse oximetry. A touch screen interface allows recent results to be viewed as longitudinal graphs as well as medication and measurement alerts to be delivered via a remote scheduler*

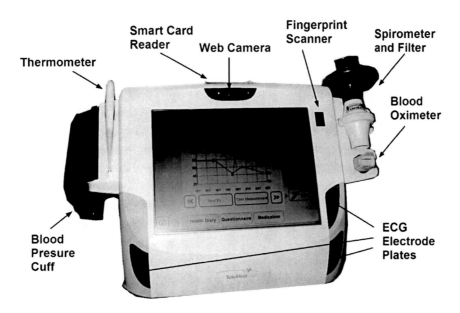

vital signs monitoring, recently there has been significant progress into using pervasive and ubiquitous networks of sensors for physiological parameter measurements. For example, sensors can be located within the environment - such as load sensors installed to the bed frame for weight measurement (Elite Care, 2008). Others can be attached to the patient when required (Leroy L. Chan, Celler, & Lovell, 2006; Warren, Yao, & Barnes, 2002; Wilson et al., 2001) while others are designed to integrate into a wearable garment for long term and continuous monitoring (Pentland, 2004) of a diverse array of body parameters. So far, vital signs monitoring using this distributed computing approach is restricted to development in the laboratory and large scale clinical deployments are yet to occur. Data privacy, mobility and continuous monitoring are characteristic features of this approach. With the remaining technical challenges such as data transfer security, sensor link reliability, system cost and sensor battery life all

expected to be resolved or contained in the future, this sensor network approach is expected to prevail as the dominant choice for vital sign monitoring due to the benefits it potentially offers.

Comprehensive activity monitoring is often referred to as activities of daily living (ADL) monitoring in the literature. ADL monitoring systems contribute to wellness monitoring by building and profiling the daily activity pattern of a subject and using it as a baseline for comparison against irregular patterns. Such systems are useful in detecting the onset of problems that are only revealed over a longer period of time. For instance, gradual and unintentional changes in appetite in an otherwise healthy patient may suggest a digestive disease, while increased episodes of wandering can be signs of the onset of dementia.

According to Kutzik, Glascock, Lundberg and York (2008), ADL monitoring systems can take on two distinct design approaches: maximalist and minimalist. The maximalist approach aims to build an infrastructure which supports a diverse network of hardware devices such as sensors, data repeaters, network coordinators and data sinks. This extensive network of devices is designed to collect as complete a data set as possible related to the daily activities of patients. These data are then processed by algorithms and translated into useful information for caregivers such as sleeping patterns, usage of toilet and bathroom facilities, eating patterns, social interaction, time spent with care-givers, activity level, etc.. Most often these can be combined with the vital sign monitoring results in order to design the best care plan tailored for the individual patient. The minimalist approach, on the other hand, employs hardware and software that are designed to monitor specific tasks and/or disease conditions.

Research in this area in terms of impact of ADL monitoring on health status remains embryonic. One of the first technology demonstrators of remote monitoring of the free-living elderly occurred in the early 1990's in Australia as a result of research at UNSW (Celler et al., 1995). More recently a single-subject study was conducted in Japan (Suzuki et al., 2004) to first build up the daily living pattern of the subject by a network of wired sensors that measured movement, human presence, door and window openings, stove usage, television and washing machine usage and sleep occurrence. Subsequent daily patterns were compared with a normal template and any dramatic change in behavior could be ascertained. Similarly, the PlaceLab at the Massachusetts Institute of Technology (Massachusetts Institute of Technology, 2003) is an apartment-style research facility hosting a rich sensing infrastructure of over 300 sensor types and is another typical example of the maximalist approach. ADL-related parameters that can be detected include light, air quality, ambient temperature and humidity, sound, motion, identity, use of appliances, door movements, etc.. Some of these parameters may

not immediately find their place in providing care to patients but the philosophy of the maximalist approach is to perform excessive measurements. Another study (Philipose et al., 2004) tested the detection of fourteen different ADL by placing over 100 radio frequency identification (RFID) tags in a test house. The subjects were made to wear a specifically designed glove containing an RFID reader and a radio front-end for data transmission to a data sink. When an activity was performed, the subject interacted by touching different RFID-tagged objects, thus providing a record of the time and sequence of the objects used. A probabilistic inference engine was used to estimate the different ADLs performed.

Perhaps the project largest in scale that applied ADL monitoring technologies to residential aged care was the Oatfield Estates project by Elite Care (Stanford, 2002). Each resident and staff on the estate wore an identification badge that could be tracked by embedded readers throughout the buildings. In other words, location tracking and wandering prevention became part of the ADL monitoring system. Residents were also monitored for weight and sleeping pattern changes by specially designed load cells placed under each bed leg. The system also allowed staff and residents to manually enter other activity information into the database.

It can be seen that the main challenge of ADL monitoring systems is the appropriate use of collected data to produce useful information. Technologies and approaches related to this area include data mining, machine learning, artificial intelligence and knowledge management. It may also be obvious to the reader that ADL monitoring systems share similar infrastructure to smart home systems. Research has shown that there are a many positives in blending the two systems. This will be addressed in the section on future research directions.

# WIRELESS SENSOR NETWORKS FOR WELLNESS MONITORING

Wireless sensor technologies provide a ubiquitous, non-invasive and cost effective way to continuously and autonomously monitor one's physiological parameters as well as ADL. While these systems may not replace every aspect of the conventional wellness monitoring approach, they allow data to be collected from areas previously inaccessible such as location information with room-level granularity. There are three major sub-systems in a wireless sensor, technology-based, wellness monitoring system:

- WSNs: collects relevant data from the subject and the subject's interaction with their environment. These data are wirelessly transmitted in either raw or processed format back to a central server for further conditioning, classification and knowledge inference.
- Data conditioning, feature extraction and data fusion: Continuous data streaming from multiple sensors over the network means there is flood of information. Data cleaning and noise reduction is critical to ensure only data with an acceptable level of noise and quality is processed to extract waveform features. This sub-system acts on individual data channels to extract relevant information. It also applies data fusion techniques across multiple channels to identify signal interactions. For example, with RFID locator technology, signal interaction can be used to infer the length of time spent toileting, the time spent dispensing medications to a particular subject, etc.
- Data fusion, knowledge management and decision support: This sub-system is heavily based on advanced software modeling of the subject data. Based on a normal pattern of ADL for a particular subject, the

system will be able to identify consistent discrepancies from this template and from these deviations infer changes in functional health state.

This section will focus on describing the first sub-system, the architectural design of WSNs. As described in the previous section, this is the most advanced area in terms of research and development. The latter two areas are relatively embryonic due to the lack of appropriate hardware systems to acquire the necessary signals and build the necessary knowledge bases.

## Sensor and Wireless Network Design

A sensor network system is comprised of wireless sensor nodes, which contain one or more sensor types used to collect data from either a person or the surrounding environment. The collected data is firstly processed locally, such as digital filtering, formatting, noise cleaning, etc.. Data is then transmitted via the RF section of the sensor. There are two main features to be considered when implementing the wireless network, namely, the network topology and protocol. For the network protocol, pros and cons of WLAN (IEEE 802.11 b/g), Bluetooth (IEEE 802.15.1) and ZigBee (based on IEEE 802.15.4) will be discussed; in terms of network topology, two typical designs will be evaluated - star and mesh network topologies.

Design and deployment of multiple types of low-cost sensors heavily impacts the utility of the monitoring system. In the next section we introduce a range of sensor types, discussing usage implications, size, power, cost and longevity.

## Types of Sensors

In one common classification approach, sensors can be categorized into three groupings; ambient environmental sensors, body area network (BAN) sensors, and location and usage sensors. Ambient environmental sensors are used to monitor the ambient condition of a given geographical environment. Some of the widely used sensors are:

- Passive Infrared (PIR) sensors are used commonly to detect the presence of moving infrared emitters. They are very reliable in terms of detecting heat sources (therefore human presence) but cannot recognize the identity of the subject present in the environment, nor are they accurate enough to detect the presence of multiple persons (Ohta, Nakamoto, Shinagawa, & Tanikawa, 2002).
- Ambient light sensors can be used to correlate the sleeping behavior of the subject in reference to circadian rhythms.
- Ambient temperature sensors provide a reference reading of the current temperature settings. Room temperatures could be used for example to build up the temperature preference for an individual subject over a period of time.

The second category of sensors are BAN sensors. These sensors include various types of monitoring transducers with wireless communication capability. The main differentiating point of these sensors is that they must be worn by the subject. They include:

- **Triaxial-accelerometry:** a sensor that measures the acceleration of the body in three-dimensions. Performing continuous acceleration measurements can be used to determine the ambulation and activity-level of a subject, as well as falls propensity and falls risk. It has been demonstrated that such technologies can classify postural orientation (sitting, standing, lying) with a reasonable accuracy (Mathie, Coster, Lovell, & Celler, 2004; Mathie, Coster, Lovell, Celler et al., 2004). Also the signal magnitude area of the acceleration signals

can be used as an estimate of energy expenditure (activity level) (Voon, Celler, & Lovell, 2008).. Determining activity level of the monitored subject provides an indication of both physical and cognitive health status (Virone et al., 2008). Moreover, we have demonstrated that such algorithms can be effectively coded in real-time, thus relieving the need to transmit large continuous streams of data over a WSN for further processing (Karantonis, Narayanan, Mathie, Lovell, & Celler, 2006).

- **ECG sensing:** it is commonly accepted that in order to accurately diagnose cardiac disease that a 12-lead ECG recording is mandated. However this is only possible in a clinical setting. As a compromise, ECG systems used in the WSN environment are normally single lead recordings using 2 or 3 attached electrodes. By applying advanced signal processing techniques, various types of arrhythmias and conduction abnormalities can be determined (Tsipouras, Fotiadis, & Sideris, 2005) even from a single lead recording.
- **Body temperature:** continual monitoring of the body temperature of an elderly patient can provide timely and accurate information that reflects the onset of infection and/or disease. In hospital wards and nursing homes this manual task is both repetitive and time consuming, so a WSN approach is beneficial.

The third category of sensors relate to location detection. These types of sensors are developed to track the location and specific movements of a subject, including their interaction with other objects, people or resources:

- **Location sensor:** Location tracking is one of the most important sensor types as it generates useful data for assessing functional health. An example is the social activity level, where the times of interaction between subject, health professionals and care givers can be tracked. One common technique adapted by wireless sensor networks is to implement a set of reference nodes around the target area, for example a nursing home environment. These nodes form a reference grid and a mobile location sensor determines the Received Signal Strength Indicator (RSSI) value from the reference nodes. It is assumed by the mobile sensor that the strongest signal it receives from the reference node is the closest therefore approximating its location within the reference grid via triangulation (Adamodt, 2006). In this instance the subject must wear the mobile sensor and in a similar way, health care professionals and other important objects (medication and meal trolleys) must also have mobile sensors attached. Another way of monitoring location is to implement a grid of pressure sensors on the floor. The advantage is that a very accurate movement path of the subject can be determined. Disadvantages include cost, difficulty of installation and handling the presence of multiple persons in the same area (Mori, Noguchi, Takada, & Sato, 2004).

- **Usage sensors:** Many of these devices are ON/OFF switches or passive RFID tags. They are installed on major objects such as the toilet, shower, fridge, stove, cabin doors, etc. and directly monitor the use of various facilities.

## Sensor Design Considerations

- **Space:** one of the most important constraints on sensor design is space limitation, especially for wearable sensors. A fully functional wireless sensor must accommodate A/D conversion, digital processing, wireless transceiver and power management within a small space, typically 40mm x 40mm x 20mm (L x W x H).

- **Power Consumption:** while the ambient environmental sensors are fixed on the wall and may possibly run from mains power, it is often not desirable as it will be an extra burden for installation. For the body area sensors, they have to be wireless and last as long as possible. Weeks-long is the minimum requirement where months-long is preferable. The ZigBee protocol has well defined power profiles, with transmission power less than 1 mW (0 dBm). It is common for many ZigBee-based sensors to last years-long because sensors like smoke alarms are in sleep mode for more than 99.9% of the time and only wake up on an alert condition.

- Longevity is another key element in the WSN environment. Due to the large number of sensors, the network may not be functional if the failure rate is high. In theory, sensors should last for years without human intervention. For active mobile sensors, the rechargeable battery is one of the failure points because the battery performance tends to degrade after multiple recharges.

- Cost is usually not considered as a main design constraint, however a balance between performance and cost should met, for example, temperature sensors will not require a high precision analogue to digital conversion (ADC) nor fast processing speed, therefore choosing a cheaper microcontroller may be more suitable.

## Sensor Design Architecture

The block diagram in figure 2 illustrates a typical architecture of a wireless sensor. As an illustrative example, a wireless single-lead ECG wireless sensor will be presented.

*Figure 2. A generic sensor block diagram illustrates the major sub-systems used in a wireless sensor*

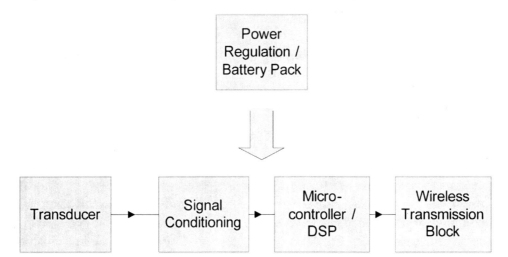

- Power Regulation / Battery: In a wireless patient monitoring environment, power regulation has to be as efficient as possible to avoid undue power wastage. The voltage regulator has to provide either 5V and / or 3.3V to the different integrated circuits. Also because most of the current-generation wireless sensors use single cell Lithium-ion rechargeable batteries, over-charge and over-discharge protection circuitry has to be implemented to ensure optimal battery life.

- Transducer: The transducer acts as the interface between the environment and the sensor. Possibly the biggest barrier to adoption and usage of physiological measurement devices involves the usability and compliance issues associated with attaching sensor to the body to transducer the biological phenomena into electrical signals that can then be further processed. In the case of an ECG, ionic currents (carried by ions in solution) in physiological media (tissues and organs of the body) must be converted into electronic currents (carried by electrons) in metallic conductor. Conventional biopotential electrodes in

use today consist of a metallic conductor in contact with the tissue of interest (e.g., the skin, when recording body surface potentials such as the ECG) via an electrolyte solution. Due to the presence of the electrolyte solution, such electrodes are sometimes referred to as "wet electrodes" to distinguish them from the less conventional "dry electrodes" which make contact with the tissue without the aid of an electrolyte solution. In nearly all cases of ambulatory ECG monitoring, these conventional or wet electrodes are used, with a pre-gelled disposable Ag/AgCl pellet attached by an adhesive pad.

- Signal Conditioning: This module is used amplify, filter and perform feature extraction and artifact rejection on the signal. For a single-lead ECG in an ambulatory subject, it is expected that the recorded signal will be severely compromised by artefacts introduced by muscle activity, movement and electrical noise (Redmond, Lovell, Basilakis, & Celler, 2008). Typically the QRS events within the ECG will be detected using a real-time algorithm in order to derive the heart rate. One common

*Table 1. A comparison of various wireless protocols*

| | WLAN (IEEE 802.11g) | Bluetooth (2.0 with EDR, Class 2) | ZigBee (2006) |
|---|---|---|---|
| Battery life | Hours | Days | Years |
| Range | 32m* | 10m | 10m |
| Bandwidth | 50Mbps | 3Mbps | 250kbps |
| Scalability (nodes) | Moderate | Poor | Excellent |

\* Typical home router with stock antenna in indoor environment

approach in the literature is to use a sliding window technique based to derive the heart rate and hence classify the heart arrhythmia status (Raju, 2007; Tsipouras et al., 2005).

- Wireless Transmission: This module contains the wireless RF transceiver (processor) and antenna. The wireless transceiver handles lower level RF packet formation and transmission. The microcontroller typically communicates with the RF transceiver via an I2C or SPI protocol and transmits data via a program interface provided by the chip vendor.

## Wireless Protocols

There are three major wireless communication protocols currently utilized by WSN projects. They are WLAN, Bluetooth, ZigBee. They all exist in the 2.4 GHz frequency band. This section will briefly described their features, characteristics, advantages and disadvantages in different applications. This information derived from commercial product specifications is summarized in Table 1.

### WLAN (IEEE 802.11 b/g)
WLAN has the highest bandwidth and longest transmission distance among the three wireless protocols and because it is widely used by computer related products, the implementation cost is relative cheap. Just based on these features, WLAN seems to be the best choice to be adapted

by WSNs. However, in RF transmission given a particular RF frequency band, the bandwidth and transmission range is directly proportional to the transmission power. Generally, the transmission power at a WLAN antenna is of the order of 10 to 30 mW (10 to 15 dBm). In general this level is too high to be implemented by small rechargeable wireless sensors. Moreover, individual sensors will never require the large bandwidth provided by WLAN.

While WLAN is not a suitable choice for wireless sensors, it is certainly more ideal for higher level gateways and servers. As the gateways in a star network topology (see below) collect data streamed from multiple sensors and transmit it higher level machines therefore have higher demands in terms of network bandwidth and transmission range. Another plus for WLAN is its dominant implementation in the computer world. As such it is well supported by operating systems from Microsoft Windows to embedded Linux systems, with a consequently low development and manufacturing cost due to its wide adoption.

### Bluetooth (IEEE 802.15.1)
Bluetooth is a mature Personal Area Network (PAN) protocol commonly found in hand-held devices. It has good power consumption compared to WLAN and excellent bandwidth given its low power consumption profile.

The network architecture of Bluetooth is a star network topology, which means the slave nodes cannot communicate with each other directly. Even though Bluetooth supports "scatternet" formation

*Figure 3. Bluetooth scatternet topology*

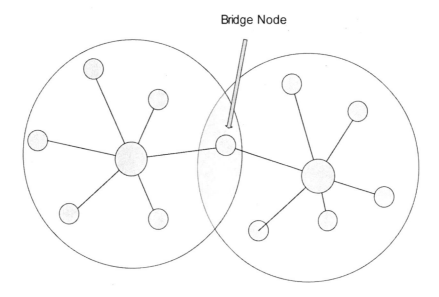

to create a mesh-like network topology (Figure 3) the routing algorithm is not well implemented (and subsequently solved by ZigBee) (Labiod, Afifi, & De Santis, 2007).

There are two major drawbacks for Bluetooth to be implemented as the WSN transmission protocol. Firstly, Bluetooth devices have to perform the "Discovery and Association" process in order to establish connection with the super node. This process can take up to ten seconds (Sandhu, Agogino, & Agogino, 2004). This is acceptable for WSNs comprised of static sensors that do not require substantial or real-time re-association. However this is certainly not suitable for mobile patient monitoring sensors, as these sensors could move within and out of the RF coverage within the association period, degrading the system performance. Another problem is a super node can only associate with up to 7 slave nodes at the same time, which will cause scalability problems if a large number of leaf nodes are present within a small area. Apart from these limitations, Bluetooth is an inexpensive and mature technology. It is certainly suitable as the protocol for small, ad hoc sensor networks.

**ZigBee (Based on IEEE 802.15.4)**

The ZigBee protocol is an upper layer architecture based on top of the IEEE 802.15.4 stack. Strictly speaking, ZigBee is not IEEE 802.15.4 rather it is a network layer application of the IEEE 802.15.4 protocol. It provides sufficient transmission distance and data rate for sensor networks while consumes relatively extremely low energy.

ZigBee supports both star and mesh topologies, which enables a versatile design of the network architecture. It is developed for home automation and has many inherent advantages compared to Bluetooth and WLAN. For example, well-defined routing protocols enable ZigBee sensors to form a reliable mesh network with redundancy. Also the 16 bit short address and 64 bit MAC address means there is essentially no node limit for a particular wireless sensor network (up to 64000 for a coordinator). Because the WSN can take full advantage of ZigBee's low power consumption and well defined network layer stack, ZigBee is widely implemented by sensor network projects.

## Wireless Network Implementation

There are two major topologies utilized in WSN design, namely mesh network and star network topologies.

### Mesh Network

A wireless mesh network (WMN) is a common topology adapted by WSNs (Figure 4). There is no central gateway in the WMN, each node within the network connects to other nodes residing within each others' RF coverage (Groth & Skandier, 2005). In a WSN environment, each node in the network is responsible to not only collect and send out data but also responsible to relay data sent by others. Such a model of data transmission is called multi-hop routing. The advantage of the WMN is it provides a degree of network redundancy because data is routed dynamically. Failure of a node will not cause a systematic failure of the network; instead data will be routed through the next possible path. However in the case of large data traffic, it is possible for a particular node to receive a large influx of data and because the limited bandwidth of Bluetooth and ZigBee, the network may congest and data may be lost. Therefore WMNs are more suitable for a relative static WSN that does not have burst data traffic, for example a static ambient environmental condition (temperature, light, humidity) monitoring sensor network.

The CodeBlue project by Harvard University is an example of WSNs for medical care. It utilizes motes (mobile sensors) with mesh network topology and the ZigBee wireless protocol. It has a wide range of sensors including pulse oximetry and wireless two-lead ECG (Shnayder, Chen, Lorincz, Fulford-Jones, & Welsh, 2005). Code-Blue also defines a framework of packet routing, sensor communication and software implementation protocols.

*Figure 4. Mesh network topology*

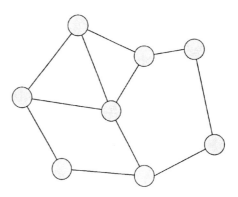

### Star Network

A star network (Figure 5) is a simple network topology with a central (super) node responsible to receive and transmit data to and from each leaf node. Hence complicated routing methods are not needed. In the wireless sensor environment there is no communication between sensors nodes and the network performance is increased because data packets are not passing through other nodes. Instead it is always the super node and a leaf node involved in communications. The star network also eliminates the possible network congestion in a mesh network as the super node could be designed to have a higher output bandwidth than the leaf node. For example, in the SensorNet@ BSL project at the University of New South Wales, Australia a gateway was designed that had both ZigBee and WLAN interfaces. ZigBee was used by the gateway to communicate with the sensors while the collected data could be transmitted to a higher level server via WLAN (L. L. Chan, Zhang, Narayanan, Celler, & Lovell, 2008). The drawback of such topology is it suffers single point of failure, namely if the super node fails, the entire network is out of service.

*Figure 5. Star network topology*

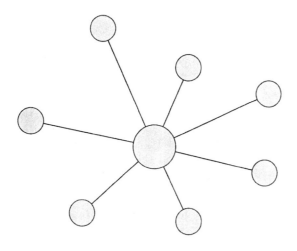

## Hybrid Network Topology

Sometimes it is practical to combine different types of network topologies in order to improve the scalability and stability, manageability and bandwidth of the network. For example, in a mesh / star network hybrid, sensors can communicate to the super node directly while it is within the coverage of the super node. While the sensor is out of range, it should be able to communicate with other leaf-node sensors and ultimately send data to the super node via multi-hop routing.

In a large geographical area like a hospital, tree (hierarchal) topology could be implemented (Figure 6). A star / mesh network hybrid sensor network could be considered as a leaf-node of the tree network. Each leaf-node monitors a small area such as a single or several rooms. Higher-level hierarchies may include a hospital ward or a level of a building. Data is processed and merged at each lower level then transmitted to the next upper hierarchy via a fast network protocol, wired (Ethernet) or wireless (WLAN). Eventually data from different sections of the site converge at the central server.

## FUTURE RESEARCH DIRECTIONS

Based on the current literature, nearly all wellness monitoring systems, whether commercial or research, focus on either vital signs monitoring or ADL monitoring. It is becoming clear that to adequately support the needs of health monitoring in residential aged care both elements need to be integrated.

A continuous wellness monitoring system (SensorNet@BSL) currently under further development at University of New South Wales is built with this goal in mind. The initial version of the system operates on a three-layer architecture, consisting of a central server controlling multiple WLANs with each WLAN coordinating multiple Zigbee-based WSNs. The three-layer architecture system design offers flexibility in terms of expanding the sensor network almost indefinitely to suit the facility area and need. It can be applied equally efficiently to a single household and a well-established, multi-storey residential aged care facility. Its complete wireless nature means that the system can be installed into places with minimal building structural change and with maximal ease. Vital signs monitoring is performed via the collection of physiological parameters such as ECG, heart rate, postural orientation, energy expenditure and body temperature. ADL information is obtained by analyzing unobtrusive data such as the resident's interaction with the environment, usage of facilities, interaction with caregivers, time spent on certain activities, etc. Currently, the system is undergoing additional technology modifications to prepare for major clinical evaluations in several commercial residential aged care facilities around Australia. Figure 7 illustrates a typical deployment of the SensorNet@BSL project. Figure 8 shows hardware layouts of the various WSN components while figure 9 shows sample data collected from this deployment.

Similar wellness monitoring systems developed around the world over the last decade include the House_n Group project (Intille, 2002;

*Figure 6. Possible network topology for coverage of large areas*

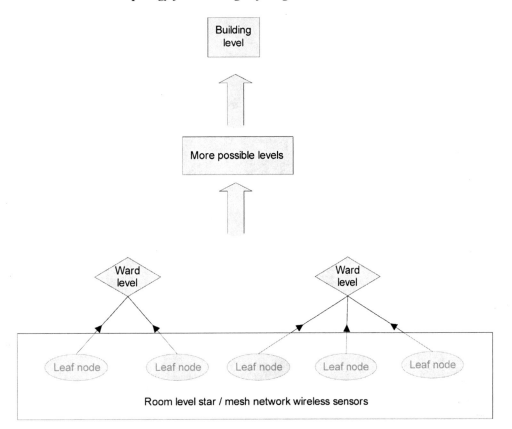

Tapia, Intille, & Larson, 2004) which studied the qualitative and quantitative relationships between users and surrounding objects. Based on collected data the system was trained to build a Bayesian network model for residential monitoring. The Welfare Techno-Houses project in Japan (Tamura, Togawa, Ogawa, & Yoda, 1998; Yamaguchi, Ogawa, Tamura, & Togawa, 1998) consisted of thirteen houses equipped with infrared sensors and magnetic switches on the doors to monitor both physical activity and physiological signals with the goal of improving the quality of life for both the elderly and their caregivers. The CareNet project in the United Kingdom (Williams, Doughty, & Bradley, 1998) provided the "Hospital at Home" service by collecting the patient's physiological data as well as analyzing the lifestyle of the patient by sensors embedded in their environment.

Another anticipated trend of wellness monitoring systems for residential aged care is the possible integration with smart home systems. Both systems can leverage on the data collected by a single sensor network to achieve separate outcomes. For instance, a light sensor detecting the light intensity of a room can be used by the smart home system to decide if lighting in a particular area should be adjusted. The same piece of information can be used by a wellness monitoring system to record the number of times a patient wakes up at night to use the bathroom and infer the health status of the patient.

A limited number of larger scale smart home projects implemented in North America and Europe over the past decade have factored in their design a wellness monitoring component. An example of such is the Aware Home Research

*Figure 7. A mock living environment of an Australian aged care facility and the operation of SensorNet@ BSL. The end server, the bridge units and the sensor units form the three-level architecture. The end server communicates with the bridge units via WLAN while the WSN connections between the bridge units and sensor units are ZigBee-based. Sensor units are either placed in the environment (static) or can be carried around (mobile). As a mobile sensor unit moves to a new geographical area served by a different bridge unit, the control of the sensor unit is handed over to the new bridge unit such that the room-level location of the mobile unit at any time is known to the end server*

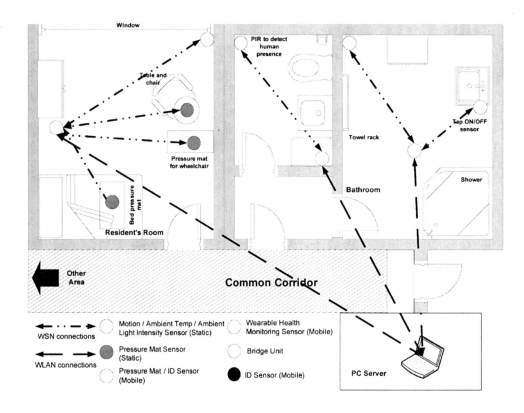

*Figure 8. The SensorNet@BSL hardware platform. Left: the modular design of the universal sensor mother board to which different sensor daughter boards can be attached to modify functionality. Middle: the middle layer ZigBee / WLAN bridge acts as the super node. Right: a sensor daughter board attached to the mother board. The illustrated daughter board has a PIR, a temperature and a light intensity sensor incorporated into the printed circuit board*

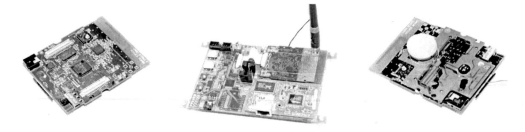

*Figure 9. Sample data from tri-accelerometry sensor with derived energy expenditure level*

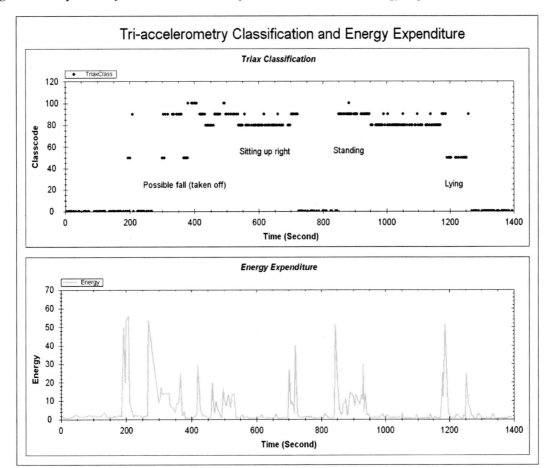

Initiative at the Georgia Institute of Technology (Kidd et al., 1999) which involved a three-storey smart home to support elderly occupants with context awareness and ubiquitous sensing, location tracking and lost object tracking capabilities. The Millennium House project pioneered by British Telecom and the Anchor Trust (Perry, Dowdall, Lines, & Hone, 2004) used infrared sensors and magnetic switches on doors to study the behavior pattern of the occupant and alert the caregiver should an abnormality be detected. This intelligent system also supported independent living of the elderly by warning them about dangerous events, or checking if they need external assistance.

## CONCLUSION

Statistics highlight the fact that the world population is aging, and this phenomenon is becoming an issue for developed countries. To maintain and improve quality and continuity of care, extra resources must be allocated for maintaining elderly health. The rise of information technologies carries the promise of providing ubiquitous wellness monitoring for functional health assessment in residential aged care facilities with higher quality and at a reduced cost. Among these, the technologies involved in constructing pervasive WSNs have been shown to improve the diversity of the parameters that can be measured in vital signs monitoring and enhance data availability to authorized healthcare personnel. WSNs are also proved to be beneficial in ADL management by monitoring residents' interaction with their environment and alert caregivers when abnormal living patterns are detected.

When designing a WSN for wellness monitoring purposes, many factors need to be considered. Each sensor type has its specific area of application such as ambient environmental monitoring, body signal measurement or location tracking. Sensors must be chosen to fit the type and environment of use while at the same time satisfy requirements such as size, power consumption, cost and longevity for a particular application. In general, a wireless sensor node consists of a transducer unit managed by a microprocessor which provides signal preconditioning capability and acts as an interface to the wireless transceiver front-end. The whole sensor node is most likely powered by a rechargeable battery that enhances mobility of the node. The wireless communication protocol and network topology must also be chosen carefully to optimize battery life, transmission range, throughput and scalability.

Raw data collected by the sensors are often pre-processed, either by the sensor node or the data sink, before further transmissions to optimize limited bandwidth usage and enhance network availability. Data must also be processed to detect and alert for corruption and artifact.

Perhaps the biggest future challenge that has only started to be addressed is the need for data fusion from multiple sensors. These data must feed into knowledge management systems that by way of machine learning and other inference methods can compare changes against normal templates for particular subjects and thus identify a decline in functional health status. The current state of research is that WSN are only now being deployed to provide the necessary baseline data from which the knowledge management systems can be developed.

It is envisioned that future wellness monitoring systems will not only incorporate capabilities to monitor both vital signs and ADL but also integrate seamlessly with smart home systems to provide a truly intelligent environment to cater for all aspects of daily living.

## REFERENCES

Adamodt, K. (2006). [Location Engine]. *Application Note, AN042*, CC2431.

Australian Bureau of Statistics. (2006). *4102.0 - Australian Social Trends, 2006*. Retrieved from http://www.abs.gov.au/ausstats/abs@.nsf/Latestp roducts/6F443192D27B9360CA2571B00013D9 54?opendocument

Australian Bureau of Statistics. (2008). *3222.0 - Population Projections, Australia, 2006 to 2101*. Retrieved from http://www.abs.gov.au/ausstats/ abs@.nsf/mf/3222.0

Australian Government. (2007a). *Clinical IT in Aged Care Product Trial - Trial of a Medication Management System - Report*. Retrieved from http://www.health.gov.au/internet/main/ publishing.nsf/Content/aging-rescare-econnect-med-mgt-trial.htm

Australian Government. (2007b). *Clinical IT in Aged Care Product Trial - Trial of a System for Monitoring Clinical Well-Being - Report*. Retrieved from http://www.health.gov.au/internet/ main/publishing.nsf/Content/1E896B258E583 DF8CA2573B5007C788D/$File/Clinical%20 Monitoring.pdf

Australian Institute of Health and Welfare. (2008). *Australia's health 2008*. Retrieved from http://www.aihw.gov.au/publications/index.cfm/ title/10585

Celler, B. G., Basilakis, J., Budge, M., & Lovell, N. H. (2006). A Clinical Monitoring and Management System for Residential Aged Care Facilities. In *Proceedings of the 28th IEEE EMBS Annual International Conference*, (pp. 3301).

Celler, B. G., Earnshaw, W., Ilsar, E. D., Betbeder-Matibet, L., Harris, M., & Clark, R. (1995). Remote monitoring of the elderly at home. A multidisciplinary project on aging at the University of New South Wales. *International Journal of Bio-Medical Computing, 40*, 147–155. doi:10.1016/0020-7101(95)01139-6

Chan, L. L., Celler, B. G., & Lovell, N. H. (2006). *Development of a Smart Health Monitoring and Evaluation System.* Paper presented at the TEN-CON 2006, IEEE Region 10 Conference.

Chan, L. L., Zhang, J. Z., Narayanan, M. R., Celler, B. G., & Lovell, N. H. (2008, February 13-15). *A Health Monitoring and Evaluation System for Assessing Care Needs of Residents in Aged-Care Facilities.* Paper presented at the IASTED Biomed. Eng., Innsbruck, Austria.

Elite Care. (2008). *Elite Care.* Retrieved 2009, 2008, from http://www.elitecare.com/

Eurostat/US Bureau of the Census. (2008, 03/09/2008). *People by age classes.* Retrieved 28/01/2009, from http://epp.eurostat.ec.europa.eu/portal/page?_pageid=1996,39140985&_dad=portal&_schema=PORTAL&screen=d etailref&language=en&product=REF_TB_population&root=REF_TB_population/t_popula/t_pop/t_demo_pop/tps00010

Golant, S. M. (2008). The Future of Assisted Living Residences. In Golant, S. M., & Hyde, J. (Eds.), *The Assisted Living Residence* (pp. 3–45). Baltimore: The John Hopkins University Press.

Groth, D., & Skandier, T. (2005). *Network+ Study Guild.* Indianapolis: Wiley Publishing Inc.

Hogan, W. (2007). *The Organisation of Residential Aged Care for an Aging Population.* The Centre of Independent Studies Limitedo.

Hyde, J., Perez, R., & Reed, P. S. (2008). The Old Road Is Rapidly Aging. In Golant, S. M., & Hyde, J. (Eds.), *The Assisted Living Residence* (pp. 46–85). Baltimore: The Johns Hopkins University Press.

Intille, S. S. (2002). Designing a Home of the Future. *IEEE Pervasive Computing / IEEE Computer Society [and] IEEE Communications Society, 1*(2), 76–82. doi:10.1109/MPRV.2002.1012340

Japan Statistics Bureau & Statistics Center. (2008, April 15). *Population by Age (Single Year), Sex and Sex ratio - Total population, Japanese population,* October 1, 2007. Retrieved 28/01/2009, from http://www.e-stat.go.jp/SG1/estat/ListE.do?lid=000001026128

Karantonis, D. M., Narayanan, M. R., Mathie, M., Lovell, N. H., & Celler, B. G. (2006). Implementation of a Real-Time Human Movement Classifier Using a Triaxial Accelerometer for Ambulatory Monitoring. *Information Technology in Biomedicine. IEEE Transactions on, 10*(1), 156–167.

Kidd, C. D., Orr, R., Abowd, G. D., Atkeson, C. G., Essa, I. A., MacIntyre, B., et al. (1999). *The Aware Home: A Living Laboratory for Ubiquitous Computing Research.* Paper presented at the Proceedings of the Second International Workshop on Cooperative Buildings, Integrating Information, Organization, and Architecture.

Kutzik, D. M., Glascock, A. P., Lundberg, L., & York, J. (2008). Technological Tools of the Future. In Golant, S. M., & Hyde, J. (Eds.), *The Assisted Living Residence.* Baltimore: The Johns Hopkins University Press.

Labiod, H., Afifi, H., & De Santis, C. (2007). *Wi-Fi Bluetooth Zigbee and WiMax.* Dordrecht: Springer. doi:10.1007/978-1-4020-5397-9

Lovell, N. H., Celler, B. G., Basilakis, J., Magrabi, F., Huynh, K., & Mathie, M. (2002). *Managing chronic disease with home telecare: a system architecture and case study*. Paper presented at the Proceedings of the Second Joint EMBS/BMES Conference.\.

Massachusetts Institute of Technology. (2003). *PlaceLab: A House_n + TIAX Initiative*. Cambridge, MA: Author. Retrieved from http://architecture.mit.edu/house_n/placelab.html

Mathie, M. J., Coster, A. C., Lovell, N. H., & Celler, B. G. (2004). Accelerometry: providing an integrated, practical method for long-term, ambulatory monitoring of human movement. *Physiological Measurement, 25*(2), R1–R20. doi:10.1088/0967-3334/25/2/R01

Mathie, M. J., Coster, A. C., Lovell, N. H., Celler, B. G., Lord, S. R., & Tiedemann, A. (2004). A pilot study of long-term monitoring of human movements in the home using accelerometry. *Journal of Telemedicine and Telecare, 10*(3), 144–151. doi:10.1258/135763304323070788

Mori, T., Noguchi, H., Takada, A., & Sato, T. (2004). Sensing Room: Distributed Sensor Environment for Measurement of Human Daily Behavior. In *First International Workshop on Networked Sensing Systems (INSS2004)*, (pp. 40-43).

Ohta, S., Nakamoto, H., Shinagawa, Y., & Tanikawa, T. (2002). A health monitoring system for elderly people living alone. *Journal of Telemedicine and Telecare, 8*(3), 151–156. doi:10.1258/135763302320118997

Pentland, A. (2004). Healthwear: Medical technology becomes wearable. *Computer, 37*(5), 42–49. doi:10.1109/MC.2004.1297238

Perry, M., Dowdall, A., Lines, L., & Hone, K. (2004). Multimodal and ubiquitous computing systems: supporting independent-living older users. *Information Technology in Biomedicine. IEEE Transactions on, 8*(3), 258–270.

Philipose, M., Fishkin, K. P., Perkowitz, M., Patterson, D. J., Fox, D., & Kautz, H. (2004). Inferring activities from interactions with objects. *Pervasive Computing, IEEE, 3*(4), 50–57. doi:10.1109/MPRV.2004.7

*Popular Mechanics*. (2004, 06). Robots Help Japan Care For Its Elderly. Retrieved 30/01/2009, 2009, from http://www.popularmechanics.com/science/technology_watch/1288241.html

Raju, M. (2007). *Heart-Rate and EKG Monitor Using the MSP430FG439* [Electronic Version].

Redmond, S. J., Lovell, N. H., Basilakis, J., & Celler, B. G. (2008). *ECG quality measures in telecare monitoring*. Paper presented at the Proc. 30th Annual Int. Conf IEEE EMBC08, 20th-24th Aug, Vancouver Canada.

Sandhu, J. S., Agogino, A. M., & Agogino, A. K. (2004). *Wireless Sensor Networks for Commercial Lighting Control: Decision Making with Multi-agent Systems*.

Shnayder, V., Chen, B., Lorincz, K., Fulford-Jones, T. R. F., & Welsh, M. (2005). Sensor Networks for Medical Care. In *Proceedings of the 3rd international conference on Embedded networked sensor systems*, (pp. 314-314).

Srovnal, V., & Penhaker, M. (2007). *Health Maintenance Embedded Systems in Home Care Applications*. Paper presented at the Systems, ICONS '07, Second International Conference on.

Stanford, V. (2002). Using Pervasive Computing to Deliver Elder Care. *IEEE Pervasive Computing / IEEE Computer Society [and] IEEE Communications Society*, 10–13. doi:10.1109/MPRV.2002.993139

Suzuki, R., Ogawa, M., Otake, S., Izutsu, T., Tobimatsu, Y., & Izumi, S. (2004). Analysis of activities of daily living in elderly people living alone: single-subject feasibility study. *Telemedicine Journal and e-Health, 10*(2), 260–276. doi:10.1089/tmj.2004.10.260

Tamura, T., Togawa, T., Ogawa, M., & Yoda, M. (1998). Fully automated health monitoring system in the home. *Medical Engineering & Physics, 20,* 573–579. doi:10.1016/S1350-4533(98)00064-2

Tapia, E., Intille, S. S., & Larson, K. (2004). Activity Recognition in the Home Using Simple and Ubiquitous Sensors. In Pervasive Computing (pp. 158-175).

Tsipouras, M. G., Fotiadis, D. I., & Sideris, D. (2005). An arrhythmia classification system based on the RR-interval signal. *Artificial Intelligence in Medicine, 33*(3), 237–250. doi:10.1016/j.artmed.2004.03.007

US Census Bureau. (2008, 13/08/2008). *Projected Population by Single Year of Age, Sex, Race, and Hispanic Origin for the United States: July 1, 2000 to July 1, 2050.* Retrieved 27/01/2009, from http://www.census.gov/population/www/projections/downloadablefiles.html

Virone, G., Alwan, M., Dalal, S., Kell, S. W., Turner, B., & Stankovic, J. A. (2008). Behavioral Patterns of Older Adults in Assisted Living. *IEEE Transactions on Information Technology in Biomedicine, 12*(3), 12. doi:10.1109/TITB.2007.904157

Voon, R., Celler, B. G., & Lovell, N. H. (2008). *The use of an energy monitor in the management of diabetes: a pilot study.* Diabetes Technology and Therapeutics.

Warren, S., Yao, J., & Barnes, G. E. (2002). Wearable sensors and component-based design for home health care. *Annual International Conference of the IEEE Engineering in Medicine and Biology - Proceedings, 3,* 1871-1872.

Williams, G., Doughty, K., & Bradley, D. A. (1998). A systems approach to achieving CarerNet- an integrated and intelligent telecare system. *Information Technology in Biomedicine. IEEE Transactions on, 2*(1), 1–9.

Wilson, L. S., Ho, P., Bengston, K. J., Dadd, M. J., Chen, C. F., Huynh, C., et al. (2001). *The CSIRO hospital without walls home telecare system.* Paper presented at the Intelligent Information Systems Conference, The Seventh Australian and New Zealand 2001.

Wolf, D. A., & Jenkins, C. (2008). Family Care and Assisted Living. In Golant, S. M., & Hyde, J. (Eds.), *The Assisted Living Residence.* Baltimore: The Johns Hopkins University Press.

Wylde, M. A. (2008). The Future of Assisted Living: Residents' Perspectives 2006-2026. In Golant, S. M., & Hyde, J. (Eds.), *The Assisted Living Residence.* Baltimore: The Johns Hopkins University Press.

Yamaguchi, A., Ogawa, M., Tamura, T., & Togawa, T. (1998). *Monitoring behavior in the home using positioning sensors.* Paper presented at the Engineering in Medicine and Biology Society, 1998. Proceedings of the 20th Annual International Conference of the IEEE.

## ADDITIONAL READING

Barger, T. S., Brown, D. E., & Alwan, M. (2005). Health-status monitoring through analysis of behavioral patterns. *Systems, Man and Cybernetics, Part A, IEEE Transactions on, 35*(1), 22-27.

Bulusu, N., & Jha, S. (Eds.). (2005). *Wireless sensor networks.* Norwood: Artech House, Inc.

Camp, J., Robinson, J., Steger, C., & Knightly, E. (2006). *Measurement driven deployment of a two-tier urban mesh access network.*

Chaudhuri, S., & Dayal, U. (1997). An Interview of Data Warehousing and OLAP technology. *SIGMOD Record*, *26*(1), 65–74. doi:10.1145/248603.248616

Deshpande, A., Guestrin, C., & Madden, S. (2005). Using probabilistic models for data management in acquisitional environments. *Proc. Biennial Conf. on Innovative Data Sys. Res.(CIDR)*, 317–328.

EL-Darieby, H., Morgan, Y., & Adbdulhai, B. (2008). A Wireless Mesh Network-based Platform for ITS [Electronic Version], Farschi, S., Pesterev, A., Nuyujukian, P. H., Mody, I., & Judy, J. W. (2007). Bi-Fi: An Embedded Sensor/System Architecture for Remote Biological Monitoring. *IEEE Transactions on Information Technology in Biomedicine*, *11*(6), 611–618.

Fayyad, U., Piatetsky-Shapiro, G., & Smyth, P. (1996). From Data Mining to Knowledge Discovery in Databases. *AI Magazine*, *17*(3), 37–54.

Forouzandeh, F. F., & Mohamed, O. A. (2008). *Ultra Low Energy Communication Protocol for Implantable Body Sensor Networks*.

Fulford-Jones, T. R. F., Wei, G. Y., & Welsh, M. (2004). A portable, low-power, wireless two-lead EKG system. *Engineering in Medicine and Biology Society, 2004. EMBC 2004. Conference Proceedings. 26th Annual International Conference of the, 1*.

Georgios, K., Eleni, K., & Stefanos, G. (2007). *Securing Medical Sensor Environments: The CodeBlue Framework Case*. Paper presented at the Proceedings of the The Second International Conference on Availability, Reliability and Security.

Han, J., & Kamber, M. (2000). *Data Mining: Concepts and Techniques*. San Diego: Academic Press.

Hayes, T. L., Pavel, M., Schallau, P. K., & Adami, A. M. (2003). Unobtrusive Monitoring of Health Status in an Aging Population. *Proceedings of The 2nd International Workshop on Ubiquitous Computing for Pervasive Healthcare Applications. UbiHealth*.

Hiramatsu, K., Hattori, T., Yamada, T., & Okadome, T. (2006). *A Simple Probabilistic Analysis of Sensor Data Fluctuations In the Real World*. Paper presented at the 20th International Conference on Advanced Information Networking and Applications.

Hori, T., Nishida, Y., Aizawa, H., Murakami, S., & Mizoguchi, H. (2004). *Sensor network for supporting elderly care home*. Paper presented at the Sensors, 2004. Proceedings of IEEE.

IEEE. (2003a). IEEE standard for information technology - telecommunications and information exchange between systems - local and metropolitan area networks specific requirements part 15.4: wireless medium access control (MAC) and physical layer (PHY) specifications for low-rate wireless personal area networks (LR-WPANs), IEEE Std 802.15.4-2003 (pp. 0_1-670).

IEEE. (2003b). *Low-Rate Wireless Personal Area Networks: Enabling Wireless Sensors with IEEE 802.15.4*. IEEE Press.

Karl, H., & Willing, A. (2005). *Protocols and architectures for wireless sensor networks*. West Sussex: John Wiley & Sons Ltd. doi:10.1002/0470095121

Kelly, D., McLoone, S., Dishongh, T., McGrath, M., & Behan, J. (2008). *Single access point location tracking for in-home health monitoring*. Paper presented at the Positioning, Navigation and Communication, 2008. WPNC 2008. 5th Workshop on.

Kotanen, A., Hannikainen, M., Leppakoski, H., & Hamalainen, T. D. (2003). *Experiments on local positioning with Bluetooth*. Paper presented at the Information Technology: Coding and Computing [Computers and Communications], 2003. Proceedings. ITCC 2003. International Conference on.

Lee, D.-S., Lee, Y.-D., Chung, W.-Y., & Myllyla, R. (2007). *Vital Sign Monitoring System with Life Emergency Event Detection using Wireless Sensor Network*. Paper presented at the Sensors, 2006. 5th IEEE Conference on.

Lin, C. C., Chiu, M. J., Hsiao, C. C., Lee, R. G., & Tsai, Y. S. (2006). Wireless Health Care Service System for Elderly With Dementia. *Information Technology in Biomedicine. IEEE Transactions on, 10*(4), 696–704.

Monton, E., Hernandez, J. F., Blasco, J. M., Herve, T., Micallef, J., & Grech, I. (2008). Body area network for wireless patient monitoring. *Communications, IET, 2*(2), 215–222. doi:10.1049/iet-com:20070046

Mori, T., Suemasu, Y., Noguchi, H., & Sato, T. (2004). *Multiple people tracking by integrating distributed floor pressure sensors and RFID system*. Paper presented at the Systems, Man and Cybernetics, 2004 IEEE International Conference on.

Rashvand, H. F., Salcedo, V. T., Sanchez, E. M., & Iliescu, D. (2008). Ubiquitous wireless telemedicine. *Communications, IET, 2*(2), 237–254. doi:10.1049/iet-com:20070361

Ristic, L. (Ed.). (1994). *Sensor Technology and Devices*. Norwood: Artech House, Inc.

Ross, P. E. (2004). Managing care through the air [remote health monitoring]. *Spectrum, IEEE, 41*(12), 26-31.

Shorey, R., Ananda, A., Chan, M. C., & OOI, W. T. (Eds.). (2006). *Mobile, Wireless, and Sensor Networks: technology, applications, and future directions*. Hoboken: John Wiley & Sons, Inc.

Wakamiya, N., & Murata, M. (2004). Scalable and robust scheme for data fusion in sensor networks. *Proceedings of International Workshop on Biologically Inspired Approaches to Advanced Information Technology (Bio-ADIT)*, 112–127.

Witten, I., & Eibe, F. (2005). *Data Mining: Practical Machine Learning Tools and Techniques*. San Diego: Academic Press.

Wood, A., Stankovic, J., Virone, G., Selavo, L., Zhimin, H., & Qiuhua, C. (2008). Context-aware wireless sensor networks for assisted living and residential monitoring. *Network, IEEE, 22*(4), 26–33. doi:10.1109/MNET.2008.4579768

Yang, G. Z., Lo, B., Wang, J., Rans, M., Thiemjarus, S., & Ng, J. (2004). *From Sensor Networks to Behaviour Profiling: A Homecare Perspective of Intelligent Building*. The IEE Seminar for Intelligent Buildings.

Zhao, Q., & Bhowmick, S. (2003). *Association Rule Mining: A survey*. CAIS, Nanyang Technological Universityo. Document Number.

## KEY TERMS AND DEFINITIONS

**Activities of Daily Living Monitoring:** This provides an assessment of a person's basic functional status by measuring the person's capability to perform daily, normal activities for self-care.

**Data Fusion:** The act of combining data from multiple data sources with a view to improve accuracy and in some cases to provide inferences.

**Network Protocol:** A common communication standard shared by all the computing nodes that participate in a network.

**Network Topology:** The physical arrangement and logical interconnection between participating computing nodes in a network.

**Residential Aged Care:** The provision of health care services to the elderly at their place of residence.

**Ubiquitous Networks:** The deployment of a large number of computing nodes in a physical environment such that the nodes are as transparent to the user as possible.

**Telehealth:** The delivery of health care services over distance using telecommunication infrastructures.

**Wellness Monitoring:** The complete assessment of a person's well-being by measuring the person's physiological conditions and through activities of daily living monitoring.

**Wireless Sensor Networks:** Networks composed of sensor nodes spatially distributed in an environment and physically connected using wireless communication techniques aiming at measuring certain parameters of interests.

*A previous version of this chapter was originally published in International Journal of Healthcare Delivery Reform Initiatives, Vol. 1, Issue 4, edited by M. Guah, copyright 2010 by IGI Publishing (an imprint of IGI Global).*

# Chapter 2

# Smart Homes to Support Elderly People:
## Innovative Technologies and Social Impacts

**Arianna D'Ulizia**
*CNR - Istituto di Ricerche sulla Popolazione e le Politiche Sociali, Italy*

**Fernando Ferri**
*CNR - Istituto di Ricerche sulla Popolazione e le Politiche Sociali, Italy*

**Patrizia Grifoni**
*CNR - Istituto di Ricerche sulla Popolazione e le Politiche Sociali, Italy*

**Tiziana Guzzo**
*CNR - Istituto di Ricerche sulla Popolazione e le Politiche Sociali, Italy*

## ABSTRACT

*Today the biggest challenge of our aging society is to enable people with impairments to have a better quality of life maintaining their independence. The chapter explores how technology can support elderly and disabled people in their home. Firstly, a classification of Smart Home Systems in Safety systems, Environmental control systems, Energy-control-systems, Reminder systems, Medication Dispensing systems, Communication and Entertainment systems is presented. For each of these systems some examples of different technological solutions presented in the literature are described. Moreover, an analysis of social and economic impacts of the use of these technologies on the society is presented. Finally, some studies about the perception and acceptance of these technologies by user are given.*

## INTRODUCTION

Society is facing the challenge of demographic changes: today, society is composed more and more by elderly people.

DOI: 10.4018/978-1-61520-765-7.ch002

According to United Nation Population Division (UNDP) (*Population Division, Department of Economic and Social Affairs, United Nations Secretariat*) one out of every ten persons is now 60 years old or above; by 2050, one out of five will be 60 years or older; and by 2150, one out of three persons will be 60 years or older. Italy is the country with more elderly people in Europe: almost one Italian out five is more 65 years and over 80 are about the 5% of the total population (Istat, 2006).

This phenomenon implies that it is necessary to face problems tied to an ageing society (Koch, 2005) such as:

- increased demand of healthcare,
- demand for accessibility of care outside hospitals (at home),
- need of efficiency and quality in healthcare with limited financial resources,
- difficulties of recruiting staff for home healthcare services.

Today the biggest challenge is to help people not only to live longer, but also assuring them more years of health and independence. Several elderly people have some limitations in performing daily activities. The disabilities connected with oldness are mainly about reduced mobility and physical abilities, sensory acuity and altered mental clarity. Moreover, several elderly people have lost consort and friends and their families live away. These factors can bring to the lack of independence and safety and toward social isolation.

Nowadays, the governments, in conjunction with different kinds of organization and companies, are searching new models and systems for health and social care that improve the services quality optimising costs.

Information and communication technologies (ICT) run parallel to these societal changes and can play an important role in dealing with these challenges. Innovative technologies are emerging as a support for reacting to problems related to oldness, bringing care outside hospitals and increasing health services into the elderly people homes.

In particular, smart homes (also known as home automation or residential automation) address the promotion of the independent living by using assistive technologies for higher quality of daily life, maintaining a high degree of autonomy and dignity.

This chapter aims at giving a comprehensive analysis of both the innovative ICT systems used in smart homes and the social and economic impacts that these systems have on the society.

In the first section a classification of systems used in smart homes has been made, analysing their functionalities and properties. In the second section, social and economic impacts of smart home technologies are discussed. Finally, in the third section the users' acceptance of these technologies is faced, starting from existing studies about the perception that users have on these technologies.

## CLASSIFICATION OF SMART HOME TECHNOLOGIES

Smart Homes are defined by Cheek as "a collective term for information and communication technology in homes where components communicate through a local network" (Cheek, 2005). These technologies allows to remotely monitor, alarm and execute actions in order to assist elderly or impaired people in their daily activities, according to the different planned needs.

Celler et al. (1999) categorize Smart Home Systems or tools into three categories: first, second and third generation systems.

First-generation systems include personal alarm systems and emergency response telephones. These systems generate alarms with the intervention of the patient who can press a wireless pendant alarm worn around the neck or wrist and connect with a control centre (Celler et al. 1999).

Second-generation systems monitor health status changes and generate alarms automatically. For example, Smart Shirt is a wearable system (like a shirt) that allows to measure heart rate, electrocardiogram results, respiration, temperature and blood pressure, alerting doctors in case of problems. (Bowie, 2000). Another second-generation system, developed by Medtronic (www.medtronic.com), allows to monitor the patients by an antenna over the implanted cardiac devices that transmit data, visualized on a monitor, and sent to a Medtronic Care Link Network; in this manner doctors and family members can access these data by a clinician's Website.

Third-generation systems allow elderly and disabled people to connect themselves with other people in similar conditions through Internet, establishing a virtual community to deal with loneliness and isolation and to have emotional support. (Celler, 1999).

As stated by Laberg (2005), several devices can be integrated into a smart home, such as safety, environmental control systems, communication, energy-control systems, and entertainment.

Starting from an analysis of these devices, we have extended the concepts introduced by Laberg proposing a rough classification of first, second and third generation systems according to the functionality they have in a smart home. This classification includes:

- *Safety systems,* that automatically generate alarms and alerts when significant changes are observed in vital signs,
- *Environmental control systems,* that control and plan lock of doors, windows and lights,
- *Energy-control-systems,* that provide appliances for monitoring and controlling the heating and energy generators,
- *Reminder systems,* that include doctor's appointments and medicine reminders,
- *Medication Dispensing systems,* that monitor for example blood pressure, pulse, fever and then dispense requested medications when needed,
- *Communication and Entertainment systems,* which help the elderly and disabled people to be connected with other elderly

or disabled people, to watch television and to play with interactive games.

In the next sections, we provide a description of each class of these systems.

## Safety Systems

Safety systems or alarm systems play a very important role in smart home applications. If an elderly person has an accident, sometimes she/he doesn't have enough time or possibility to ask help: safety monitoring systems can save their life. For example, in case of collapse, panic or loss of consciousness, passive alarms are the best solution. These alarms send information (e.g. about vital signal such as pulse, blood pressure, etc.) to an evaluation system that automatically sends an alarm signal to the emergency service station (Kannan et al., 2008).

Another serious health problem for elderly people is for example arterial hypertension: smart homes provide measurement and monitoring technologies to evaluate patients' health status at home exemplifying health care through home tele-monitoring of blood pressure. Clinical applications include: emergency interventions, audio or video triage, tele-consultations, remote diagnosis and treatment.

Other systems monitor elderly people mobility and their interactions with the environment using sensors. These detect the location of the elderly person and record their time stay or measure the time spent for movements. Nì Scanaill et al. (2006) described several sensors employed in smart homes: pressure sensors (pads placed under mattresses or chairs to detect if they are used), pressure mat (pats to detect movement), smart tiles (to detect the direction in which the elderly person walks), passive infrared sensors (to detect movement if there are heat variations. False alarms can be due to wind or excessive heat), sound sensors (to determine if some activities are carried out), magnetic switches (switches used in doorframes or friges to detect movement), active infrared sensors (to estimate size and direction when elderly people passe through doors) and optical/ultrasonic system (to measure the speed and direction passing through doors).

Celler et al. (1994) presented the first system to monitor mobility. This system uses: (i) magnetic switches placed in the doors to detect the presence in a room by recording the movements, (ii) infrared sensors to determine the specific position of elderly people in room, and (iii) generic sound sensors to detect the type of activity. Collected data were transmitted via the telephone network to a monitoring and supervisory center.

## Environmental Control Systems

People with physical disabilities have difficulties in controlling appliances such as: to turn on/off lights, to answer the telephone, to control television and so on.

Environmental control systems are hardware or software systems that allow to operate electronic devices at home by remote control. These systems enhance the ability of disabled or elderly people to execute actions such as to turn on/off lights, radio, and television, to answer phone calls, to unlock doors and windows.

Generally, the technologies used to control the appliances of environmental control systems are based on (Ability Research Centre, 1999):

- Infrareds, they are wavelengths of light beyond the visible spectrum. They allow to control several appliances such as television, video, stereo. Their advantages consist in the portability and low installation costs. The limitation is that the device must be pointed at the appliances to control them.
- X-10 technology: it is based on the X-10 Power Line Carrier (PLC) signalling "language" that enables control signals to be transmitted in the house over existing

220/240v electrical lines. The advantage of this technology is its wide accessibility. The limitation is the low level of reliability that precludes its use for people with disabilities.
- Radio frequency (RF) transmission: it uses radio waves to transmit the output power of a transmitter to an antenna. When the antenna is not closely situated to the transmitter, special transmission lines are required. The advantage is that it has a greater range than infrared and does not require line of sight between devices. The limitation is that it can have interference problems.

The project INSPIRE 2004 (Infotainment management with SPeech Interaction via Remote microphones and telephone interfaces) has developed a system that allows to control via speech different devices such as lamps, TV, video recorders, fans, blinds, answering machines, etc. This system can be used via microphone or from remote locations via the telephone network. It records users' speeches, which are recognized by a commercial speech recogniser and interpreted by a key-expression matching module (Gödde et al. 2008).

Another portable system is Nemo, that can be controlled both by voice commands for people who can't walk, and by a switch with sensor control or a joystick for people who can't speak. Users have to input words belonging to training menu to train the system to recognise voice. Users receive auditory feedback that indicates if the option selected was activated. (Marsden, 1999).

The Gewa Prog III (http://www.possum.co.uk/gewa_prog.htm) is a learning infrared transmitter, which can be programmed to provide remote control of TV, video, stereo, intercom, lights, doors and other domestic appliances. It allows to control 150 commands spread over 10 different levels, by the integral keyboard or by external switches. Single switches, multifunction switches and also joysticks can be used. This system allows programming macro sequences, (e.g. by pressing a single key the system automatically performs a sequence of functions, such as to turn off the television and to answer to the telephone).

## Energy Control Systems

Energy control systems offer to users security, convenience and energy management functionalities. Automated controls are mainly about lighting, heating and air conditioning and safety and security monitoring. Sensors input and schedules allow to turn on/off an appliance automatically, only when it is needed. During the day, these systems do not open the lights but the drapes. During the night instead the light opens when a person enters in a room and turn off when no one is in the room. These systems help also to save electricity. So if people are not watching the television, the system will turn off it.

Energy control systems monitor and control the heating and air conditioning, by correcting, for example, the temperature in the rooms depending on the cold and turning off air conditioning when people are not in the house. Moreover, these systems can set off alarm when detect a fire, turn on lights to get out, open the doors and the windows to ventilate the smoke and call rescue services through auto-dialer (Kassim, 2007). In case of gas leak, the system detects it and turns off the gas main and all electric devices to avoid spark, and sounds an alarm to alert the home inhabitants. Other more advanced systems use voice automation to inform them about what is happening and what needs to be done (Chambers, 2004).

## Reminder Systems

The decline of cognitive abilities is the most common effect of aging. Memory problems are very debilitating for elderly people and their families. To provide a solution to these problems, several devices have been developed.

The Memojog project has developed an interactive communication system (see Figure 1) that utilizes current and easily available technologies, such as the Internet and GPRS mobile telephony (Morrison et al. 2004). Reminders are stored in a remote server and wirelessly transmitted from server to the Personal Digital Assistant (PDA) of the user at the appropriate time. The users or carers can add reminders remotely by using any Internet accessible device. Furthermore, the system can monitor if users react correctly to reminders. For example, if the user doesn't respond to the reminder "take medication", a phone message is sent to the carers or family members by the central server.

Hermes (Geven et al. 2008) is a mobile guide that, similarly to a memo-recorder, allows the user to record events for later re-call. The PDA or mobile phone records information about the time and place of an event. The user provides this information by speech. Afterwards, the recorded data are processed into text and the meaningful information is extracted and entered in a calendar. When the planned event is about to occur, the system remembers it to the user by a reminder.

Unlike other systems that use fixed reminders at pre-specified times, Autominder (Pollack et al. 2003) is an assistive technology system deployed on a mobile robot that uses artificial-intelligence technology to model an individual daily plan. It makes adaptive decisions about whether and when it is most appropriate to issue reminders on the strength of observation of user's behavior. Sometimes, elderly people perceive reminders as an intrusion. For this reason, it is important to give advise only at the appropriate moments.

An extension of Autominder is MAGS, the Michigan Autonomous Guidance System, (Weber et al. 2007) which introduces advanced technologies for interfacing and interacting with the user. Such technologies include:

- an adaptive user interface that customizes its elements according to the degree of both

*Figure 1. Memojog system (Morrison et al. 2004)*

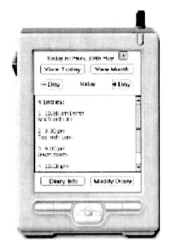 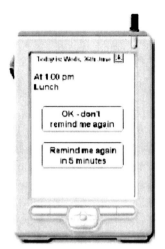

ability and disability of each user obtained by monitoring the interaction;

- preference learning techniques, that infer the preferences of a user on the base of the interactions with the system;
- advanced activity recognition and execution monitoring. The last one keeps track of planned activities and avoids conflicts within the user's daily plan, controlling whether, when, and how the system will interact with the user. The activity recognition module determines which activities are being performed by the user at any given time;
- information access engines to obtain data from the web (for example, for accessing to medical appointment calendars or weather information) and from other MAGS applications (for example, to promote social interaction).

## Medication Dispensing Systems

The elderly people, due to the decline of their cognitive abilities, can forget to take drugs, can take wrong drugs or do not take right doses to correct times. This can have serious effects on the health of these people. Consequently, technologies to remind elderly people what and when drugs have to be taken are proposed. Medication Dispensers are systems aimed at assisting elderly people in safely managing complex drug administration at home. In particular, technological solutions include:

- *Pill organizers,* that organize pills in compartments corresponding to a scheduling regime;
- *Electronic pill organizers,* that remind when take the pills through beeping, a voice, or a flashing light;
- *Personal Medication Systems,* that remind when the drug should be taken by a visual and auditory alarm, dispense the drugs if a single button is pressed, and alert carers if drugs are taken upon non-compliance.

Med-O-Wheel Smart (http://www.addoz.com) is a system that indicates with an audio alarm when to take medication and dispenses the right dosage. If the elderly person does not take the drugs, the device emits a flashing light and a warning signal. If elderly person does not take the drugs again,

*Figure 2. The context-aware pill bottle and medication monitor (Agarawala et al. 2004)*

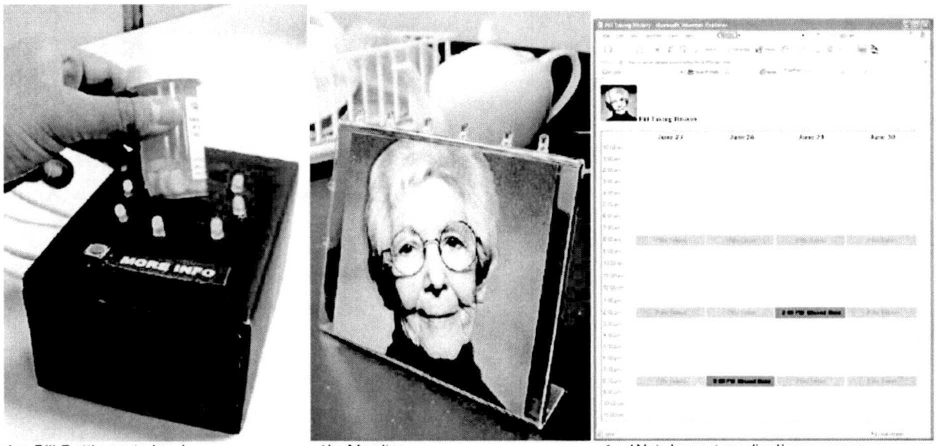

| 1a: Pill Bottle and stand | 1b: Montior | 1c: Web-based medication summary |

a radio transmitter communicates a missed dose to medical call centre or relatives.

Agarawala et al. (2004) proposed a context-aware pill bottle/stand (see Figure 3) that reminds elderly people when take drugs by dispensing them on the basis of the medication schedule. Pill bottles are augmented with RFID tags that are associated with specific prescription information filled in by a pharmacist and stored in an XML database. Moreover this device is connected with a medication monitor situated in a carer's home, which displays the status of elderly user's medication compliance and alarms if necessary.

## Communication and Entertainment systems

The social relationships with other people are important for emotional well-being of elderly people. Interaction can be carried out directly, by correspondence, by phone or by Internet. The new ICT solutions offer good tools to maintain contacts (e.g. mobile technologies or social networks), to know other people in the same condition and to find moral support. These tools play an important role to maintain and develop social relationships even if they do not replace personal contacts, but they encourage social involvement of elderly people.

Mobile technologies enable communication anywhere and anytime, allowing access to any services and creating a sense of security and safety for elderly people and their families.

Entertainment systems, such as for example intelligent television, learn user's preferences and can be remotely programmed to be available whenever wanted.

Smart Table is a system that provides a broadband communication without the need of a computer. This system provides an easy and intuitive way to communicate and avoid social isolation of elderly people. The television is used for video communication (web-cam) and the table as a user interface. Contacts can be selected on the table, which enables also the sharing images and video (http://www.propeller.com/story/2008/12/31/smart-table-communication-system-for-elderly-smart-computing-blog/).

Mynatt et al. (2001) developed a communication device, named Digital Family Portrait, which provides back-story information about distant relatives it is a useful tool for elderly people living far from the family. Elderly people need to be in touch with their closest relatives, and a tool that helps to feel that "things seems ok to Mum's house" is useful for the people.

The digital family portrait consists of a frame that displays different icons, each one representing different situations and concepts related to previous time. Time lapsing also is displayed by the system providing more information about closest time (last day), and average for remote past time (two weeks before).

## SOCIAL IMPACTS OF SMART HOME TECHNOLOGIES

The smart home technologies have several social, economic and organizational impacts. At the social level, the improvement of the quality of life, for both the sick person and those who take care of her/him, is the first and foremost impact of these technologies. The elderly person, supported and monitored continuously by smart home technologies, can therefore continue to live in her/his own social environment with safety and dignity, and even when she/he needs health care she/he can receive assistance at home, instead of into a clinic or a hospital. In this way, impaired people can perform their daily activities in an independent and autonomous way without the help of relatives or carers, reducing social problems.

The systems we have described in the previous sections guarantee to elderly people personal assistance, medical care, support in daily activities, and leisure activities. These systems provide also monitoring and risks management functionalities, avoiding incidents, by using sensors that automatically alert to a central monitoring system.

Moreover, the automation of these systems supports an independent living of elderly people. For example, the use of switches allows to set particular conditions of the house in order to help elderly people with reduced mobility to turn on/off appliances without doing it manually.

These technologies allow elderly people to live in a familiar environment without the need of going to a nursing home. The domestic attendance is often chosen in the attempt to maintain an independent life of the elderly people and to delay the hospitalisation as much as possible.

In Europe the choice of home attendance is due to the following reasons:

- a limited number of healthcare structures,
- high costs for long stay hospital care,
- ethical-cultural preferences that lead to maintain the elderly person at home with her/his family.

Today, the senile diseases, such as dementia, are considered "social diseases", because they do not involve the sick person only, but also the social network in which s/he is inserted in, and the families that are deeply involved in the care and attendance.

The progressive ageing of the population has led to reconsider the social impact of some diseases, such as for example Alzheimers, which has been having an increasing incidence in the last years. The social cost of this pathology is very high both in terms of life quality of the sick person and in terms of psychophysical health of the family. A lot of people are assisted at home and the majority of them receive attendance from relatives or friends. The strong involvement of the family in the health care and attendance of Alzheimer patients has led to refer to this disease as a "familiar disease".

Psychological, emotional, social and economic impacts that Alzheimer has on the families that live with an Alzheimer's patient are enormous. Families and friends bear psychological and financial weights, incurring often in physical and mental problems.

In this situation, smart home technologies can increase personal independence of the sick person, helping her/him to live autonomously and more safely for a longer time. These technologies help to improve the quality of life of impaired people, to mitigate difficulties of the dementia, to prevent patients from risks, to assist elderly people, and to give more years of health and independence, mainly in the first stage of the disease.

Moreover, these systems provide a great opportunity for integrating people that may risk the social exclusion: elderly people can contact other people who have the same problem in order to share experiences and to exchange opinions.

Smart homes can have also psychosocial effects on the elderly people and their carers. Firstly, they feel more involved in the care process and enhance their well-being as they feel continuously monitored by the medical centre. Patients at home can have an improved access to health care, particularly those with chronic diseases. The patients feel a sense of connection to medical staff and enhance communication regarding their health status. Relatives are more informed and secure about their parents controlling their health status in the distance (Magnusson et al., 2004).

Another important impact is the reduction of social service costs, due to the decrease of the hospitalisation days and the lower necessity of medical tools. However today, the costs of smart home technologies can be high. Furthermore, some countries do not provide economic support to elderly people who install these technologies, although they are cheaper than health care in hospitals. Then, elderly people have to use their savings or those of their families. Institutions should change the focus of healthcare aiming at the wellness of elderly person. Smart homes allow to stay at home with a better coordination of care, decreasing costs of institutionalisation (Cheek, 2005). The most important study on costs and benefits of smart homes has been carried out by Quigley and Tweed (1999). They face the problem in qualitative terms rather than monetary: "The costs and benefits to a person's quality of life are more important than the financial cost. Any system, no matter how costly that improves quality of life is probably worthwhile. The financial benefits of such a system will be recuperated in due time as the costs of care and hospital expenditure drop. Any system that does not improve

quality of life will in the long run prove costly financially because not only is there the expense of the installation but there will be a continued need for high level of care for the individual. It is in the interest of care providers and housing authorities to install and maintain such systems. It would be unreasonable to expect an old age pensioner to purchase assistive technology, as this would prove a financial strain. It may be possible for the users to contribute in some way e.g. deduction from their pension or deductions in benefits." (Quigley et al., 1999).

At the organizational level the realization of a policy that aims to favourite the home care involves different levels of government: national, regional and local (Tarricone et al., 2008).

At the national level, central administration should implement policies in order to plan, legislate and regulate home care. Moreover, it should develop and set priorities on allocating human and material resources in homogeneous way among different regions.

At the regional level, administration is in charge of allocating resources set at national level. These allocations should be based on standards that consider regional and local needs. Moreover, guidelines are needed in order to avoid gaps and problems in providing services.

At the local level, strategies for mobilizing community actions (that involve carers, health and social service workers, community volunteers, influential leaders) are expected in order to plan and implement home care. The involvement of local communities allows to initiate, ensure the reactivity, and sustain the programme.

In several European countries, home care is located between health care system and the social system, according to the kind of service (health or social). The organizational model of Italy, France, Belgium, Spain, Portugal, and United Kingdom is based on the separation of health and social components. The first is part of the health care system, the second is part of the social system. This separation is due to the fact that health is regulated by either the national health system (Italy, Greece, United Kingdom and the Nordic countries) or a national social insurance system (Austria, France, Germany and the Netherlands), while the social welfare is managed by regional or local governments.

In Denmark, Finland and Sweden, home care is provided within a single organization and the responsible institution is the municipalities. Germany and the Netherlands have an insurance-based funding that covers both health and social care services.

In Italy, home care is based on public funding provided by local health authorities; however other kinds of funding are possible. Lombardy Region, for example, has funded some people by a voucher. Accredited (both public and private) suppliers can provide services, which are paid by the voucher. The monthly vouchers are allotted considering three aspects: i) the nature of the needs (social and health problems, the complexity of the problems, ill people); ii) the kind of resources involved (professionals and technologies); iii) the intensity of care.

## PERCEPTIONS AND ACCEPTANCE OF SMART HOMES BY ELDERLY AND DISABLED PEOPLE

A very important aspect for the development of assistive technologies in smart homes is the acceptance of users. This can differ among users, age and time. Some studies, carrying out several interviews with elderly people, have found some important aspects described below.

Giuliani et al. (2005) have shown that innovative technologies are accepted by users if usefulness and perceived benefits are high. The studies of McCreadie et al. (2005) and Sanchez et al. (2005) affirmed that beyond need satisfaction, reliability is another very important aspect in the perception and consequently in acceptance of these technologies.

Meyer et al. (2002) in their study about analysis of consumer's behaviour have compared elderly and younger people. From their analysis, it is possible to gather that a common opinion of elderly people is that smart homes improve their everyday life quality by increasing comfort and security. The negative aspects, described in these studies, are the high costs, the very high complexity of the risk to damage privacy, the risk of dominance of technology and the consequent reduction of social relationship. The main problem that elderly people have in using technologies is the difficulty to acquire skill with new tools as their short-term memory is reduced. In fact, they express the need to have at their disposal more natural and easy-to-use technologies, able to improve their independence. Moreover, they wish technologies that assure more security and independence and robots that clean the home.

Vincent et al. (2002) analysed perception that users have about environmental control systems: they concluded that verbal reminders were greatly appreciated than the use of remote control by people with moderate cognitive impairments.

A study about perception and expectations of elderly people about smart home technologies installed in their homes has been performed by Demiris et al. (2004). They have carried out three focus group sessions with 15 older adults participants to assess their perceptions about these technologies. Participants expressed some concerns about the privacy. They would prefer the use of cameras that do not identify people but only shadows and movements in order to maintain anonymity. Some people expressed the need of a human presence because technologies alone are not useful enough. An aspect, emphasized by elderly people, was the lack of usability of some devices. According to them, some interfaces do not take into account the functional limitations of ageing such as: loss of vision or tactile sense, hearing impairment, memory or balance loss, difficulty in using computer mouse or small buttons. They expressed the need for training sessions for elderly people that are low skilled with technologies. Moreover, some people are technophobes: sensors that do not require to be controlled by users could be more useful. This concern has been contradicted by Collins et al. (1992) who, in their survey of 2500 older people, have shown that there is not relationship between age and technophobia. This has been explained also by Selwyn (2004), who has shown, by interviews, how technologies are less accepted by elderly people than younger people because the last ones have more pleasure in using them.

All these studies show how people generally have positive perceptions towards smart home technologies. They perceived these technologies as tools that can improve or make safer their lives. Elderly people are favourable disposed to accept these technologies as support of their daily life but some concerns are perceived in negative way. In order to increase the acceptance of these technologies by users is fundamental (for designers) to take into account the issues discussed in this section and make devices user-friendly, not intrusive, reliable and low-cost.

New technologies can improve the quality of life of disabled people, only if they are developed according to criteria that allow everyone to use them. Smart home systems are effective if they are understood and accepted by users. Usability is a fundamental requirement. There is therefore the need to have technologies that are more simple and easy to use, in line with actual and concrete needs of users.

The coordination among the different actors of the supply chain is of primary importance for the development of this market. The common aim should be to make smart technologies usable for all people and to satisfy user expectations.

To support this strategy, interfaces between people and home environment should be user-friendly, multi-modal, context-aware, intelligent, and interactive. Home environment integration and automation enable a reduction of commands to be given and simplify the human computer interac-

tion. Multimodal interaction is a good solution to improve the efficiency of Smart Home systems for elderly care, because it offers improved flexibility, usability and interaction efficiency, allowing the user to interact through input modalities, such as speech, handwriting, hand gesture and gaze, and to receive information by the system through output modalities, such as speech synthesis and smart graphics and others modalities, opportunely combined. The studies of Oviatt et al. (2000) demonstrate in fact, that multimodal systems enhance the accessibility, usability, flexibility and efficiency compared to unimodal ones. As elderly people can have the necessity to use different modality of interaction according to their disabilities, multimodal interfaces provide a helpful support for Smart Home usability.

## CONCLUSION

In this chapter we have analysed different systems used in smart homes. We have proposed a classification of these systems, into six main categories: *safety systems* that monitor health status of users and their mobility; *environmental systems* that control by remote electronic devices; *energy control systems* that monitor and manage temperature; *reminder systems* that remind when take medicines; *medication dispensing systems* that dispense drugs in a safety way; *communication and entertainment systems* that enable communication with other people by Internet or other devices, and entertainment by intelligent televisions.

These technologies can have several social and psychological impacts on elderly people enabling to live with more independence and dignity. Some studies about user's perception and acceptance of these technologies have underlined some issues and limitations. Future directions of research should take into account these concerns. User's acceptance of technology, in fact, is a very important aspect to consider for achieving the success and diffusion into the society of smart home technologies.

Today, smart home technologies have to address several challenges. The biggest one is to meet individual needs of each person (patient or elderly people). For example, people with hearing impairments have different problems compared to people with cognitive or visual impairments. Therefore, they can meet limitations in using technologies that are not designed to take into account the kind of impairment (Cheek, 2005). It is very important to design a user-friendly systems for the elderly people who often are not able to use electronic devices.

Another challenge to address is the privacy. The technologies that we have described in this chapter cause some ethical questions. Monitoring is very important for security and safety of elderly people but these technologies are very intrusive for users' privacy. These ethical questions about privacy of users become more severe when these systems are installed in a normal family evoking the idea of "Big Brother".

Moreover, it is necessary to hint that smart homes support but they do not replace human care. In fact, several elderly people perceive remote services, provided only by telematic networks and not by human care, as a replacement of human carers by technologies, causing social isolation and exclusion.

For these reasons, designers were suggested to provide guidelines that consider social and ethical issues. Moreover, the necessity arises to promulgate laws, devoted to protect privacy and to define measures avoiding social exclusion and promoting the socialization (Abascal, 2004).

## REFERENCES

Abascal, J. (2004). Ambient Intelligence for people with disabilities and elderly people. *SIGCHI Workshop on Ambient Intelligence for Scienti_c Discovery (AISD). ACM 2004,* Vienna.

Ability Research Centre. (1999). *Environmental Control System for People with Spinal Injuries.* A report on Research Undertaken by the Ability Research Centre.

Agarawala, A., Greenberg, S., & Ho, G. (2004). The Context-Aware Pill Bottle and Medication Monitor. In *Video Proceedings and Proceedings Supplement of the UBICOM 2004 Conference,* Sept. 7-10, Nottingham, England.

Bowie, L. (2000). *Smart Shirt Moves From Research to Market: Goal is to Ease Healthcare Monitoring.* Georgia Institute of Technology. Retrieved March 10, 2003 from http://www.news-info.gatech.edu/news_release/sensatex.html

Celler, B. G., Hesketh, T., Earnshaw, W., & Ilsar, E. (1994). An instrumentation system for the remote monitoring of changes in functional health status of the elderly at home. In *Proceedings of the 16thAnnual International Conference of the IEEE EMBS,* (vol. 2, pp. 908–909).

Celler, B. G., Lovell, N. H., & Chan, D. K. Y. (1999). The potential impact of home telecare on clinical practice. *MJA, 171,* 518–521.

Chambers, C. (2004). *Smart Home How Home Automation Works and what it can do.* http://islab.oregonstate.edu/koc/ece399/f04/explo/chambers.pdf

Cheek, P. (2005). Aging Well With Smart Technology. *Nursing Administration Quarterly, 29*(4), 329–338.

Collins, S. C., Bhatti, J. Z., Dexter, S. L., & Rabbitt, P. M. (1992). Elderly people in a new world: attitudes to advanced communications technologies. In Boumqa, H., & Graafmans, J. A. M. (Eds.), *Gerontechnology.* Amsterdam: IOS Press.

Demiris, G., Rantz, M. J., Aud, M. A., Marek, K. D., Tyrer, H. W., Skubic, M., & Hussam, A. A. (2004). Older adults' attitudes towards and perceptions of 'smart home' technologies: a pilot study. *Med. Inform. Taylor & Francis Healthsciences, 29*(2), 87–94. doi:10.1080/146392304 10001684387

Geven, A., Tscheligi, M., Sorin, A., & Aronowitz, H. (2008). Presenting a speech-based mobile reminder system. In Proceedings of SiMPE 2008. Amsterdam, Netherlands.

Gödde, F., Möller, S., Engelbrecht, K.-P., Kühnel, C., Schleicher, R., Naumann, A., & Wolters, M. (2008). Study of a Speech-based Smart Home System with Older Users. In *International Workshop on Intelligent User Interfaces for Ambient Assisted Living*.

Guilliani, V., Scopeletti, M., & Fornara, F. (2005). Elderly People at Home: Technological Help in Everyday Activities. In *IEEE, International Workshop on Robots and Human Interactive Communication*. Retrieved from http://www.dinf.ne.jp/doc/english/Us_Eu/conf/csun_99/session0260.html

ISTAT. (2006). Popolazione comunale per sesso, età e stato civile - Anni 2002-2005. *Informazioni, 29*.

Kannan, G., & Vijayakumar, S. (2008). Smart Home Testbed for Disabled People. *Mobile and Pervasive Computing, CoMPC*.

Kassim, M. R. M. (2007). Design, development and implementation of smart home systems using rf and power line communication. In *The 2nd National Intelligent Systems And Information Technology Symposium (ISITS'07),* Oct 30-31, 2007, ITMA -UPM, Malaysia.

Koch, S. (2005). Home telehealth - Current state and future trends. *International Journal of Medical Informatics*.

Laberg, T. (2005). Smart Home Technology; Technology supporting independent living - does it have an impact on health? In E-health 05, Tromsø, Norway, 23 -24 May.

Magnusson, L., Hanson, E., & Borg, M. (2004). *A literature review study of Information and Communication Technology as a support for frail older people living at home and their family carers.* Technology and Disability.

Marsden, R. (1999). *What's new in Computer Access and Environmental Control Units (ECU's) at Madenta, Inc.*

McCreadie, C., & Tinker, A. (2005). The Acceptabiliy of Assistive Technology to Older People. *Ageing and Society, 25*, 91–110. doi:10.1017/S0144686X0400248X

Meyer, S., & Schulze, E. (2002). Smart Home and the Aging User. Trends and Analyses of Consumer Behaviour. In *Symposium "Domotics and Networking", Miami*, 11/19-12.

Morrison, K., Szymkowiak, A., & Gregor, P. (2004). Memojog - an interactive memory aid incorporating mobile based technologies. In S. Brewster & M. Dunlop (Eds.), MobileHCI, September 13-16, Glasgow, UK, (LNCS 3160, pp. 481-485). Berlin: Springer-Verlag.

Mynatt E.D., Rowan, J., Jacobs, A., & Craighill, S. (2001). Digital Family Portraits: Supporting Peace of Mind for Extended Family Members. *SIGCHI 2001 3*(1), 333-340.

Ni Scanaill, C., Carew, S., Barralon, P., Noury, N., Lyons, D., & Lyons, G. M. (2006). A Review of Approaches to Mobility Telemonitoring of the Elderly in Their Living Environment. Annals of Biomedical Engineering. *The Journal of the Biomedical Engineering Society, 34*(4).

Oviatt, S. L., & Cohen, P. R. (2000). Multimodal interfaces that process what comes naturally. *Communications of the ACM, 43*(3), 45–53. doi:10.1145/330534.330538

Pollack, M. E., Brown, L., Colbry, D., McCarthy Colleen, E., Orosz, C., & Peintner, B. (2003). *Autominder: An Intelligent Cognitive Orthotic System for People with Memory Impairment.* Robotics and Autonomous Systems.

Quigley, G., & Tweed, C. (1999). *Costs benefits analysis for assistive technologies. Research report on EPSRC GR/M05171.* Belfast, UK: Queen's University of Belfast.

Sanchez, J., Calcaterra, G., & Tran, Q. Q. (2005). Automation in the Home: The Development of an Appropriate System representation and its effects on reliance. In *Proceedings of the Human Factors and Ergonomics Society 49th Annual Meeting (HFES'05).* Santa Monica, CA: Human Factors and Ergonomics Society.

Selwyn, N. (2004). The Information Aged: A Qualitative Study of Older Adults' Use of Information and Communications Technology. *Journal of Aging Studies, 18*, 369–384. doi:10.1016/j.jaging.2004.06.008

Tarricone, R., & Tsouros, A. D. (2008). *Home Care in Europe.* World Health Organisation.

Vincent, C., Drouin, G., & Routhier, F. (2002). Examination of new environmental control applications. *Assistive Technology, 14*(2), 98–111.

Weber, J. S., Clippingdale, B., & Pollack, M. E. (2007). The Michigan Autonomous Guidance System. In *Proceedings of the 2nd International Conference on Technology and Aging.*

# Chapter 3
# Nursing Home

**Shuyan Xie**
*The University of Alabama, USA*

**Yang Xiao**
*The University of Alabama, USA*

**Hsiao-Hwa Chen**
*National Cheng Kung University, Taiwan*

## ABSTRACT

*A nursing home is an entity that provides skilled nursing care and rehabilitation services to people with illnesses, injuries or functional disabilities, but most facilities serve the elderly. There are various services that nursing homes provide for different residents' needs, including daily necessity care, mentally disabled, and drug rehabilitation. The levels of care and the care quality provided by nursing homes have increased significantly over the past decade. The trend nowadays is the continuous quality development towards to residents' satisfaction; therefore healthcare technology plays a significant role in nursing home operations. This chapter points out the general information about current nursing home conditions and functioning systems in the United States, which indicates the way that technology and e-health help improve the nursing home development based on the present needs and demanding trends. The authors' also provide a visiting report about Thomasville Nursing Home with the depth of the consideration to how to catch the trends by implementing the technologies.*

## INTRODUCTION

Nursing home is a significant part of long-term care in the health care system. Nursing homes provide a broad range of long-term care services – personal, social, and medical services designed to assist people who have functional or cognitive limitations in their ability to perform self-care and other activi-

ties necessary to live independently. This survey release some information about nursing home, including general introduction of nursing homes in the United States, resident information, quality of life, services that are providing, governmental regulations, and developing trends. Objectives of this chapter are providing the broad information about current nursing homes in the United States to help understand the positive and negative situations that confront to nursing homes. Furthermore, our

DOI: 10.4018/978-1-61520-765-7.ch007

nursing home visiting report points out the real residents' experience and opinions on their life qualities, needs and attitudes on technologies. Based on this information we introduce more technological innovations to improve nursing home development.

## PART I: NURSING HOMES IN THE UNITED STATES

### General Information

A nursing home, a facility for the care of individuals who do not require hospitalization and who cannot be cared for at home, is a type of care of residents. It is a place of residence of people who require constant nursing care and have significant deficiencies with activity of daily living ("Analysis of the National Nursing Home Survey (NNHS)," 2004).

People enter nursing homes for a variety of reasons. Some may enter for a brief time when they leave the hospital because they need sub-acute care, such as skilled nursing care, medical services, and therapies ("Analysis of the National Nursing Home Survey (NNHS)," 2004). Others, however, need long-term care (LTC). LTC is generally defined as a broad range of personal, social, and medical services that assist people who have functional or cognitive limitations in their ability to perform self-care and other activities necessary to live independently ("Analysis of the National Nursing Home Survey (NNHS)," 2004).

In the United States, nursing homes are required to have a licensed nurse on duty 24 hours a day, and during at least one shift each day, one of those nurses must be a Register Nurse ("Analysis of the National Nursing Home Survey (NNHS)," 2004). A registered nurse (RN) is a health care professional responsible for implementing the practice of nursing in concert with other health care professionals. Registered nurses work as patient advocates for the care and recovery of the sick and maintenance of the health ("Nursing Facts: Today's Registered Nurse - Numbers and Demographics," 2006).

In April, 2005 there were a total of 16,094 nursing homes in the United States. Some states having nursing homes that are called nursing facilities (NF), which do not have beds certified for Medicare patients, but can only treat patients whose payments sources is Private Payment, Private Insurance or Medicaid ("Medical & You handbook," 2008). Medicare is a social insurance program administered by the United States government, providing health insurance coverage to people who are aged 65 and over, or who meet other special criteria (Castle, 2008). Medicaid is the United States health program for eligible individuals and families with low incomes and resources. It is a means-tested program that is jointly funded by the states and federal government, and is managed by the states. Among the groups of people served by Medicaid are eligible low-income parents, children, seniors, and people with disabilities. Being poor, or even very poor, does not necessarily qualify an individual for Medicaid ("Overview Medicaid Program: General Information," 2006).

### Services

### Baseline Services

Those services included in the daily rate. The following basic services should be made available to all the residents:

- Lodging-a clean, healthful, sheltered environment, proper outfitted;
- Dietary services;
- 24-hour-per-day nursing care;
- pharmacy services;
- diagnostic services;
- the use of all equipment, medical supplies and modalities used in the care of nursing home residents, including but not limited

to catheters, hypodermic syringes and needles, irrigation outfits, dressings and pads, etc.("Durable medical equipment: Scope and conditions," 2006).

- general household medicine cabinet supplies, including but not limited nonprescription medications, materials for routine skin care, dental hygiene, care of hair, etc., except when specific items are medically indicated and prescribed for exceptional use for a specific resident ("Durable medical equipment: Scope and conditions," 2006).
- assistance and/or supervision, when required, with activities of daily living, including but not limited to toileting, bathing, feeding and assistance with getting from place to place ("Home Health Service," 2003).
- use of customarily stocked equipment, including but not limited to crutches, walkers, wheelchairs or other supportive equipments, including training in their use when necessary, unless such items are prescribed by a doctor for regular and sole use by a specific resident ("Durable medical equipment: Scope and conditions," 2006).
- activities program, including but not limited to a planned schedule of recreational, motivational, social and other activities together with the necessary materials and supplies to make the resident's life more meaningful ("Home Health Service," 2003).
- social services as needed;
- provision of optician and optometrist services (""Home Health Service," 2003,).
- physical therapy, occupational therapy, speech pathology services, audiology services and dental services, on either a staff or fee-for-services basis, as prescribed by a doctor, administered by or under the direct supervision of a licensed and currently registered physical therapist, occupational therapist, speech pathologist, qualified audiologist or registered dentist ("Home Health Service," 2003).

**Adult Day Health Care (ADHC)**

ADHC program provides the health care services and activities provided to a group of persons, who are not residents of a residential health care facility, but are functionally impaired and not home bounded (Castle, 2008). Require supervision, monitoring, preventive, diagnostic, therapeutic, rehabilitative or palliative care or services but not require continuous 24-hour-a-day inpatient care and services to maintain their health status and enable them to remain in the community ("Home Health Service, 2003,) (Castle, 2008).

## Behavioral Intervention Services

This program must include a discrete unit with a planned combination of services with staffing, equipment and physical facilities designed to serve individuals whose severe behavior cannot be managed in a less restrictive setting (Castle, 2008). The program shall provide goal-directed, comprehensive and interdisciplinary services directed at attaining or maintaining the individual at the highest practicable level of physical, affective, behavioral and cognitive functioning (Castle, 2008).

## Clinical Laboratory Service

Clinical laboratory means a facility for the microbiological, immunological, chemical, hematological, biophysical, cytological, pathological, genetic or other examination of materials derived from the human body, for the purpose of obtaining information for the diagnosis, prevention or treatment of disease, or the assessment of a health condition, or for identification purposes ("Home Health Service, 2003,) (Castle, 2008).

Such examinations shall include procedures to determine, measure, or otherwise describe the presence or absence of various substances, components or organisms in the human body ("Home Health Service, 2003,) (Castle, 2008).

## Coma Services

A resident admitted for a coma management shall be a person who has suffered a traumatic brain injury, and is in a coma (Castle, 2008). This resident may be completely unresponsive to any stimuli or may exhibit a generalized response by reacting inconsistently and non-purposefully to stimuli in a nonspecific manner (Castle, 2008).

## Government Regulations

All nursing homes in the United States that receive Medicare and/or Medicaid funding are subject to federal regulations. People who inspect nursing homes are called surveyors or called as state surveyors ("NURSING HOMESHOMES: Federal Monitoring Surveys Demonstrate Continued Understatement of Serious Care Problems and CMS Oversight Weaknesses," 2008).

The Center for Medicare & Medicaid (CMS) is the component of the Federal Government's Department of Health and Human Services that oversees the Medicare and Medicaid programs ("Overview Medicaid Program: General Information," 2006). A large portion of Medicaid and Medicare dollars is used each year to cover nursing home care and services for elderly and disabled. State governments oversee the licensing of nursing homes ("Overview Medicaid Program: General Information," 2006). In addition, State have contract with CMS to monitor those nursing homes that want to be eligible to provide care to Medicare and Medicaid beneficiaries ("Overview Medicaid Program: General Information," 2006). Congress established minimum requirements for nursing homes that want to provide services under Medicare and Medicaid ("NURSING HOMESHOMES: Federal Monitoring Surveys Demonstrate Continued Understatement of Serious

Care Problems and CMS Oversight Weaknesses," 2008). CMS also publishes a list of Special Focus Facilities- nursing homes with "a history of serious quality issues." The US government Accountability Office (GAO), however, has found that state nursing home inspections understate the numbers of serious nursing home problems that present a danger to residents ("NURSING HOMES" 2008). CMS contracts with each state to conduct onsite inspections that determine whether its nursing homes meet the minimum Medicare and Medicaid quality and performance standards. Typically, the part of state government that takes care of this duty is the health department or department of human services ("NURSING HOMES" 2008) (*Inspectors Often Overlook Serious Deficiencies at U.S. Nursing Homes*, 2008).

A report issued in September of 2008 found that over 90% of nursing homes were cited for federal health or safety violations in 2007, with about 17% of nursing homes having deficiencies causing "actual harm or immediate jeopardy" to patients (Pear, 2008).

Nursing homes are subject to federal regulations and also strict state regulations (*Inspectors Often Overlook Serious Deficiencies at U.S. Nursing Homes*, 2008). The nursing home industry is considered one of the two most heavily regulated industries in the United States (the other being the nuclear power industry) (Wolf, 2003).

As for the state and federal regulations that affect health care IT, CMS interpreted HIPAA's security aspects to cover CIA--confidentiality, integrity, and availability. To date, most of the emphasis has been on confidentiality to reduce citizens' fears that employers, insurers, or governmental agencies could use their personal health data against them (Sloane, 2009). The federal government left the implementation details surrounding HIPAA up to the states to oversee, however, because the states themselves manage the Medicare reimbursements, typically through third-party insurance companies. The result, unfortunately, really does look like a quilted patchwork of confusing and conflicting regulations (Sloane, 2009). Therefore, when information technology steps into the nursing homes, there are some concerns caused by the regulation complications.

## Quality of Life

### Resident-Oriented Care

Resident oriented care is designed as the place that nurses are assigned to particular patients and have the ability to develop relationships with individuals (Shields, 2005). Patients are treated more as family members. Using resident-oriented care, nurses are able to become familiar with each patient and cater more to their specific needs, both in emotional and medical aspects (*Home Care and Nursing Home Services*).

According to various findings residents who receive resident-oriented are experience a higher quality of life, in respect to attention and time spent with patients and the number of fault reports (Boumans, 2005). Although resident-oriented nursing does not lengthen life, nursing home residents may dispel many feelings of loneliness and discontent (Boumans, 2005).

"Resident assignment" refers to the extent to which residents are allocated to the same nurse. With this particular system one person is responsible for the entire admission period of the resident (Shields, 2005). However, this system can cause difficulties for the nurse or care-giver when one of the residents they are assigned to pass away or move to a different facility, since the nurse may become attached to the resident(s) they are caring for (Shields, 2005;*Home Care and Nursing Home Services*).

Therefore, three guidelines must be assessed: structure, process and outcome. Structure is the assessment of the instrumentalities of care and their organization (Pear, 2008); Process being the quality of the way in which care is given (Shields,

2005); Outcome is usually specified in terms of health, well-being, patient satisfaction, etc. (Shields, 2005); Using these three criteria, find that they are strengthened when residents experience resident oriented care (Shields, 2005; *Home Care and Nursing Home Services*) (Boumans, 2005). Communication is also heightened when residents feel comfortable discussing various issues with someone who is experienced with their particular case. In this particular situation nurses are also better able to do longitudinal follow up, and this insures the implementation of more lasting results (Shields, 2005; Boumans, 2005).

### Task-Oriented Care

Task oriented care is where nurses are assigned specific tasks to perform for numerous residents on a specific ward (Shields, 2005). Residents in this particular situation are exposed to multiple nurses at any given time. Because of the random disbursement of tasks, nurses are declined the ability to develop more in depth relations with any particular resident (Shields, 2005). Various findings suggest that task-oriented care produces less satisfied residents (Shields, 2005). In many cases, residents are disoriented and unsure of whom to disclose information to and as a result decide not to share information at all (Shields, 2005).

Patients usually complain of loneliness and feelings of displacement.

"Resident assignment" is allocated to numerous nurses as opposed to one person carrying the responsibility of one resident (Shields, 2005). Because the load on one nurse can become so great, various nurses are unable to identify with gradual emotional and physical changes experienced by one particular resident (*CMS*, 2008). Resident information has the ability to get misplaced or undocumented because of the numerous amounts of nurses that deal with one resident (Shields, 2005; *CMS*, 2008).

## Options

Current trends are to provide people with significant needs for long term supports and services with a variety of living arrangements (*Home Care and Nursing Home Services*). Indeed, research in the U.S as a result of the Real Choice Systems Change Grants, shows that many people are able to return to their own homes in the community. Private nursing agencies (Nursing Agency, also known as Nurses Agency or Nurses Registry) is a business that provides nurses and usually health care assistants (such as Certified Nursing Assistants) to people who need the services of healthcare professionals. Nurses are normally engaged by the agency on temporary contracts and make themselves available for hire by hospitals, care homes and other providers of care for help during busy periods or to cover for staff absences; "Assisted Living Facilities (ALF)," 2007) may be able to provide live-in nurses to stay and work with patients in their own homes.

When considering living arrangements for those who are unable to live by themselves, potential customers consider it to be important to carefully look at many nursing homes and assisted living; Assisted living residences or assisted living facilities (ALFs) provide supervision or assistance with activities of daily living (ADLs), coordination of services by outside health care providers, and monitoring of resident activities to help to ensure their health, safety, and well-being ("Assisted Living Facilities (ALF)," 2007). Assistance may include the administration or supervision of medication, or personal care services provided by a trained staff person ("Assisted Living Facilities (ALF)," 2007), facilities as well as retirement homes, where a retirement home is a multi-residence housing facility intended for the elderly ("Assisted Living Facilities (ALF)," 2007). The usual pattern is that each person or couple in the home has an apartment-style room or suite of rooms. Additional facilities are provided within the building. Often this includes facilities for meals, gathering, recreation, and some form of health or hospice care (*Inspectors Often Overlook Serious Deficiencies at U.S. Nursing Homes*, 2008), keeping in mind the person's abilities to take care of themselves independently. While certainly not a residential option, many families choose to have their elderly loved one spend several hours per day at an adult daycare center, which is a non-residential facility specializing in providing activities for elderly and/or handicapped individuals (Boumans, 2005). Most centers operate 10 - 12 hours per day and provide meals, social/recreational outings, and general supervision (*Inspectors Often Overlook Serious Deficiencies at U.S. Nursing Homes*, 2008).

Beginning in 2002, Medicare began hosting an online comparison site intended to foster quality improving competition between nursing homes (Boumans, 2005).

## Culture Change

Nursing homes are leading to the way they are organized and direct to create a more resident-centered environment, making it more home-like and less hospital like (*Home Care and Nursing Home Services*). In these homes, nursing home units are replaced with a small set of rooms surrounding a common kitchen and living room. The design and decoration are more home style. One of the staff giving care is assigned to be the "household" (*Home Care and Nursing Home Services*). Residents have way more choices about when and what they want to eat, when they want to wake up, and what they want to do during the day. They also have access to more companionship such as pets, plants (Shields, 2005). Due to the residents' diversity, the nurses and staff are learning more about different cultural difference, and meet more of the residents needs. Many of the facilities utilizing these models refer to such change as the "Culture Shift" or "Culture Change" occurring in the Long Term Care industry (Shields, 2005).

*Table 1. Nursing home residents by age and gender (Carrillo, 2006)*

| Age Group | Total | Men | Women |
|---|---|---|---|
| 64 or Younger | 175,000 | 54% | 64% |
| 65 to 84 | 643,000 | 34% | 66% |
| 85 or older | 674,000 | 18% | 82% |

Due to the nursing shortage problem, more and more nursing homes are heading the tendency to have more technology involve. Robot nurses are proposed to be part of the nursing home's asset in the near future ("Robots may be next solution to nursing shortage," 2003).

## Resident Characteristics

Nursing home residents are among the frailest Americans. In 2005, nearly half of all residents had dementia, and more than half were confined to a bed or wheelchair. In 2004, nearly 80 percent of residents needed help with 4 or 5 activities of daily living (bed mobility, transferring, dressing, eating, and toileting) ("Analysis of the National Nursing Home Survey (NNHS)," 2004).

Most nursing home residents are female, especially at older ages, shown in Table 1 (Carrillo, 2006). Widowhood is a key predictor of nursing home use – at time of admission, over half of nursing home residents were widowed, and only 1 in 5 was married or living with a partner (Carrillo, 2006).

The number of nursing home residents has remained approximately constant since 1985, but as a proportion of the population likely to need long-term care, it actually has declined ("The 65 and Over Population: 2000-Census 2000 Brief,"; "Nursing Home Data Compendium ", 2007). Over the past 20 years, the age 65 to 84 population increased by more than 20 percentage and the age 85+ population increased by more than 80 percentage, shown in Figure 1.

As the percentage of older people living in nursing homes has declined, the number of stays has grown because of increasing use for short-term post-acute care (*CMS*, 2008). There were close to 3.2 million total nursing home stays in Medicare and Medicaid certified facilities during 2005, up from 3 million in 2000 ("Nursing Home Data Compendium ", 2007).

Projecting future trends is difficult, since nursing home usage is driven by care preferences as well as life expectancy and disability trends ("Nursing Home Data Compendium ", 2007). Current estimates are that 35% of Americans age 65 in 2005 will receive some nursing home care in their lifetime, 18% will live in a nursing home for at least one year, and 5% for at least five years ("The 65 and Over Population: 2000-Census 2000 Brief,"; Kemper, Komisar, & Alecixh, 2005). Women, with longer life expectancy and higher rates of disability and widowhood, are more likely that men to need nursing home care, and especially likely to need lengthy stays (Kemper et al., 2005).

## Concerns on Nursing Home Quality

### Nursing Home Abuse

It seems that a lot of information that we have received are positive and promising, however, negative news would never too small to negligent. Here is a piece of news from New York Times: nursing home inspectors routinely overlook or minimize problems that pose a serious, immediate threat to patients, said by congressional investigators in a new report (Pear, 2008a).

In the report, the investigators from the Government Accountability Office claim that they have

*Figure 1. AARP Public Policy Institute analysis of 2004 NNHS*

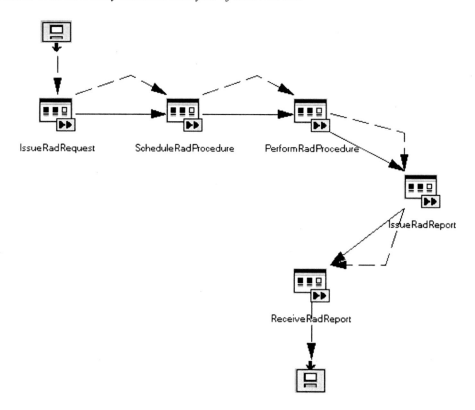

IssueRadRequest    ScheduleRadProcedure    PerformRadProcedure

IssueRadReport

ReceiveRadReport

found widespread "understatement of deficiencies," including malnutrition, severe bedsores, overuse of prescription medications, and abuse of nursing home residents (Pear, 2008a).

Nursing homes are typically inspected once a year by state employees working under a contract with the federal government, which sets stringent standards (Pear, 2008b). Federal officials try to validate the work of state inspectors by accompanying them or doing follow-up surveys within a few weeks.

It released that Alabama, Arizona, Missouri, New Mexico, Oklahoma, South Carolina, South Dakota, Tennessee and Wyoming were the nine states most likely to miss serious deficiencies (Pear, 2008a).

More than 1.5 million people live in nursing homes. Nationwide, about one-fifth of the homes

were cited for serious deficiencies last year (Pear, 2008a). "Poor quality of care -- worsening pressure sores or untreated weight loss -- in a small but unacceptably high number of nursing homes continues to harm residents or place them in immediate jeopardy, that is, at risk of death or serious injury," the report said (Pear, 2008b).

There are several studies point out similar quality problems that occur in nursing homes. As to logical thoughts, nursing homes must meet federal standards as a condition of participating in Medicaid and Medicare, which cover more than two-thirds of their residents, at a cost of more than $75 billion a year (Pear, 2008b). Later section in this survey, there is an illustration on more details about the financial part and dilemmas that bother nursing homes.

## Study of Residents Experience in Nursing Homes

There has been increasing interest in the quality of care in nursing homes. Nursing homes should protect resident's integrity and autonomy, and it should be the place that residents can thrive (Anderson, Issel, & McDaniel, 2003). The relationship between management practice (communication openness, decision making, relationship-oriented leadership and formalization) and resident outcome (aggressive behavior, fractures) should be paid attention on. Several studies (Anderson, 2003, 2003) show that lack of competent personnel and nursing home residents with more complex caring needs leads to insufficient care. There are correlations between satisfaction, commitment, stress and quality of care as perceived by staff. Reports from family members are often positive but have also led to implementation of emotion-oriented care in some homes. Despite this, while generally positive, the overall assessment of nursing homes by family members has not improved (Harris & Clauser, 2002; Redfern, Hannan, Norman & Martin, 2002; Finnema, de Lange, Droes, Ribbe & Tilburg, 2001).

The quality of care as assessed by competent nursing home residents has been studied by some authors (Polit & Beck, 2004). They found that the residents were mostly satisfied with the extent to which their wishes were met in regards to meals, shower routines, opportunities to listen to radio and TV, and their feeling of safety. The greatest difference between what residents wanted and what they experienced concerned the opportunities they had for close social relationships (Anderson, 2003).

Understanding how residents in nursing homes regard living is important and has implications for nursing care and practice. In the study "Residents are Safe but Lonely", it describe the experiences of a group of nursing home residents (Anderson, 2003). The two research questions were: How do the residents experience care? How can nurses help the residents to have a good life in the nursing home (Anderson, 2003)?

The analyses were conducted by using a qualitative content analysis method [48]. The main finding was that the experience of being 'safe but lonely' characterizes residents' experiences of living in a nursing home (Anderson, 2003).

The residents at the nursing home emphasized that moving into the nursing home had made them feel safer than they felt when living in their private home (Anderson, 2003). Many residents told of feeling insecure and anxious when they lived at home. They were afraid that something adverse might happen to them and that they would not be able to get help when they needed it (Harris & Clauser, 2002). The informants stressed that having people in the vicinity at all times was one of the substantial benefits of living in a nursing home. However, most of them have a feeling of a lack of trust in the foreign nurses (Anderson, 2003). These nurses had weak language skills which led to problems with communication and understanding both for the residents and the nurses and in turn led to feeling of insecurity for the residents (Anderson, 2003). Another thing was "haste". The nurses were too busy to attend to the residents properly, so the informants did not feel that they were respected and regarded as unique individuals. This gave them a feeling of insecurity. All informants, however, stressed the importance of safety as the greatest benefit of living in a nursing home (Harris & Clauser, 2002).

The informants gave their particular nursing home more credit than they appeared to think that nursing homes were generally given in the mass media (Harris & Clauser, 2002). They felt that they were cared for, but that at the same time the standard of their care would have been even better if there had been more nursing personnel. Feelings of loneliness and sadness are felt strongly by the residents. The days were long, boring, and empty, and informants felt uncared for (Harris & Clauser, 2002). Even though the activities are organized sometimes, it is far from what they have expected.

The nurses do not see, nor do they meet the residents' social needs. Some informants pointed out that a language barrier made communication with some of the nurses difficult (Harris & Clauser, 2002). According to those residents, the lack of personnel led to loneliness among the residents because the nurses had little time to chat with the residents (Harris & Clauser, 2002).

Residents felt that this lack of respect was expressed as nonchalance (Harris & Clauser, 2002). It gave the residents a feeling of not being understood. Several informants stressed that they could not discuss their problems with the nurses because the nurses did not understand what they said and thus did not understand their needs. Other informants said that they used humor to solve language problems and that by the combined use of hands and words they could communicate what they wanted from the nurses (Harris & Clauser, 2002).

As to the feeling a lack of reliability, it is reported that the nurses often did not follow up on agreements such as making training appointments and other agreements related to care (Redfern et al., 2002). The informants stressed that if a nurse had promised the resident something, he or she should attend to this immediately or at an agreed time. This was not always the case, and the residents felt frustrated at having to wait for 'eternities' for what they had been promised. This, the informants agreed on, was an aspect of their care that could be improved (Finnema et al., 2001).

A central phenomenon in this study is the resident's feelings of being met with respect. Several of the informants mentioned their feelings of being met with respect as a fundamental aspect of good nursing care (Finnema et al., 2001). To be met with respect means that the person is being met with appreciation for the unique human being he or she is. Residents in a nursing home have an unexpressed right to be taken care of in such a way that he or she feels comfortable and is regarded as a human being (Redfern et al., 2002). A resident is a human being with unique integral

qualities and capabilities (Redfern et al., 2002). If residents are met in this way, hopefully they experience that more of their social needs are met so that they will not experience such a high degree of loneliness.

The fact is that only competent residents were counted into this report, and 70-80% of the residents in nursing homes suffer from a dementia disease (Finnema et al., 2001). Residents suffering from dementia may have a different experience of living in a nursing home (Polit & Beck, 2004).

Even if the informants mentioned positive factors in their experience of living in the nursing homes, they also mentioned deficiencies in the care they experienced (Polit & Beck, 2004). Nurses are therefore faced with the huge challenge of providing holistic care that addresses both the social as well as the physical needs of the residents (Finnema et al., 2001). Therefore, some nursing homes start reform and try to design different daily activities for their residents.

## Daily Activities

There are more and more people receiving long term care in an institutional setting and that population is going to continue to grow with the aging of the "baby boomers."So it is important to find out the what the residents 'daily life, which is a way to spark more ideas to improve the nursing homes quality. It has been proven that when people move into nursing homes they lose a sense of control and feel a sense of isolation. Activities are one the best ways to fight these feelings and give a sense of empowerment back to the people. The variety of programs available in any nursing home depends on the health and interests of the residents. After doing research, basically, it comes up with a fairly wide range of activities in nursing homes that are designed to meet the needs of the residents.

A broad range of programs is directed by the activities coordinator (Daily Activities, 2008). A home certified for Medicare and Medicaid must have someone designated as an activities coordinator (Daily Activities, 2008). The planning and implementation of activities comes from requests by residents, families, staff, and volunteers (Daily Activities, 2008). The activities are usually posted on a calendar of events that is available to each resident. Through the web reveal, here are some of the examples:

- Monthly birthday parties. Parties to which all residents are invited. Families and friends may be invited to participate (Fun Times, 2008).
- Celebrations of various holidays, both secular and religious. Holidays are particularly difficult times for those away from their own homes, families, and friends. Valentine's Day, Halloween, Christmas, Hannukah, Easter, and Memorial Day are a few examples (Daily Activities, 2008; Fun Times, 2008; Activities, 2008).
- Musical events can be enjoyed actively or passively depending on the abilities of the residents. Many homes have sing-alongs in which the residents request their favorite songs and sing along with a leader. Again, the involvement of families, and friends is crucial to the success of such a program. Sometimes concerts are given by a church or school group or friend of the nursing home. Hopefully, the public is invited to attend, for this allows the residents to provide a source of pleasure to their community (Daily Activities, 2008; Fun Times, 2008).
- Games foster both one-to-one relationships and group activity. Bingo is a favorite for many, but bridge, chess, and other games for smaller groups usually are available. Volunteers and families often are the ones to stimulate resident interest in a game and they may be able to help arrange suitable opponents. Contests sometimes are run with work games, and tournaments

are arranged for bridge or game players (Daily Activities, 2008; Fun Times, 2008; Activities, 2008).

- Outdoor activities include gardening, cookouts, or just enjoying time in the sun alone or with a friend. Often the staff does not have the time to take the immobile residents outside (Fun Times, 2008; Activities, 2008).
- Trips and tours to community events. Some homes have a special resident fund from the sale of arts and crafts made and sold by the residents to finance transportation rentals and ticket purchases. Friends or volunteers may donate to the fund or sometimes the nursing home sets aside money. Transportation can be a problem for those in wheelchairs, but the activities coordinator usually can find volunteer drivers who are taught to cope with the special needs of disabled people. Some communities have special vans that transport residents in wheelchairs. Trips outside the home offer variety and mental stimulation (Activities, 2008).
- Nursing home newsletter, especially if published by residents. This is an especially valuable method of expression and uses resident talent that otherwise may lie idle. Poetry, history, birthdays, and resident and staff personality profiles are all topics that can be included (Fun Times, 2008; Activities, 2008). As we know, lots of elders are losing their ability to read as they are getting old, and therefore, it will be great if they can introduce the electronic reading device or arrange a "story time" when one of the caregivers read the news to the residents.
- Resident discussion groups. Sometimes a resident is an expert on a particular subject and will be the group leader. Other times a volunteer may offer to lead a discussion group. Topics may include current events,

literature, and religion. The residents choose the topics and those interested attend.

- Exercise fun and physical fitness. Community leaders often volunteer to lead yoga or other exercise sessions. Even wheelchair-bound residents find satisfaction in exercising on a regular basis.
- Books. Volunteers may run a book service, taking a cart of books to the room of immobile residents. There may be a central library or small bookcases on each floor. Talking books for the blind may be part of the service. Families, friends, and volunteers can buy, bring, and hand out books. Many people help with reading to those unable to see well.
- Coffee or cocktail hours. Policies vary from home to home, but social hours provide a time of resident interaction. It is a particularly nice time for volunteers, family, and friends to join the residents (Daily Activities, 2008; Fun Times, 2008; Activities, 2008).
- Arts and crafts programs. They separate from occupational therapy, and are frequently offered by the activities' coordinator.
- Religious services. Every Medicare- and Medicaid-certified nursing home must, by federal regulation, provide the opportunity for residents to attend religious services of their preference. Many nursing homes welcome denominational groups to provide religious services in the home for those who wish to attend. Again, this often provides an opportunity for families and friends to join the resident in worship. The organization of such services is usually handled by the activities' coordinator (Activities, 2008).

## Nursing Home Financial Regulations

### Billing Model

Nursing home billing model is very like hospitals (Webb, 2001). Staff are housed in accessible nursing homes. Residents live in utilitarian, hospital-like rooms with little or no privacy and they sleep on hospital beds and are usually referred to as "patients" by the staff. Hospital pricing models are also used. (Webb, 2001) Residents are charged daily flat rates for semiprivate or private rooms just like a hospital. Extra services and supplies are added to the bill. This pricing model assumes that all residents require the same supervision and care. Of course this is not true (Webb, 2001).

A lot could be done to improve the current system. For example, if family or friends were to help in the care of loved ones, these services could be deducted from the bill (Webb, 2001). A number of residents are also capable of helping with the care of fellow residents or they might help with the facility services such as cleaning, food preparation, social needs, and laundry and so on. These cost savings could be passed on to all residents (Webb, 2001).

State and Federal governments pay about 70% of nursing home costs and for about 85% of all residents the government pays part of or all of their costs (More Can be Done, 2002). Because the government pays such a large portion, nursing homes structure their care delivery system around the government payment system (More Can be Done, 2002).

Government reimbursement is based on nursing hours and aide hours per patient, plant costs, wages, utilities, insurance, ancillary services, etc. and basically follows a hospital model (Webb, 2001). Because government programs typically are burdened with massive stationery inertia, the current pricing model will be around for a long time (Webb, 2001; More Can be Done, 2002).

## Payment Sources

### Medicare

Medicare is the government health insurance plan for all eligible individuals age 65 and older. Because of its universal availability almost everyone over age 65 in this country is covered by Medicare. There are about 40 million Medicare beneficiaries nationwide (ELJAY, 2006).

Medicare will pay for 20 days of a skilled nursing care facility at full cost and the difference between $114 per day and the actual cost for another 80 days (ELJAY, 2006). Private Medicare supplement insurance usually pays the 80 day deductible of $114 per day, if a person carries this insurance and the right policy form. However, Medicare often stops paying before reaching the full 100 days. When Medicare stops, so does the supplement coverage (ELJAY, 2006).

To qualify for Medicare nursing home coverage, the individual must spend at least 3 full days in a hospital and must have a skilled nursing need and have a doctor order it (ELJAY, 2006). The transfer from a hospital must occur within a certain time period (ELJAY, 2006).

### Medicaid

Medicaid is a welfare program jointly funded by the federal government and the states and largely administered by the states (Caring for the Elderly, 1998). In 1998, Medicaid paid for 46.3% of the $88 billion received by all US nursing homes (Caring for the Elderly, 1998). Although the bias is only to cover eligible patients in semiprivate rooms in nursing homes, a recent court decision is forcing the States to consider more Medicaid funding for home care and assisted living (Caring for the Elderly, 1998). To receive a Medicaid waiver for alternative community services, the patient must first be evaluated for 90 days in a nursing home. There is a certain requirement for Medicaid to cover residents' nursing home care.

In order to qualify for nursing home Medicaid, an applicant must meet the "medical necessity" requirement, which generally requires a medical disorder or disease requiring attention by registered or licensed vocational nurses on a regular basis ("National Health Accounts,"). The Director of Nursing in the nursing home or an applicant's medical doctor should be able to assess whether someone meets the medical necessity requirement ("National Health Accounts,").

Once it is determined that there is a medical necessity for nursing home care, the applicant must meet two financial tests: the income test and the resources test. The general rule is that in order to qualify for Medicaid nursing home care, an unmarried applicant cannot have more than $1,737.00 in monthly income (for the 2005 calendar year) and no more than $2,000.00 in resources or assets. If both spouses apply, the incomes are combined and the income cap is twice the cap for the individual. The resource limitations for a married couple, both of whom apply, is $3,000.00. However, the limitations are not as stringent when the applicant is married and his or her spouse is not institutionalized ("National Health Accounts,").

### Insurance

Insurance is an alternative source of funding for long term nursing home care. From virtually nothing 10 years ago, insurance paid 5% of nursing home receipts in 1998 (Sloan & Shayne, 1993). This percentage is increasing every year. The government is also sending a clear message it wants private insurance to play a larger role. This began with the recommendation of the Pepper Commission in 1992 and continued with the HIPAA legislation in 1996 and on to the offering in 2003 of long-term care insurance for federal workers, military, retirees and their families ("National Health Accounts,"; Sloan & Shayne, 1993).

There are several bills now pending in Congress allowing full deduction of premiums and the pass-through of premiums in cafeteria plans. These tax breaks are meant as an incentive for the purchase of insurance.

Medicare covers about 12% of private nursing home costs while Medicaid covers about 50%. The Veteran's Administration nursing home operations bring total government support of nursing home costs to about 70% of the total. Such a large reliance on government support has made nursing homes vulnerable to vagaries in state and Federal reimbursement policies towards nursing homes (Sloan & Shayne, 1993).

## Current Problems For Nursing Homes

### Funding Shortfalls

The majority of nursing home income comes from government reimbursement (Polit & Beck, 2004). The industry claims that many of its nursing homes are losing money on government payments causing yearly net business losses. For those homes that make profit, there's not margin enough for improving infrastructure or hiring more or better qualified staff to improve quality of care (Polit & Beck, 2004). Quality of care eventually suffers with inadequate income. On the other hand, critics contend the current revelations of poor care with many nursing homes across the country stem not from lack of income but from greedy owners not willing to apply profits to improvement in care. The national chains, in particular, are accused of retaining profits to bolster stock prices in an effort to fund acquisitions (*Staff Turnover and Retention*, 2007; Peter, 2001).

### Staffing

A recent report from the Government Accounting Office cites widespread understaffing by nursing homes both in levels of nurses and certified nurse's assistants (Mukamel & Spector, 2000). Staffing in these cases is below government-recommended adequate standards (Mukamel & Spector, 2000). Recently states such as California have mandated higher staffing ratios for hospitals and skilled nursing homes. But in most cases there is not additional money to cover the cost of more staff. So mandated staffing ratios will probably have little effect on the problems facing nursing homes and may actually increase their problems (Mukamel & Spector, 2000).

### Turnover of Aides

There's no question that tight labor markets over the past decade have made it difficult to recruit and retain workers. But turnover of qualified aides is so high. Nursing homes claim they can't afford to pay for the higher level of wages and benefits necessary to retain aides who will stay around for a while (*Staff Turnover and Retention*, 2007).

### Shortage of Nurses

Next is the problem of nurses. There is currently a nationwide shortage of nurses. Nursing homes are willing to pay the salary to attract nurses but in many areas there aren't enough nurses to meet demand (Peter, 2001). Nursing homes, as well as hospitals are using innovative work schedules to meet staffing requirements but in many cases, nurses are overloaded with too many patients. In other cases, less qualified workers are substituting for nurses (Peter, 2001). These shortages and high turnover affect the quality of care that a nursing home can provide (Peter, 2001).

### Elder Abuse and Lawsuits

It shouldn't come as a surprise with the problems of funding and staffing that reported incidents of patient neglect and abuse are on the rise (Williams, 2003). Of particular concern is the more frequent occurrence of abuse. Abuse is not only just physical assault or threats but it can also be such things as improper use of restraints, failure to feed or give water, failure to bathe, improper care resulting in pressure sores or allowing a patient to lie too long in a soiled diaper or bed linen. Lawsuits are increasing in number. (Williams, 2003; Webb, 2001)

There is a great concern at the Federal and state levels to control abuse (Webb, 2001). So far, aside from proposing tougher laws to penalize the industry, there appears to be little effort in finding a way to improve the nursing home system of care delivery (Webb, 2001).

## PART II: E-HEALTH AND NURSING HOMES

E-health is a type of telemedicine that encompasses any "e-thing" in health field; that is, any database or encyclopedia containing information pertinent to health, medicine, or pharmacy that is accessible via internet (Breen & Zhang, 2008).

It is a typical form commonly referenced and understood as that consists of internet-based services such as WebMD.com, Medlineplus.gov, and Mentalhelp.net. Telemedicine involves the use of telecommunications technologies to facilitate clinical healthcare delivery and exchange at a distance (Thompson, Dorsey, Miller, & Parrott, 2003). This delivery method was initially designed to specifically benefit patients (Breen, & Matusitz, 2006; Wootton, 2001). E-health is a subunit of the "telemedicine umbrella" (Breen & Zhang, 2008).

Because of the distance barrier that telemedicine and e-health services are able to transcend, Matusitz and Breen (Breen, & Matusitz, 2006) were convinced, through their published research, that telemedicine would be particularly beneficial in secluded towns and communities deficient in adequate healthcare services, such as bucolic regions, in mountains, on islands, and in locations of arctic climate (Breen & Zhang, 2008).

Given the efficacy of telemedicine services noted by these scholars in their work in both metropolitan and more rural or remote regions, it makes logical sense that such e-health services would prove valuable when actively used by nursing staff in a variety of nursing homes, regardless of the structure and organization of the nursing home (e.g., nursing home chains in urban and rural areas, for-profit or non-profit homes, etc.) (Matusitz & Breen, 2007). E-health provides a faster and easier alternative, as well as a more cost-effective means, to accessing healthcare information, as opposed to more traditional and costly physical interactions between doctors and patients. Besides the fact that the use of e-health services is rapidly rising with, according to Matusitz and Breen (Breen, & Matusitz, 2006) 88.5 million American adults on average seeking on-line health information daily, studies have also been published that identify the quantity of and frequency of use among specific medical practitioners in a variety of specialties and settings: psychiatry, pathology, dermatology, cardiology, in intensive care units, and in emergency rooms where surgery is performed (Matusitz & Breen, 2007; Thompson, Dorsey, Miller, & Parrott, 2003). More relevantly, many of these relate to types of care needed and applied in nursing home settings. WebMD.com is preferred by most medical practitioners (Matusitz, 2007). One of the most important financial advantages found within the WebMD.com site (Our Products and Services) for medical practitioners in particular is that "its products and services streamline administrative and clinical processes, promote efficiency and reduce costs by facilitating information exchange, and enhance communication and electronic transactions between healthcare participants" (Our Products and Services). Further, WebMD.com (Our Products and Services) offers, free-of-charge, disease and treatment information, pharmacy and drug information, and an array of forums and interactive e-communities where practitioners and consumers can correspond using specialized e-messages. WebMD.com (Our Products and Services) doesn't stop there in its free provisions and benefits to medical practitioners and its potential assets to nursing home settings in particular (Breen & Zhang, 2008).

E-health should be readily accepted and generally understood by the professional medical population, especially in nursing home settings across metropolitan, suburban, and rural sectors. Mitka (2003) also reported that telemedicine services, particularly e-health applications, improved delivery of psychiatric care to residents of rural nursing homes (Breen & Zhang, 2008).

## Health IT Acceptance in Long-Term Care

Nursing homes are often depicted as laggards when it comes to embracing technology tools. But an analysis by the American Association of Homes and Services for the Aging shows that they are more than holding their own.

Nearly all nursing homes at the time had electronic information systems for MDS data collection and billing, and 43% maintained electronic health record systems, according to analysts, who studied data from the 2004 National Nursing Home Survey. By comparison, 25% of doctor offices and 59% of hospitals handled EHRs (O'Connor, 2008).

## Staff Survey

There are various factors determining the acceptance of health IT applications by caregivers in long-term care facilities, including social influence factors such as subjective norm and image understandable level and demographic variables including age, job level, long-term care work experience and computer skills in regard to their impact on caregivers' acceptance of health IT applications.

A nationwide survey, being applied a modified version of the extended technology acceptance model (TAM2) to examine the health IT acceptance in long-term care, reveals a positive results: Although it is suggested that the effect of the Technology Acceptance Model on professionals and general users (King & He, 2006) and

on people from different cultures (Schepers & Wetzels, 2007) is different, the survey results clearly suggest that the caregivers' acceptance of IT innovations in long-term care environment at the pre-implementation stage. In fact, the caregivers show high levels of acceptance of health IT applications. In order to ensure the successful introduction of a new health IT application into a long-term care facility, a positive environment should be established with support from facility managers and RNs for the introduction of the new innovation. As computer skills directly impact on the caregivers' perceived ease of use and intention to use an application, effort should be made to understand the caregivers' computer skills, and provide adequate training and support to improve their skills if necessary. "Our findings also suggest that improving the caregivers' understanding of the importance of the introduced system for nursing care will improve their acceptance of the new innovation" (Yu, Li, & Gagnon, 2009). In this survey, it appears that 66.4% of the participants would be able to adapt to a health IT application with reasonable training and support 34% of caregivers' intention to use an introduced IT application before any hands-on experience with the system established (Yu et al., 2009).

## Health Information Technology in Nursing Homes

Information technology (IT) has significant potential to reduce error and improve the quality and efficiency of health care (Bates et al., 2001; Institute of Medicine [IOM], 2001). Some researchers also believe that computer systems can be used to reduce error and improve the reporting of adverse incidents in health care settings (Wald & Shojania, 2001). Since

October 1998, all state licensed nursing homes have been required to electronically transmit data generated by the federally mandated Resident Assessment Instrument (RAI) via state public health agencies to the Centers for Medicare and

Medicaid Services (CMS) (Mor et al., 2003). Advanced features in the software were available to most (87% to 98%) of the facilities; however, most features were not being used all the time. There are huge potentials addressing the technology applications with various aspects such as enhancing the administrator's ability to manage the facility, tracking quality, and monitoring multiple performance indicators.

HIT is used to collect, store, retrieve, and transfer clinical, administrative, and financial health information electronically (General Accounting Office, 2004). The IOM publication To Err is Human (Kohn, Corrigan, & Donaldson, 1999) drew attention to the potential for HIT to improve quality of care and prevent medical errors across the health care system. The focus of HIT development and implementation has been mainly on acute and ambulatory care settings (American Health Information Management Association [AHIMA], 2005; Hamilton, 2006; Kramer et al., 2004).

Commonly found HIT systems provide computerized physician order entry (CPOE), electronic health records (EHR), and point of care (POC) to access data for entry and retrieval (e.g., reviewing records, entering orders at the bedside or in the examination room; Hamilton, 2006). In addition, electronic systems for management operations such as patient scheduling and reimbursement have been available for longer and are used frequently (AHIMA, 2005; Baron, Fabens, Schiffman, & Wolf, 2005; Poon et al., 2006). An EHR is an electronic formatting of medical records documenting the patient's medical history, written orders, and progress notes. CPOE is a system making information available for physicians at the time an order is entered (Bates et al., 1998; Bates et al., 1999). POC is a technology automating the care provider's procedure, visit notes, and educational materials at the place of care (Anderson & Wittwer, 2004). Although the implementation of HIT in the long-term care sector is recognized to be lagging behind the acute and

ambulatory settings (AHIMA, 2005; Hamilton, 2006), there is a wide range potentials for nursing homes such as functions covering domains such as financial management, administration, ancillary care, support, and resident care (McKnight's LTC News, 2005).

## Technology Streamlines Long-Term Care Operations

Technology's role in nursing homes has been greater importance as these types of facilities serve more older adults. Most of them are expanding their focus on the best ways to deploy technology to improve residents' quality of care. In this section, we explored some equipments/devices that favor nursing homes, skilled nursing facilities (SNFs) and assisted living facilities.

### Fall Management

This care issue includes technologies aimed at decreasing the occurrence of resident falls, as well as technologies that alert caregivers and reduce injury when falls occur (Burland, 2008). Products include grab bars, non slips mats and socks, and differnt types of alarms.

What fall management options are currently available? According to Gillespie SM, Friedman SM (2007), the major two categories are as following:

- *Technologies aimed at reducing the risk of a fall:*
  - Anti-slip footwears are socks and slippers with anti-slip material incorporated on the bottom.
  - Anti-slip matting and materials provide a slip resistant surface to stand on in slippery areas such as tubs and bathroom floors.
  - Grab bars provide stability and support in bathrooms and other areas.

- Wheelchair anti-rollback devices prevent a wheelchair from rolling away when residents stand or lower themselves into a chair.
- Chair, bed, and toilet alarms signal a caregiver when a resident who is at risk for falling attempts to leave a bed, chair, wheelchair, or toilet unattended.
- Rehabilitation equipment and programs geared toward the restoration and maintenance of strength, endurance, range of motion, bone density, balance, and gait. Some examples include unweighting systems that enable residents to perform gait training in a supported reduced weight environment, systems that can test balance, and treadmills.

- *Technologies aimed at reducing the risk of injury when falls occur:*
  - Hip protectors are designed to protect the hip from injury in the event of a fall.
  - Bedside cushions may help reduce the impact of a fall if a resident rolls out of bed.
  - Technologies that notify caregivers when a resident has fallen: Fall detection devices use technologies that sense a change in body position, body altitude, and the force of impact to determine when a fall has occurred.

## Medication Management

Products geared toward enabling residents to manage and adhere to their medication regime with greater independence (Field, 2008).

- Medication Applicators enable the user to apply lotions and ointments on hard to reach areas such as the back and feet. They typically consist of a sponge or pad that is attached to a long handle (Lilley RC 2006).
- Medication Reminder Software is installed on Personal Digital Assistants (PDA's), personal computers, or mobile phones to provide reminders to take or administer medication at predetermined time. Some of these applications have the ability to manage complex medication regimens and can store medication and medical histories(Wolfstadt, 2008).
- Pill Organizers keep dry medications and vitamins arranged in compartments to assist with medication compliance and protocol adherence. Compartments are labeled for weekly or daily dosage frequencies and may be marked in Braille for individuals with visual impairments (McGraw, 2004).
- Multi-Alarm Medication Reminders and Watches are programmed to remind the user to take medications at predetermined time schedules. They typically come in the form of a specialized watch, pager or pocket device, or medication bottle cap (Lilley RC 2006).
- Multi-Alarm Pill Boxes serve two purposes; to store medication and provide reminder alerts to take medications at prescribed times. Most alerts come in the form of an audible tone at specific times of the day or predetermined hourly intervals (Lilley RC 2006). These pill boxes also offer compartments to help organize medications by day of the week and time of day.
- Personal Automatic Medication Dispensers are programmable, locked devices that will automatically dispense a dose of dry medications at predetermined times. These devices also act as multi-alarm medication reminders that alert the resident when it is time to take their medication with audible alarms, lights, text and voice messages(Lilley RC 2006).

- Talking Medication Bottles contain recording mechanisms that enable a caregiver or pharmacist to record a message that can be played back anytime by the user. The recorded message verbally identifies bottle contents and provides reminders concerning the medication protocol (Lilley RC 2006).

- Automated Medication Dispensing Cabinets provide computer controlled storage, dispensation, tracking, and documentation of medication distribution on the resident care unit. Monitoring of these cabinets is accomplished by interfacing them with the facility's central pharmacy computer. These cabinets can also be interfaced with other external databases such as resident profiles, the facility's admission/discharge/transfer system, and billing systems (MacLaughlin, 2005).

- Automated Medication Dispensing Carts offer secure medication dispensation and tracking at the bedside or wherever a resident may be located during their medication time. These carts feature a wireless computer terminal with tracking software to audit access to the system and control electronically locked medication drawers (Lilley RC 2006).

- Barcode Medication Administration utilizes barcode scanning technology to match the resident with his/her medication order at the point of administration. If any variables of the "5 Rights of Medication Administration" do not match correctly, the administering nurse will be notified via a combination of warning tones and text messages. In many cases, this technology is used to complement automated medication distribution systems (Greenly, 2002).

## Assistance Call

This care issue, also known as nurse call or emergency call, includes technologies that enable a resident to summon assistance by means of a transmitter that they can carry with them or access from somewhere in their living area (Alexander, 2008).

- Wired Systems: These systems rely on wires for communication between the main components of the system. Some wired systems allow for the addition of wireless features, such as wireless call stations, wireless phones, pagers, and locator systems. However these systems are not fully wireless and are categorized here as wired systems (Michael, 2000).

- Wireless Systems: These systems require no wiring for installation. All components of the system communicate wirelessly through radio waves (Douglas Holmes, 2007).

- Telephone Based Systems: These systems use telephone lines to alert caregivers to a resident need. When a resident is in need of assistance, they press a wireless transmitter that they wear (typically a pendant or wristband) or a wall mounted transmitter that sends a signal to dialing device. The dialing device automatically sends a signal to a central CPU that alerts staff to the resident need.

## Bathing

This care issue includes products that focus on bath safety, enable residents to be more independent with bathing tasks, and that make bathing tasks easier for caregivers (Barrick, 2008).

According to Gill and Han (2006), products that enable residents to access showers and tubs more independently and safely:

- Barrier Free and ADA Compliant Showers offer accessible features that enable residents to enter and exit the shower, sit, and access controls with greater ease and safety.
- Tub and Shower Chairs can be placed inside of a tub or shower and provide a seating surface while showering.
- Transfer Benches are placed in a tub and provide a seating surface that extends over the side of the tub, thereby easing transfers, eliminating the need to step over the side of the tub, and providing a place to sit while showering.
- In-Tub Bath Lifts are powered devices that are placed in a tub, creating an adjustable height surface for transfers.
- Mobile Commode/Shower Chairs serve several roles. They can be pushed in to barrier free and roll-in showers, thereby providing a means of transporting the resident to the showering area (self propelled or pushed by a caregiver). They provide seating during showers, and act as a commode or raised seat for toileting.
- Grab Bars provide stability and support in bathrooms and other areas.
- Anti-slip Matting and materials provide a slip resistant surface to stand on in slippery areas such as tubs and bathroom floors.

Products that enable residents to perform bathing tasks more independently:

- Wash Mitts offer a washing solution for those with decreased fine motor skills and an inability to handle a washcloth.
- Long Handled Brushes and Sponges enable residents with limited range to wash hard to reach areas such as their back, feet, and head.
- Rinse-Free Bathing Products enable residents to wash their body and hair without the need for running water or transferring in to a tub or shower (Gill TM, 2006).

According to Moller, Julie etc. (2003), products that assist caregivers with the transfer of residents to showers and tubs:

- Height Adjustable Bathtubs can be raised and lowered to assist with transfers and place the tub at a comfortable working height for caregivers.
- Side-Opening Bathtubs provide a side opening that facilitates transfers in and out of the tub.
- Bath Lifts fully support the resident during bathing as well as transfers in and out of a tub. Depending on the resident's trunk support and sitting balance, bath lifts are offered that enable the resident to be transferred and bathed in a seated or recumbent (reclined) position.
- Shower Trolleys and Gurneys enable caregivers to transport and shower fully dependent residents that need full body support at a comfortable working height.
- Showering Cabinets allow caregivers to shower residents while standing outside of the cabinet and provide the resident with some privacy. Showering cabinets open in the front to provide access to mobile commode/shower chairs or assist with transfers on to a sliding seat.
- Mobile Commode/Shower Chairs serve several roles. They can be pushed in to barrier free and roll-in showers, thereby providing a means of transporting the resident to the showering area (self propelled or pushed by a caregiver). They also provide seating during showers and act as a commode or raised seat for toileting (Moller, 2003).

According to Wendt (2007), products that assist caregivers with bathing tasks:

- Shampooing Basins and Rinse Trays allow caregivers to wash residents' hair in bed, a chair, or a wheelchair.
- Rinse-Free Bathing Products enable caregivers to wash and shampoo residents without the need for running water or transferring residents into to a tub or shower.
- Height Adjustable Bathtubs can be raised and lowered to assist with transfers and place the tub at a comfortable working height for caregivers.

## Detailed Examples

### A study of Remote Monitoring Test

Understanding senior's attitudes toward technology and their willingness to adopt technological solutions that help them remain independent longer, which presents a significant challenge to the aging industry. (Reilly & Bischoff, 2008; "Intelligent remote visual monitoring system for home health care service," 1996) until recently, limited information regarding the practical impact if remote monitoring systems on the elderly has been available. Fortunately, as the technology development, a recent study has yield new data about this remote monitoring test ("Intelligent remote visual monitoring system for home health care service," 1996). The April 2008 study consulting firm at four Philadelphia-based NewCourtland Eleder Services communities measured the effectiveness of senior technology and captured the perceptions of residents, family member, and staff employing it (Reilly & Bischoff, 2008).

Results of the study indicate that users had a very positive attitude toward the remote monitoring technology. The two greatest advantages of the system, according to the residents' responses, were the assistance it provided to get help quickly in the event of an emergency, such as a fall or sudden illness, and the added benefit of enabling them to live independently for a longer period of time (Reilly & Bischoff, 2008). They conducted

a survey for all the residents, and 100 percent of the survey respondents either "strongly agreed" or "agreed" with the two statements. Among those surveyed, only one resident reported a concern about intrusiveness (Reilly & Bischoff, 2008).

The staff study indicated similar sentiments about the system's ability to provide better care to their residents ("Intelligent remote visual monitoring system for home health care service," 1996). "We thought at first that adapting to the technology would be a major issue for our residents, but clearly it was not," says Kim Brooks, NewCourtland's vice president of housing and community-based services. "The results of the survey demonstrate that even seniors with little or no prior exposure to this technology can readily adapt to it (Reilly & Bischoff, 2008)."

A remote monitoring system, typically consisting of small wireless electronic sensors, monitors daily living activities ("Intelligent remote visual monitoring system for home health care service,"). The sensors are placed in stratefic areas of the residents, including walls, to detect movements within the rooms; on the kitchen cupboards and refrigerator doors, to monitor whether the resident is eating regularly; and tilt sensors on the medicine boxes to monitor medication usage. The sensor in the bed can detect when a resident gets in or out of bed, toilet sensors monitor toilet usage, and home- or away sensors tell when the resident leaves or return to her residence (Reilly & Bischoff, 2008; "Intelligent remote visual monitoring system for home health care service," 1996).

A call pendant can be used as an emergency call button, which may be worn or carried by the resident. Besides, if the sensor detects abnormal activity, the system calls will help and automatically alters a caregiver via phone. A cancel button clears in-home alerts or emergency calls (Reilly & Bischoff, 2008).

There is a central computing component in the nursing home—that receives all information transmitted by the sensors (Reilly & Bischoff, 2008). Based on information that is received, the base station will determine if there is a need to call for help, for example. In such a case, the base station will first sound an "in-home alert." If the resident is okay, a cancel button can be pressed to discontinue the alert. If it is an emergency and the in-home alert is not cancelled, the system will automatically proceed through a user-defined call list, via the telephone line, until a responder accepts responsibility to check on the user. If no contacts in the personal caregiver network can be reached, an automated call can be placed to facility security services (Reilly & Bischoff, 2008).

Forty-three of 54 residents were interviewed, and the response of the seniors who participated indicated that the peace of mind they obtain from knowing that they will receive help by using the new technology (Reilly & Bischoff, 2008). Only one of the residents commented as a doubt attitude to the remote monitoring method at the beginning, since they ran the risk by leaving the nurse/caregiver always "invisible". After realizing the success on for awhile, she became happy and satisfied with the new system (Reilly & Bischoff, 2008).

Mitzi Boegly, a 97-year-old resident who was interviewed for the study, said that she welcomed having the sensor technology in her apartment—especially after she used it to summon help after a fall. "It gives you a feeling of security knowing that if something happened to you, you can get help right away. I go to bed at night with peace of mind," she said. The NewCourtland staff responses indicate that they also feel the sensor technology has improved the residents' basic security and safety (Reilly & Bischoff, 2008).

"The study shows our staffs appreciate the system's ability to improve the efficacy of care delivery by directing it quickly to where it is most needed," says Brooks. At the same time, she adds, the staff's responses suggest a need for additional training, better reporting tools, and extensions into prognostics for chronic conditions (Reilly & Bischoff, 2008).

From such a successful testing, we feel that it is promising to adapt this technology system in nursing homes. As to earlier mentioned that the shortage of nurse in the Unite State, while the continuous increasing of demands for caregivers, the installment of remote monitoring system definitely will be helpful for regulate such a lack. One thing, we need concern is about the cultural and situational difference in different areas. Research indicates that in most of northern United States that people are generally more open minded, and easier to accept new methods ("Intelligent remote visual monitoring system for home health care service," 1996). So that in the later sections will release the indication on the attitudes of nursing home residents here in Alabama, by conducting the personal interviews to different nursing homes.

## Carpet Sensor in Bedroom

Due to the frequent accident happening on the seniors during the night time, a new technology has been applied to the carpet to make sure their safety in year 1997, making it as big as a rug. Result: floors that can sound an alert when a nursing-home patient falls or when a nighttime intruder enters (Otis, 2007). It proves that such carpet has been commonly used in health care organizations, especially in nursing homes. Developed by Messet Oy, a five-person company in Kuopio, Finland, with the Technical Research Center of Finland's VTT Automation Institute in Tampere, the room-size sensors are being tested in nursing homes in Helsinki and Tampere, says Messet Chairman Keijo Korhonen (Otis, 2007). The sensor is a thin polypropylene lamination that goes under carpeting or floor tiles (Otis, 2007). Inside the 0.002-inch-thick structure are tiny pillows of foamed plastic (Otis, 2007). These function as "electrets," a type of electromagnet used in some microphones. When a weak current is flowing through the top surface, the pillows respond to the slightest changes in pressure by generating an electrical signal (Otis, 2007). Messet says that the structure is so sensitive that it can detect the breathing of a person lying on the floor — through the carpet. This talking carpet is welcomed by the patients as well as the healthcare providers.

## Scheduling Software

Using specialized software to schedule the nursing staff at St. Joseph Convent retirement and nursing home is easy and affordable. It's also a time-saver. Marilyn Fuller says she couldn't do without it ("St. Joseph", 2007). Fuller, a scheduler at St. Joseph Convent, a home for 170 retired nuns, uses the Visual Staff Scheduler Pro by Atlas Business Solutions to ensure shift coverage, track and reduce overtime, view staff availability and contact information, and define custom shifts. "The software has helped eliminate mistakes and questions in the schedule and provides an accurate report on cost effectiveness by showing me a complete picture of how many hours each staff member is scheduled each week," Fuller said ("St. Joseph", 2007).

The scheduler software eliminates the opportunity for staff to make changes to the work schedule. Only Fuller and the director of nursing can edit the schedule, but each unit can access a copy ("St. Joseph", 2007).

The Visual Staff Scheduler Pro software by Atlas Business Solutions is a quick and flexible tool that makes staff scheduling easy and very affordable ("St. Joseph", 2007).

## Seating System

Since 1994, recliner and wheelchair design, developing cushioning and posturing appliances to make the patient comfortable, has been introduced to health care industry (David, 1994). Chairs were designed to fit the largest size potential users and modified on-site with pillows, cushions, foam pads, gel seats and, most recently, active pneumatic technology (David, 1994). This has its obvious limits, especially to whose are small.

Such a high-tech seating system encountered a roadblock in nursing homes: Their funding mechanisms haven't advanced to keep up with developments in equipment (David, 1994). These new seating systems have been developed for use in more intensive rehabilitation environments and haven't reached long-term care yet, largely because of high cost and reimbursement difficulties (David, 1994). A higher level of seating care becomes available and is widely used nowadays, because there is a change in how therapy services are being provided to nursing homes (David, 1994). As nursing homes contract for physical and occupational therapy, they are being exposed to newer technology. Subacute care is educating staff and creating advocates for more comprehensive seating solutions (David, 1994).

Intelligent surface technology, according to BCA, allows surfaces which come in contact with the body to automatically change shape to facilitate comfort, fit, and safety (David, 1994). It first measures load distribution on the body, then calculates the most comfortable surface shape, and changes the shape of the surface to optimize comfort (David, 1994).

"There is a dichotomy in seating," explained by Sprigle, PhD, biomedical engineer at the Center for Assistive Technology, State University of New York at Buffalo, and an expert on therapeutic seating design. "involving two concepts that are always in opposition -- support and mobility." (David, 1994). By optimizing support and then allowing that support to change as a patient moves in a chair, intelligent surface technology is bringing new comfort and safety to long-duration seating.

## Telecommunication

The use of telemedicine technology provides an opportunity to bridge the geographic distance between family and nursing home residents

(Debra, 2006). Several studies have focused on using communication technologies in community settings (Demiris, 2001). Videophone technology has been used to enhance communication between home-bound patients and healthcare providers. Several studies confirm the feasibility of using videophone technology in a community setting with few technological challenges (Debra, 2006) Generally, home-based research has found that the technology is accepted by the general public and is easily managed in the home setting. "These interventions have been demonstrated to be cost-effective and satisfactory overall to users." (Whitten, 2001; Parker, Demiris, Day, Courtney, & Porock, 2006) While most studies have focused on home care, a few have been tried in the nursing home setting (Debra, 2006).

A video link between a resident and family may also allow staff to use the technology to communicate with the family, enhancing their relationship with distant caregivers. A facility may consider a shared phone for the facility to decrease resident cost and allow family members the opportunity to connect not only with the resident but also with the entire care team (Debra, 2006). Nursing home providers may want to be prepared to accommodate family members experienced with various forms of telecommunications and engage them in the life of the resident, regardless of their geographic distance. Facilities should consider participating in projects that evaluate this and other technology designed to enhance and improve resident and family care (Johnson, Wheeler, Dueser, & Sousa, 2000).

## Heart Guard

Heart disease is the frequent cause of death and early diagnosis is essential to save lives. Monitoring the heart's rhythm and electrical activity using an electrocardiogram (ECG) provides vital information about abnormalities and gives clues to the nature of a problem (Hoban, 2003). Some cardiac conditions need long-term monitoring inconvenient for patients as it requires them to be away from their everyday environment for indeterminate periods of time (Hoban, 2003).

Six years ago, Latvian company Integris Ltd, a specialist in the development of mobile wireless telemedicine ECG recording devices, came up with the concept of an inexpensive, real-time heart activity monitor for personal use. After years research and tests, 3489 HEART GUARD was born (Hoban, 2003).

According to Integris, we know that "The HEART GUARD system comprises a lightweight, simple to use, matchbox-size device with five electrodes that are strategically placed on the wearer's chest. The wireless device transmits data in real time directly to the patient's pocket computer or desktop PC for instant interpretation by the system's unique software" (Hoban, 2003). The low-cost device is discreet enough to be worn 24 hours a day, recording, analyzing and reporting not only the rhythm and electrical activity of a patient's heart but also his physical activity and body positions, as they go about their daily life (Hoban, 2003).

"Effectively, it is an early warning system," explains Juris Lauznis, Director of Integris, the project's lead partner. "If HEART GUARD detects a problem, patients are alerted by means of vibration or a buzzer, prompting them to check their PC for further information and advice. At the very least, the device will help to monitor and manage a patient's condition and it could even save a life." (Hoban, 2003).

Currently HEART GUARD is being developed for home use only, with patients monitoring their own condition and only contacting a doctor or hospital if the system identifies a cause for concern (Hoban, 2003). HEART GUARD also has applications in a number of other areas, including telemedicine, sports medicine, patient rehabilitation following cardiac surgery or a heart attack and as a low-cost ECG monitoring system in hospitals and nursing homes with limited budgets (Hoban, 2003), which will be extremely beneficial for the elders that want to live home with the monitoring system in the nursing home.

With the 30-month project completed and clinical trials of the prototype successfully concluded by Kaunas Medical University's Institute of Cardiology, the Lithuania Academy of Physical Education and the Research Institute of Cardiology at the University of Latvia, the next steps are to satisfy the EU's strict compliance requirements for medical devices and then source a company to manufacture and distribute the system (Hoban, 2003). If successful, the first commercial HEART GUARD devices could be on the market and saving lives by the end of 2008 or early 2009 (Hoban, 2003).

## The Latest Innovations Regarding to HIT

According to long-term care (LTC) health information technology (HIT) Summit, touting the trends and innovations in HIT for long-term care, the latest innovations include handheld devices for care documentation by staff; easy-to-use touch screens with graphic icons to assess the documentations and care by direct care staff; hands-free, eyes-free voice documentation of assessment and care for certified nursing assistants; and software for electronic prescription processing from electronic physician order systems (O'Connor, 2005). Other technologies include managing medication passes to robotic medication dispensing, capturing quality data electronically for benchmarking and ongoing quality improvement, and operational and management information systems to assist in management functions (Harrison, 2002).

According to COMTEX News Network (2009), two of the latest innovations include electronic patient monitoring and e-prescribing devices. Some of the latest technologies include products Vigil Dementia System, which features intelligent software and sensors to detect unexpected behavior, such as extended time out of bed, leaving a room, or incontinence. Others are the monitors for fall prevention, wireless call with location tracking, Wi-Fi coverage for staff communications using voice-over Internet protocol phones, and use of mobile devices necessary for electronic health record (EHR) data entry.

In the past, it was a paper-compliant process done at the end of a shift and was not always the most accurate (Andrews, 2009). Facilities moving toward point-of-care systems (like touch pads in the hallways near care delivery) for nursing assistants are seeing more accurate documentation that is impacting their reimbursement rates because it is reflecting what is actually being delivered.

## Challenges to Success

Wilt admits that training presented one of the biggest challenges to HIT implementation. Employees needed to develop proficiency in computer use, a process that may last for several years. This is one of the more significant barriers to implementation (O'Connor, 2008). A lot of time are needed to spend in training and support to make the communities successful.

Nursing homes' adoption of technology has been slow. We have learned studies from the AHCA and the California HealthCare Foundation. Responses to the December 2006 AHCA and National Center for Assisted Living study "A Snap-Shot of the Use of Health Information Technology in Long Term Care" indicated that 46% of long-term care facilities continued to do the majority of their work on paper or were just beginning to use computers. Only 1% reported being paperless, and only 2% considered themselves fully computerized and just beginning to communicate or communicating fully with outside healthcare providers (O'Connor, 2008).

## Concern of Standards

In terms of other challenges, the issue of standards creates a concern. According to Andrews (2009), the technology integration has been a challenge mostly because there are standards out there, but they give the implementers of them great flexibility in how to go about using them. It enables to improve the monthly nursing summary that shared between the nurses and doctors by providing an electronic exchange between our two clinical systems. This has improved access to information and hopefully influenced decision making properly.

"Many nursing homes are adopting a wait-and-see approach until software products are certified by the Certification Commission for Healthcare Information Technology (CCHIT) using the Health Level Seven (HL7)-approved LTC EHR-S functional profile", says Eileen T. Doll, RN, BS, NHA, president of Efficiency Driven Healthcare Consulting, Inc. in Baltimore. HL7 is an American National Standards Institute standard for healthcare-specific data exchange between computer applications (Sloane, 2006).

Proper integration of technology is essential. True streamlining occurs when the clinical and administrative sides are fully integrated in all aspects—no duplicate entry, no data inconsistency, and integrated processes. Duplications are reduced or eliminated when common information is shared among care settings and information systems (Sloane, 2006). Reduced duplication also improves accuracy, with less likelihood that the same piece of information is different in other systems.

One thing that helps with standardization is the LTC HIT Collaborative. CAST, the American Association of Homes and Services for the Aging, the NCAL, and the AHCA are partners in ensuring that the LTC sector is represented and the national HIT standards cater to the unique requirements of LTC applications (Sloane, 2006).

## Nursing Home Size

How large must nursing homes be to make various technologies cost-effective? What can be done for smaller homes interested in technology but unable to invest as much as larger operations? According to Majd Alwan, PhD, director of the Center for Aging Services Technologies (CAST) in Washington, DC, and a member of the LTC HIT Summit, "It really depends on the size of the facility, where they are in the process, whether they have the basic infrastructure in place or not, whether they are part of a chain or not, the management's position, etc. Generally speaking, if shown a return on investment potential, including return in terms of quality and competitive advantage, providers should be willing to invest," Even so, smaller homes should not be discouraged. "The best approach is to have a plan and to take EHR implementation in stages," he says. "Plan one application or module at a time based on the organization's tolerance for change, leadership, and financial resources. If resources are limited, start with one or two smaller applications that will make an impact, such as the nursing assistant documentation/kiosk touchpad, and keep building."

For smaller homes interested in technology, Alwan explains that most companies price technology based on usage, so smaller providers pay less than larger providers. "Many smaller homes choose not to host and manage their software and data," he says. "With software as a service, even the smallest [nursing home] providers can benefit."

## The Future of Technology

After thorough research work, we believe that resident access to the electronic documentation will continue to be an area providers will eventually offer for their residents. We think that technologies that connect the resident and family closer together will continue to be the most requested items. Innovative technology enables residents and their families to access basic information such as lists of problems, medications, allergies, contact information, and lab reports. The ability to make this easy to use for all will be the challenge but we see an opportunity with telehealth devices that are coming onto the market today for other uses that will eventually be extended to the SNF environment ("Telehealth can improve quality of life," 2009).

As mentioned earlier, a variety of exciting technologies are on the drawing board, including advanced total quality systems that integrate several basic components already in existence, such as nurse call, wandering management, fall prevention, resident tracking, resident assessment, electronic medication administration record, and electronic treatment administration record systems. Also in the works are advanced fall prevention systems, advanced beds with embedded sensors, and comprehensive interoperable EHRs that allow sharing health information securely across different settings.

Resistance to change presents one of the biggest challenges to technology integration in the nursing home environment. The industry has been manual and paper-based for so long, it requires a cultural shift to a technology base. We believe that communication is the key to overcoming this challenge. We look forward to seeing technology beyond EHR systems. According to CosmoCom Showcases Telehealth at World Health Care Congress (2009), in the near future, we will see current high-tech devices integrated with EHRs. Telehealth is an emerging and important technology for the future. Technology is needed to upgrade all equipment used in SNFs as well as changing the homes to meet the cultural change required for a higher quality of life.

## PART III: REPORT ON THOMASVILLE NURSING HOME VISITING

In this part, we will report our visiting a nursing home in south Alabama.

## Background

Thomasville Nursing Home is a well known nursing home in south Alabama, which is equipped with standardized facilities. It is a religious nonmedical health care institution with SNF/NF (dually certificated). Five residents are interviewed and four filled out the questionnaire. Three nurses, two social workers, and the administrator are also interviewed by giving out some brief opinions on the technology involved in the nursing home daily bases. Figures 2 (a) and (b) shows the outside photos of the nursing home.

## Research Purpose

Know the actual conditions in Nursing Home in Alabama rural areas. Research are specific in the residents room decoration, overall quality on the residents' living conditions, residents satisfaction on Nursing Home care, and staff, residents' attitudes about technology applying.

## Outcomes

In Thomasville nursing home, what makes residents happy or unhappy? What are their special wishes? In this report, three themes emerged from resident responses: community, care, supportive relationships. In addition to residents' daily happiness in nursing homes, quality life includes another great factor: technology involvement.

## Community

As in any community, nursing home residents focus on their living space, neighbors, and what is happening. For some residents, having others around affords conversation and companionship, especially when their roommate is or becomes a friend. The nursing home provides a sense of "fellowship, friendship, and care." In contrast, other residents may be uncomfortable with the number of people and the amount of activity level within

*Figure 2. Thomasville Nursing Home*

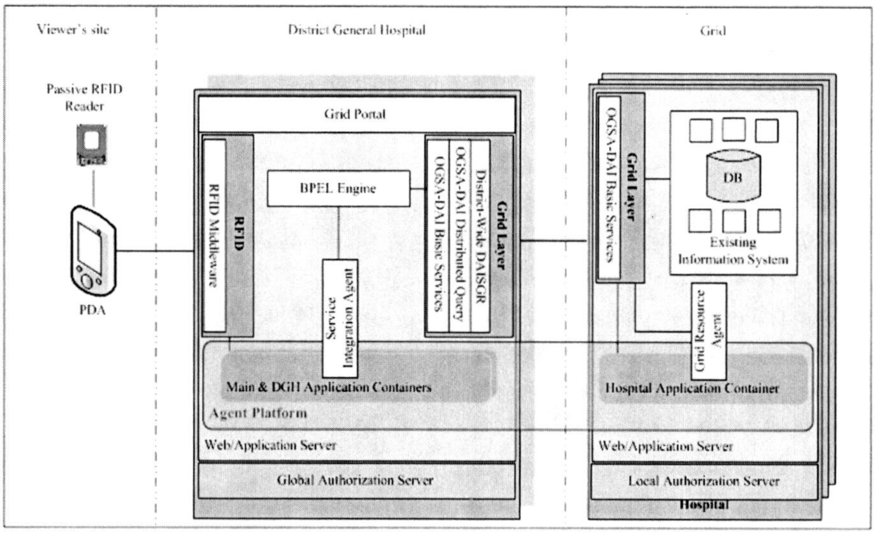

the environment. These residents are unhappy because they "always have someone around," and wish for "a private room" or "a lot of space like I had at home." So that in Thomasville Nursing Home, they offer different types of rooms for their residents, though it is more demanding on the single rooms, all of the interviewed residents are somewhat satisfied with their accommodations. Figures 3(a) and (b) shows the single- room pictures. To some residents, there is a sensor pad underneath the bed sheet to secure residents' safety. Though pets are not allowed, some of the patients still feel like to have a kitty or puppy toy around with them. "TV is another important accompanier to stay away from lonely, which helps us kill time and catch up with the everyday ongoing" said couple of the residents. In the single room, some of the residents feel that they have their own privacy and their own time.

Residents enjoy going to the dining room and visiting with their tablemates. They are happy when the food is good, there are snacks at night, and they celebrate birthdays together. They are unhappy when the coffee is not freshly brewed, the same foods are served too often, or the food is not cooked to their personal taste. Residents'

special wishes include "to have food and meat like I had on the farm," "for someone to bring food from outside for my birthday," and "to have a Residents enjoy going to the dining room and visiting with their tablemates. They are happy when the food is good, there are snacks at night, and they celebrate birthdays together. They are unhappy when the coffee is not freshly brewed, the same foods are served too often, or the food is not cooked to their personal taste". Residents' special wishes include "to have food and meat like I had on the farm," "for someone to bring food from outside for my birthday," and "to have a martini once in a while." The dining room (Figure 4) and activity room (Figure 5) play a significant role in their daily life in the nursing home.

The planned activities provided by nursing homes are an important part of the community. Residents like to be busy and enjoy "the chance to play bingo and laugh." Some are happy because church services are offered in their home. One of the residents says that many residents want to get into town and see new sights, and others simply would like to "get out more and see flowers and trees." Others want to go shopping or go out to lunch. Most residents are elders, and the

*Figure 3. Residents' Bed Room withh Her Toy Kitty and TV*

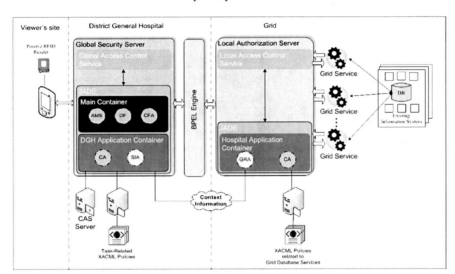

*Figure 4. Dining room for the residents*

```
1    <Subject>
2      <SubjectMatch MatchId="&function;anyURI-equal">
3        <AttributeValue DataType="&xml;anyURI"
           Scope="Attiki.DGH">&roles;physician</AttributeValue>
4        <SubjectAttributeDesignator AttributeId="&role;" DataType="&xml;anyURI"/>
5      </SubjectMatch>
6    </Subject>
```

nursing home community may be less satisfying for younger residents. A younger resident says, "There's a bunch of old people here instead of people my own age." In Thomasville, the nursing home staffs also say that they understand the different demands on the their residents, however, it is hard to satisfy everyone, say, it's a complicated process to bring the elders to the shopping in terms of their safety concern; because of the small portion of young residents in the nursing home, considering of the budget concern, it is not realistic to arrange activities for couple of them only.

Fulfilling residents' special wishes could increase their sense of community. According to the administrator, Dania, she says that one approach would be for the care planning coordinator or social worker to ask residents about special wishes when completing the quarterly or annual Myelodysplastic syndromes (MDS), a group of diseases that affect the bone marrow and blood, assessment. Many of the wishes are easy to grant through staff or family members, and that special treat could be added to the respective resident's care plan as an onetime event. Using the MDS assessment process ensures that residents with limiting physical or mental impairments would be included. Other actions to increase residents' sense of community might include providing quiet places where they can go to be alone or arranging activities targeted for younger residents that offer interactions with age-mates. Access to the Internet, with assistance in learning to use that technology, could facilitate participation in chat rooms and, perhaps, cyber friendships with peers in other facilities.

*Figure 5. Activity scene: Inauguration Day*

```
4    <Resource>
5      <ResourceMatch MatchId="&function;string-equal">
6        <AttributeValue
         DataType="&xml;string">http://localhost/active-bpel/services/RadProcProcess/IssueRadRequest
         </AttributeValue>
7        <ResourceAttributeDesignator AttributeId="&resource;resource-id" DataType="&xml;string"/>
8      </ResourceMatch>
9    </Resource>
10   ...
12   <Action>
13     <ActionMatch MatchId="&function;string-equal">
14       <AttributeValue DataType="&xml;string">execute</AttributeValue>
15       <ActionAttributeDesignator AttributeId="&action;action-id" DataType="&xml;string"/>
16     </ActionMatch>
17   </Action>
18   ...
20   <Condition>
21   <Apply FunctionId="&function;and">
22   <Apply FunctionId="&function;string-equal">
23     <EnvironmentAttributeDesignator
         AttributeId="urn:oasis:names:tc:xacml:2.0:environment:userPatientRelationship"
         DataType="&xml;string"/>
24     <AttributeValue DataType="&xml;string">currentPatient</AttributeValue>
25   </Apply>
26   <Apply FunctionId="&function;string-equal">
27     <EnvironmentAttributeDesignator
         AttributeId=" urn:oasis:names:tc:xacml:2.0:environment:status" DataType="&xml;string"/>
28     <AttributeValue DataType="&xml;yes">onDuty</AttributeValue>
29   </Apply>
30   <Apply FunctionId="&function;string-equal">
31     <EnvironmentAttributeDesignator
         AttributeId="urn:oasis:names:tc:xacml:2.0:environment:location" DataType="&xml;string"/>
32     <AttributeValue DataType="&xml;string">inPremises</AttributeValue>
33   </Apply>
34   </Apply>
35   </Condition>
```

The "Miss. Nursing Home", shown in Figure 6, who is 90 year-old, told me with a big smile and proud that she has rewarded as the Miss Nursing Home last year, which brings her a lot of confidence and self-esteem. Such rewarding games and programs are consistently held by Thomasville Nursing Home, which bring all the residents get into their fun daily life.

## Care

Residents come to nursing homes because they need help with basic activities of daily life. Many residents are happy because someone else does the housework, prepares the meals, washes the dishes, and does the laundry. They like having someone who pays attention to them and helps them meet their needs.

Having things go the resident's way is important. Residents appreciate special attention to unique interests or needs, such as having staff communicate with sign language, being able to listen to music of their choice, and having coffee with the chaplain. They need flexibility; for instance, too many baths make one resident unhappy, whereas another's special wish is to have more baths.

Residents are happy when they are satisfied with staff and believe they receive good care. They describe good care as having staff listen to what they say, having someone respond quickly to the call light, being handled gently by staff during care, receiving proper medications and

*Figure 6. "Miss Nursing Home" wears her crown*

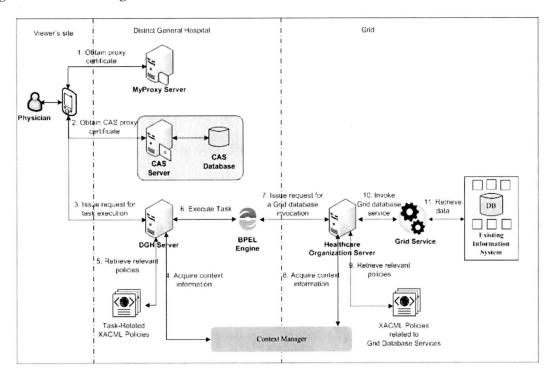

treatments, and having the doctor visit. Personal cleanliness is valued--being kept clean, having clean clothes, and having clean teeth.

Good care depends on the facility having enough qualified staff to meet resident needs. Long waits--for meals to be served, for help to the bathroom, or for the nurse--make residents unhappy, which has been changed in Thomasville Nursing Home after getting feedbacks from their residents. One of the residents says that sometimes busy staff save time by doing things residents could do for themselves. It may be faster to change a resident's briefs than to take him to the bathroom, or to push a resident's wheelchair to the dining room rather than letting her use a walker.

High staff turnover also creates problems. One resident says, "The people who help me change all the time; they don't know what they're supposed to do."

Some residents are more vulnerable than others because of cognitive impairment, hearing or vision loss, or limited mobility. A touching spe-

cial wish is that everybody be treated the same. A resident observes, "Some people who don't know where they are get left behind on answering call lights."

According to the nursing home staffs and Diane, It is important that staff seek input from residents and family members about care. Feedback about how their concerns are addressed reinforces a need for their participation. Although maintaining independence is desirable, a resident's ability to do a task warrants careful evaluation. For example, vision and fine motor skills must be considered in deciding how a resident participates in an insulin injection.

Employee recognition programs should emphasize specific staff behaviors that make a difference for residents. They saw a program in another facility where residents and family members nominate staff for a "STAR" award based on outstanding performance, and a star is attached to the employee's name tag.

## Supportive Relationships

Establishing new relationships with staff and other residents is part of settling into a nursing home community. Support from family, friends, and staff is critical to new residents' successful transition and adaptation. Family and friends, "Being with those you love", make residents happy. Their hearts will be warmed may be just by receiving a small gift, and services from family and friends, such as a cassette player from a nephew, a fish fillet from a friend, and dresses laundered with a daughter's special touch. Residents who are unhappy about relationships with family most often feel greater separation because of distance or a perceived lack of concern. Special wishes regarding family and friends usually relate to having more contact. However, one man feels that there is too much pressure on his wife and wishes for someone to help her take care of him. Another man wishes that staff would watch his wife, a resident in the same facility, more closely.

Staff members make residents happy through interactions based on respect, kindness, and concern, and by taking time to help, listen, and share their lives. Residents are happy when staff are attentive, but without fuss; when they invite them to events, but also allow them to be alone; and, in general, when they try to make things better for them. Residents appreciate a pat on the shoulder and staff coming to tell them good-bye. It is important for them to have something in common with staff; for example, boosting the same sports team. Shared laughter is a crucial happiness factor. For some residents, teasing staff and being teased, kidding, telling jokes, playing tricks on each other, and "picking on" staff add spice to the day.

In addition to the resident council, residents need an opportunity to voice concerns privately to someone who can do something about them. Residents may feel powerless or threatened by abandonment in conflicts with staff, and may need support from a family member or friend in voicing their concerns. Family members and friends who do support residents and add quality to their daily lives deserve recognition. Examples of uncomplicated acknowledgments include feedback from staff about how much a resident enjoyed a special outing or a snapshot of a resident wearing a new sweater sent by a brother in another town.

## Technology

The overall quality is satisfying, and the Thomasville nursing home has already been switch to home-like style, which makes the residents more comfortable to live than that of traditional style. From the interviews on the residents, it reveals that most of the patients are willing to accept the new technology equipments. The overall attitudes on their nursing home quality is fairly satisfied, including the hygiene, food, daily activities, and nursing home services. Two of them feel it is too hard to communicate with others, and lonely is the major issue they do not want to stay in the nursing home. All of them think that it is safer to have the advanced facilities to assist their livings, and they feel secured to have the sitting pad on the wheel chair, alarm sleeping sheet on the bed, but they reject the clips connect the cloth and the chair, which makes them feel like being framed and controlled by a string.

"Tech-Bed" is another favorite assistant at Thomasville Home. It looks and feels the same as other normal beds, so that the residents do not take it as a weird stuff. The nurses absolutely love those tech beds. "It truly is like another pair of eyes." Sensors in the zip-on, washable mattress cover provide continuous heart and respiratory rate data. Nothing attaches to the patient. A monitor sits next to the bed and picks up the signals. Hoana presets defaults, but nurses can easily program the sensors to alarm at rates specific to their patients. "We have caught someone going into atrial fibrillation, that we had checked vital signs on an hour before," Diane, the administrator, said. "It's an early warning system." Nurses at Thomasville have also picked up respiratory depression in patients receiving patient- controlled narcotics. The nursing home has monitored nurse and residents satisfaction, fall rates and cardiac arrests. Diane notes positive trends in the preliminary data.

The nurses felt that the covers provided a valuable service and they found the device easy to use, said Valerie Martinez, RN, BSN. "It's a great tool for the nurse, to help them monitor the patients when they can't be in there," Martinez said. "You can go back and trend things." The nurse can assess what the alert was for and how many times it activated.

"It allows the nurse to be more involved in the early recognition of patients that are starting to fail," said Heather Long, RN, chief operating officer of Thomasville. "It provides data that brings the nurse to the bedside."

The Tech-Bed also has a bed exit alarm, with three push-button settings for patients at different fall risks. At high risk, the bed will alert if the patient lifts his or her head or shoulders off the bed. For moderate risk patients, it waits until the patient sits up and for low risk it delays issuing an alarm until the patient actually exits the bed. Loved ones or the nurse can program the device to play a personalized, prerecorded message to get back into bed and wait for the nurse.

"It's very helpful for the elderly," Diane said. "They hear a human voice, saying 'I'm coming to get you,' and they will stop and wait."

Heather said that patients do not feel or see the sensors. Once the patient understands the system, she said, "It makes them feel more secure and safe."

All of the being interviewed are holding a positive attitudes to have made the nursing home computerized, such as EMR, monitoring equipments, and alarm system. Technology makes their work a lot easier, though it took a while to get used to it. It is useful and powerful tool to make the working place more organized. Diane says though it is getting harder to get funds from the state or federal government, the government is still sup-porting the ideas of keeping getting technology into long-term care, because it worth investing by thinking of saving money in a long run. She also points out that the facilities usages are not from patients' expenses, but from the nursing homes.

As for the e-prescribing which is another revolution for healthcare industry, Diane said lots of concerns. "Standards for e-prescribing have recently been developed, so this isn't an area of widespread adoption yet," says Diane, the administrator of Thomasville Nursing Home, "This is a complex undertaking for long-term care facilities because it requires standards to communicate between three parties: the facility, the pharmacy, and the physician."

To date, cost has been a primary inhibitor. "We as an industry have not compiled and communicated enough quantitative ROI [return on investment] data," Diane adds. "I believe that technology can improve the quality of care, reduce risk, save time, and grow the business. These data will continue to be made available and will definitively show providers that technology is good for business and good for resident care."

Thomasville nursing home has been successfully implementing electronic records management: nurses' use of clinical notes, clinical assessments, orders, and electronic medication administration records. For nursing aides, the company has implemented electronic activities of daily living documentation. "We are in the process of implementing electronic lab and integration with our Doc EMR [electronic medical record] to allow for even better communication between the teams," says Diane.

*"The biggest improvements have been on the management side of the implementation," she says. "We have been able to provide greater insight into the amount and frequency of the documentation that we have never had before. We are able to monitor more efficiently the documentation process by providing reporting capabilities that are not feasible with paper." The concern for the*

*Thomasville Home is financial support, "we hope that either the federal government or states will come up with more money to fund general high-tech operation and HIT efforts"*

It is a great visiting to Thomasville Nursing Home, which allowed us to approach the residents' real life in south United State. Those three themes are the major concern for the residents in this specific nursing home. Additionally, it is a promising future to have technology involve into the nursing homes, because the demanding is still growing, because a lot of facilities in the homes are not greatly developed, however, the residents numbers are still growing. According to the personal visiting and research, it reveals that the elders are willing to accept the new technologies for the sake of their life quality. The staffs as well as the government are taking a positive attitude in considering of long term benefits.

## CONCLUSION

This chapter provides broad information on the current and future views of nursing home in the United States, in terms of the condition and management level, residents' satisfactions and demands, government regulation and influence. The ability of e-health technology enables nursing homes to improve their quality to meet residents' needs, though there are challenges. The visiting report about Thomasville Nursing Home reaches the depth of the consideration to how to catch the trends by implementing the technologies.

## ACKNOWLEDGMENT

This work is supported in part by the US National Science Foundation (NSF) under the grant number CNS-0716211, as well as RGC (Research Grants Committee) award at The University of Alabama 2008.

## REFERENCES

*Activities*. (n.d.). Retrieved October 20, 2008, from http://www.hardingnh.com/

Alexander, G. L. (2008). A Descriptive Analysis of a Nursing Home Clinical Information System with Decision Support. *Perspectives in Health Information Management / AHIMA, American Health Information Management Association, 5*(12).

American Health Information Management Association. (2005). *A road map for health IT in long-term care*. Chicago: Author.

*Analysis of the National Nursing Home Survey (NNHS)* (2004). AARP Public Policy Institute.

Anderson, R., Issel, L. M., & McDaniel, R. R. (2003). Nursing homes as complex adaptive systems: relationship between management practice and resident outcomes. *Nursing Research, 52*(1), 12–21. doi:10.1097/00006199-200301000-00003

Anderson, S., & Wittwer, W. (2004). Using barcode point-of-care technology for patient safety. *Journal for Healthcare Quality, 26*(6), 5–11.

Andrews, J. (2009). Keeping record: long-term care may not deserve its reputation as a tech laggard. But more could be done to prepare for the electronic health record.(Information technology). *McKnight's Long-Term Care News, 30*(1), 42(43).

Assisted Living Facilities (ALF). (2007). Virginia Department of Social Services: Virginia.gov.

Baron, R. J., Fabens, E. L., Schiffman, M., & Wolf, E. (2005). Electronic health records: Just around the corner? Or over the cliff? *Annals of Internal Medicine, 143*(3), 222–226.

Barrick, A., & Rader, J. (2008). *Bathing without a battle: person-directed care of individuals with dementia*. New York: Springer Pub.

Bates, D. W., Cohen, M., Leape, L. L., Overhage, J. M., Shabot, M. M., & Sheridan, T. (2001). Reducing the frequency of errors in medicine using information technology. *Journal of the American Medical Informatics Association, 8*(4), 299–308.

Bates, D. W., Leape, L. L., Cullen, D. J., Laird, N., Petersen, L. A., & Teich, J. M. (1998). Effect of computerized physician order entry and a team intervention on prevention of serious medication errors. *Journal of the American Medical Association, 280*(15), 1311–1316. doi:10.1001/jama.280.15.1311

Bates, D. W., Teich, J. M., Lee, J., Seger, D., & Kuperman, G. J., Ma'Luf, N., et al. (1999). The impact of computerized physician order entry on medication error prevention. *Journal of the American Medical Informatics Association, 6*(4), 313–321.

Berger, L. (2006, January 13). Information technology feature: The IT payback. *McKnight's Long-Term Care News,* (pp. 34-37).

Boumans, N., Berkhout, A., & Landeweerd, A. (2005). Efforts of resident-oriented care on quality of care, wellbeing and satisfaction with care. *Scandinavian Journal of Caring Sciences, 19*(3), 11. doi:10.1111/j.1471-6712.2005.00351.x

Breen, G., & Zhang, N. (2008). Theoretical Analysis of Improving Resident Care. *Journal of Medical Systems, 32*(2), 18–23. doi:10.1007/s10916-007-9121-9

Breen, G. M., & Matusitz, J. (2007). An interpersonal examination of telemedicine: Applying relevant communication theories. *e-health. International Journal (Toronto, Ont.), 3*(1), 187–192.

Burland, E. M. J. (2008). An Evaluation of a Fall Management Program in a Personal Care Home Population. *Healthcare Quaterly, 11*(3), 137–140.

Burland, E. M. J. (2008). An Evaluation of a Fall Management Program in a Personal Care Home Population. *Healthcare Quaterly, 11*(3), 137–140.

*Caring for the Elderly: Is Adequate Long-Term Care Available.* (1998). Congressional Quarterly, Inc., CQ Researcher.

Carrillo, H., & Harrington, C. (2006). Cross the States 2006: Profiles of Long-Term Care and Independent Living. In AARP (Ed.).

Castle, N. G. (2008). Nursing Home Evacuation Plans. *American Journal of Public Health, 98*(7), 1235–1241. doi:10.2105/AJPH.2006.107532

*CMS Adds Searchable Database of Lowest-Quality Nursing Homes Nationwide to Web Site.* (2008). Kaiser Family Foundation.

Corporation, W. (2005). Our products and services. About WebMD.com.

CosmoCom Showcases Telehealth at World Health Care Congress (2009). *Health &amp; Beauty Close-Up,* NA.

*Daily Activities.* (n.d.). Retrieved October 20, 2008, from http://seniors-site.com/nursingm/index.html

David, P. (1994). *A revolution in seating - Nursing Home Technology.* Retrieved November 03, 2008.

Debra, O., & Brain, H. (2006). A promising Technology to Reduce Social Isolation of Nursing Home Residents. *Journal of Nursing Care Quality, 21*(4), 302–306.

Demiris, G., Speedie, S.M., & Finkelstein, S. (2001). Change of patients' perceptions of TeleHomeCare. *Telemedicine Journal and e-Health, 7*(3), 241–249. doi:10.1089/153056201316970948

Durable medical equipment: Scope and conditions. (2006). *CFR, 38,* 42.

*Eljay, L. (2006)*. A Report on Shortfalls in Medicaid Funding for Nursing Home Care: American Health Care Association.

Facts, N. (2006). *Today's Registered Nurse - Numbers and Demographics.* Washington, DC: A. N. Association.

Field, T., & Rochon, P. (2008). Costs associated with developing and implementing a computerized clinical decision support system for medication dosing for patients with renal insufficiency in the long-term care setting. *Journal of the American Medical Informatics Association, 15*(4), 466–472. doi:10.1197/jamia.M2589

Finnema, E., de Lange, J., Droes, R. M., Ribbe, M., & Tilburg, W. (2001). The quality of nursing home care: do the opinions of family members change after implementation of emotion-oriented care? *Journal of Advanced Nursing, 35*(5), 728–732. doi:10.1046/j.1365-2648.2001.01905.x

*Fun Times.* (n.d.). Retrieved October 20, 2008, from http://www.goldenlivingcenters.com/GGNSC

General Accounting Office. (2004). *HS's efforts to promote health information technology and legal barriers to its adoption.* Washington, DC: Author.

Gill, TM, A. H., Han L. (2006). Bathing disability and the risk of long-term admission to a nursing home. *Journal of Gerontology, 61*(8), 821–825.

Greenly, M., & Gugerty, B. (2002). How bar coding reduces medication errors. *Nursing, 32*(5), 70.

Hamilton, B. (2006). *Evaluation design of the business case of health information technology in long-term care (Final report).* Baltimore: Centers for Medicare and Medicaid Services.

Harris, Y., & Clauser, S. B. (2002). Achieving improvement through nursing home quality measurement. *Health Care Financing Review, 23*(4), 13.

Harrison, S. (2002). Telehealth skills hailed as answer to discharge delays: costs of high-tech monitoring systems compare favourably with long-term care. (news). *Nursing Standard, 17*(12), 7(1).

Hetzel, L., & Smith, A. (2001). *The 65 and Over Population: 2000-Census 2000 Brief.* Washington, DC: U.S. CENSUS BUREAU.

Hoban, S. (2003). Activities plus at Montgomery Place: the "new" active senior wants to be entertained, enlightened, and engaged--and will let you know how. *Nursing Homes, 52*(6), 52–56.

Holmes, D. (2007). An evaluation of a monitoring system intervention: falls, injuries, and affect in nursing homes. *Clinical Nursing Research, 16*(4), 317–335. doi:10.1177/1054773807307870

*Home Care and Nursing Home Services.* (n.d.). Retrieved December 12, 2008, from http://dhs.dc.gov/dhs/cwp/view,a,3,Q,613301.asp

Home Health Service. (2003). *CFR484.30, 1*(42).

*Inspectors Often Overlook Serious Deficiencies at U.S. Nursing Homes* (GAO Report). (2008). Medical New Today.

Institute of Medicine. (2001). *Crossing the quality chasm: A new health system for 21st century.* Washington, DC: National Academy Press.

(1996). Intelligent remote visual monitoring system for home health care service. InPatient, U. S. (Ed.), *United States Patient.*

Johnson, B., Wheeler, L., Dueser, J., & Sousa, K. (2000). Outcomes of the Kaiser Permanente Tele-Home Health Research Project. *Archives of Family Medicine, 9*(4), 40–45. doi:10.1001/archfami.9.1.40

St. Joseph Convent retirement and nursing home. (2007). *McKnight's Long-Term Care News, 1.*

Kemper, P., Komisar, H. L., & Alecixh, L. (2005). Long-Term Care Over What can Current Retirees Expect? *Inquiry, 42*, 15.

King, W. R., & He, J. (2006). A meta-analysis of the technology acceptance model. *Information & Management, 43*(6), 740–755. doi:10.1016/j.im.2006.05.003

Kohn, L. T., Corrigan, J. M., & Donaldson, M. S. (1999). *To err is human: Building a safer human system.* Washington, DC: National Academy Press.

Kramer, A., Bennett, R., Fish, R., Lin, C. T., Floersch, N., & Conway, K. (2004). *Case studies of electronic health records in post-acute and long-term care.* Washington, DC: U.S. Department of Health and Human Services.

Lilley, R. C. L. P., Lambden P. (2006). Medicines management for residential and nursing homes: a toolkit for best practice and accredited learning. Seattle: Radcliffe.

Lilley RC, L. P., Lambden P. (2006). *Medicines management for residential and nursing homes: a toolkit for best practice and accredited learning.* Seatle: Radcliffe.

MacLaughlin, E. J. (2005). Assessing medication adherence in the elderly: which tools to use in clinical practice? *Drugs & Aging, 22*(3), 55–231.

Matusitz, J., & Breen, G. M. (2007). Telemedicine: Its effects on health communication. *Health Communication, 21*(1), 10–21.

McGraw, C. (2004). Multi-compartment medication devices and patient compliance. *British Journal of Community Nursing, 9*(7), 90–285.

McKnight's LTC News. (2005, July). 2005 software. *McKnight's Long-Term Care News,* 43.

(2008). Medical & You handbook. InServices, M. M. (Ed.), *C. f.*

Michael, S. J. C. (2000). Wireless clinical alerts for physiologic, laboratory and medication data. In *Proceedings / AMIA 2000 Annual Symposium,* (pp. 789-793).

Mitka, M. (2003). Approach could widen access for older patients. *Telemedicine eyes for mental health services, 290*(14), 22-25.

Moller, J., Renegar, Carrie. (2003). Bathing as a wellness experience. *Nursing Homes Long Term Care Management, 52*(10), 108.

Mor, V., Berg, K., Angelelli, J., Gifford, D., Morris, J., & Moore, T. (2003). The quality of quality measurement in U.S. nursing homes. *The Gerontologist, 43*(2), 37–46.

*More Can Be Done to Protect Residents from Abuse.* (2002). U.S. General Accounting Office.

Mukamel, B. D., & Spector, D. W. (2000). Nursing home Costs and Risk-Adjusted Outcome Measures of Quality. *Medical Care, 38*(1), 32–35. doi:10.1097/00005650-200001000-00009

National Health Accounts. (n.d.). In C. f. M. a. M. S. (CMS) (Ed.).

Nursing Home Data Compendium. (2007). In CMS (Ed.): HS.gov.

NURSING HOMES. (2008). Federal Monitoring Surveys Demonstrate Continued Understatement of Serious Care Problems and CMS Oversight Weaknesses. In Office, S. G. A. (Ed.), *U (Vol. 517).* GAO.

O'Connor, J. (2005). Feds provide info on LTC tech products on market.(Technology)(Long Term Care)(Brief Article). *McKnight's Long-Term Care News,* 14(11).

O'Connor, J. (2008). Nursing homes up on technology, (NEWS). *McKnight's Long-Term Care News, 29*(12), 3(1).

Otis, P. (1997). Don't worry, The Carpet is Keep Watching. *BusinessWeek,* 1.

Overview Medicaid Program. (2006). *General Information* (In, C. M. S., Ed.).

Parker, O. D., Demiris, G., Day, M., Courtney, K. L., & Porock, D. (2006). Tele-hospice support for elder caregivers of hospice patients: two case studies. *Journal of Palliative Medicine, 9*(2), 54–59.

Patient Placement Systems Unveils Referral Automation Vision Center. (2009). *PRWeb*, NA.

Pear, R. (2008a). Serious Deficiencies in Nursing Homes Are Often Missed. *New York Times*.

Pear, R. (2008b). Violations Reported at 94% of Nursing Homes. *New York Times*.

Peter, D. (2001). *The Nurse Shortage: Perspectives from Current Direct Care Nurses and Former Direct Care Nurses* (Report).

Polit, F. D., & Beck, T. C. (2004). *Nursing Research: Principles and Methods*. Wickford, RI: Lippincott-Raven Publishers.

Poon, E. G., Jha, A. K., Christino, M., Honour, M. M., Fernandopulle, R., & Middleton, B. (2006). Assessing the level of healthcare information technology adoption in the United States: A snapshot. *BMC Medical Informatics and Decision Making, 6*, 1. doi:10.1186/1472-6947-6-1

Redfern, S., Hannan, S., Norman, I., & Martin, F. (2002). Work satisfaction, stress, quality of care and morale of older people in a nursing home. *Health & Social Care in the Community, 10*(6), 17–35. doi:10.1046/j.1365-2524.2002.00396.x

Reilly, J., & Bischoff, J. (2008). Remote Monitoring Tested. *Technology and Health Care, 34*(9), 12–14.

Robots may be next solution to nursing shortage. (2003). *Managed Care Weekly*, 102.

Schepers, J., & Wetzels, M. (2007). A meta-analysis of the technology acceptance model: Investigating subjective norm and moderation effects. *Information & Management, 44*(1), 90–103. doi:10.1016/j.im.2006.10.007

Shields, S. (2005, March 23). Culture Change in Nursing homes. *The Commonwealth Fund*.

Sloan, F., & Shayne, M. (1993). Long-Term Care, Medicaid, and the Impoverishment of the Elderly. *The Milbank Quarterly, 70*(4), 19.

Sloane, E. B. (2006). The emerging health care IT infrastructure, (Tech Talk). *24x7, 11*(12), 42(43).

Sloane, E. B. (2006). The emerging health care IT infrastructure.(Tech Talk). *24x7, 11*(12), 42(43).

Sloane, E. B. (2009). Regulatory overview.(Networking). *24x7, 14*(4), 24(22).

*Staff Turnover and Retention*. (2007). AAHSA.

Telehealth can improve quality of life. (2009). *Nursing Standard, 23*(24), 21(21).

Thompson, L. T., Dorsey, M. A., Miller, I. K., & Parrott, R. (Eds.). (2003). Telemedicine: Expanding healthcare into virtual environments. Mahwah, NJ: Handbook of health communication.

Wald, H., & Shojania, K. G. (2001). Incident reporting. In Shojania, K. G., Ducan, B. W., McDonald, K. M., & Wachter, R. M. (Eds.), *Making health care safer: A critical analysis of patient safety practices* (pp. 41–47). Rockville, MD: Agency for Healthcare Research and Quality.

Webb, A. (2001). *The Impact of the Cost of Long-Term Care on the Saving of the Elderly*. New York: International Longevity Center.

Whitten, P., Doolittle, G., & Heilmich, S. (2001). Telehospice: using telecommunication technology for terminally ill patients. *Comput-Mediat Commun, 6*(4), 43–47.

Williams, L. (2003). Medication-Monitoring Lawsuit: Case Study and Lessons Learned. *Nursing Homes/Long Term Care Management, 3*.

Wolf, A. (2003). *Behind Closed Doors.* NFPA Journal.

Wolfstadt, J. (2008). The effect of computerized physician order entry with clinical decision support on the rates of adverse drug events: a systematic review. *Journal of General Internal Medicine, 23*(4), 451–458. doi:10.1007/s11606-008-0504-5

Wootton, R. (2001). Telemedicine. *British Medical Journal, 323*, 4.

Wunderlich, G. S., & Kohler, P. O. (2001). *Improving the quality of long-term care: 4. Information systems for monitoring Quality.* Washington, DC: National Academy Press.

Yu, P., Li, H., & Gagnon, M.-P. (2009). Health IT acceptance factors in long-term care facilities: A cross-sectional survey. *International Journal of Medical Informatics, 78*(4), 219–229. doi:10.1016/j.ijmedinf.2008.07.006

*A previous version of this chapter was originally published in International Journal of Healthcare Delivery Reform Initiatives, Vol. 1, Issue 4, edited by M. Guah, copyright 2010 by IGI Publishing (an imprint of IGI Global).*

# Chapter 4

# Localization and Monitoring of People with a Near-Field Imaging System:
## Boosting the Elderly Care

**Matti Linnavuo**
*Aalto University, Finland*

**Henry Rimminen**
*Aalto University, Finland*

## ABSTRACT

*The chapter describes the state of the art and potentialities of near-field imaging (NFI) technology, applications, and nursing tools in health care. First, principles of NFI are discussed. Various uses of NFI sensor data are presented. The data can be used for indoor tracking, automatic fall detection, activity monitoring, bed exit detection, passage control, vital functions monitoring, household automation and other applications. Special attention is given to the techniques and problems in localization, posture recognition, vital functions recording and additional functions for people identification. Examples of statistical analysis of person behavior are given. Three cases of realized applications of NFI technique are discussed.*

## INTRODUCTION

Both in developing and industrialized countries, the proportion of aged people is predicted to grow remarkably (Pollack 2005). This will create a major need for resources for the elderly care. Given the prospective age proportions, the human resources for manual care will be exhausted in a decade. We have to use the appropriate technologies, even if there are questions about their humanity.

To provide efficient services in pervasive applications in health care, a proactive approach is necessary. This means that the service is made available on the basis of context, not by manual command. New sensor and analysis technologies can be effectively utilized by matching infrastructure capabilities to health care needs. Emerging technologies include, e.g. (Varshney, 2006):

DOI: 10.4018/978-1-61520-765-7.ch004

- The use of location tracking, intelligent devices, user interfaces, body sensors, and short-range wireless communications for patient monitoring.
- The use of instant, flexible, and universal wireless access to increase the accessibility of health care providers.
- The use of unobstructed communication among medical devices, patients, health-care providers, and vehicles for effective emergency management.

The main requirements of a pervasive application in elderly care are effectiveness, unobtrusiveness, and reliability. Effectiveness means that the service provides both the elderly and the care personnel with some real added value, not only a new gadget or extra work. Unobtrusiveness means that the system should not interfere in any way with the elderly or the caregiver. Reliability means that there is a possibility of the use of the system really improving living or work habits.

Many pervasive applications, especially technologies to support ambient assisted living, rely on tracking people. The applications include e.g. activity monitoring, straying detection, and a simple detection of presence (Lin, Chiu, Hsiao, Lee & Tsai Y 2006). Falling is one of the greatest health risks and also a source of insecurity for the elderly. Pervasive tracking of movement and falls in a home environment could open the way to independent living for many ageing people, and thus improve their quality of life (Perry, Dowdall, Lines, & Hone 2004).

The tracking function can be realized in various ways, depending on the application, required area, and resolution. The environment also presents different limitations and benefits to the systems intended for application. For example, the widely used GPS location system can be used to locate objects to within an accuracy of 1 to 10 m. The system, however, does not function inside build-

ings and even if it did, its accuracy is not sufficient to track people in a room-scale environment (Bahl & Padmanabhan 2000).

A contemporary home monitoring system consists of various sensors which communicate with a local base station. The sensors can be infra red motion sensors, magnetic door sensors or pressure sensors in bed or on floor. If abnormal or a lack of activity is detected, the base station generates an alert to a family member, care facility or emergency unit, whichever is suitable for the case. The resident may also wear an emergency call device for immediate help when needed. The communication is internet or subscriber line based. Often there is also a teleconferencing possibility for telemedicine applications or simply for communicating with family or friends.

On the other hand, the system in an elderly care facility consists mainly of wandering or bed exit sensors, mostly pressure sensors. Also here the resident may wear a personal emergency call. The main difference from home environment is that the assisting person is always quite near.

In addition to the mainstream sensor techniques, an emerging technique of near field imaging (NFI) can be used to replace most separate sensors. To elicit the state of the art and potentialities of NFI technology, applications, requirements, boundaries and nursing tools related to the floor based sensors are discussed in this chapter. Some case examples are also presented of systems which have been realized and relate to human tracking and tracking analysis.

## BACKGROUND

### Tracking Methods in Elderly Care

Person tracking services in elderly care should meet some major requirements (Kleinberger, Becker, Ras, Holzinger &. Muller 2007):

- They have to be ambient and unobtrusive.
- They have to be ever ready to be taken into use.
- They have to provide their services in an accessible way.

The first requirement enables both the elderly and the care personnel to accept and use the system. An ideal system would be never seen or heard. The readiness means that there are a number of services, which can easily be taken into use promptly when the inhabitant's situation requires it.

There are two basic methods for tracking people, an active method, where the person is tagged with a transmitter or a transponder, and a passive method, which observes any person. Both basic methods can be realized with several technologies (Hightower & Borriello, 2001).

Active methods are technically more advantageous, because the object to be localized is not the person themselves, but some other object, a tag, which can be optimized for detection performance. The use of a tag, however, entails a problem in elderly care: how can one ensure that the tag is always with the person to be tracked? The tag should be designed to be small, invisible, and attached to a garment or the body in a way which effectively prevents the person from forgetting to wear it. The popular wristband with an alarm button is far from an optimum tag. The advantage of active methods is that in most cases they also enable a person to be identified, which makes the tracking system more versatile.

There are a lot of component and service providers in the field of person monitoring. For example, Accutech-ICS (Wisconsin, USA), HomeTronex, LLC (Baltimore and Columbia, USA), RF Technologies® (Wisconsin, USA) and STT Condigi (Sweden, Norway, Finland and Denmark) provide components and systems for person monitoring and localization by active (tag) method.

Passive methods rely on measuring some human property. It might be movement, weight, body temperature, electrical conductivity, or a detail of the body's geometry. Measuring any of these is, in general, a more demanding task than the measurements performed by active methods. In elderly care, passive methods are advantageous because of their tagless realization. Passive method measurements very seldom allow person identification. If identification is required, other systems are used in addition to the tracking system.

Both passive and active methods must utilize some technique for actually performing the measurements for calculating the coordinates for the object being tracked. Remote measurements are performed at a distance from the object. This technique often allows a wide tracking area with relatively modest equipment but at the cost of accuracy.

A typical active localization system is built using readily available RFID tag to be carried by the person and a number of stationary position transmitter units by which the different locations are determined (STT Condigi, Finland).

The position transmitter uses short range (80 … 240 cm) 17 kHz electromagnetic field with unique position code. The tag listens to the position codes and sends them to a base station using UHF transmitter in 432-470 MHz band. The system monitoring program then utilizes monitoring rules to generate alerts.

## Practical Realizations of Floor-Based Systems

Although the active methods are widely available, the need for a tag and their limited resolution restrict their use in the elderly care. Floor-based methods offer the required resolution but require cheap sensors, which should also be suitable for installation on arbitrary floors. In the following sections, some near-field floor sensors are introduced, which rely on force, static charge, and electric field measurement.

The oldest and most referenced floor sensor system, called the Active Floor (Addlesee, Jones,

Livesey & Samaria 1997), allows the time-varying spatial weight distribution of an active office environment to be captured. In the Active Floor, a matrix of carpet tiles backed with plywood and steel plate is supported at its corners by load cells. The load cells are able to recognize weight changes of about 50 g.

The measuring technique in the Active Floor is accurate and the resulting measurement signals are clear and easy to convert to coordinates. Some tests have been done to classify persons by their walking characteristics using a hidden Markov model technique. The construction, however, is quite expensive in room-scale realizations because of the special floor structure and very expensive load cell technique.

Another force sensing technique, 'ForSe FIElds' (McElligott, Dillon, Leydon, Richardson, Fernström & Paradiso. 2002), relies on a special force-sensing material that can be screen-printed onto circuit boards. A mixture of silicon rubber and carbon granules change its electrical resistance with applied force.

The 'ForSe FIElds' system shows scalability by consisting of inexpensive modules and of a modular sensor arrangement with local computational power that can be used for building larger floor spaces.

Force measuring systems tend to be complicated and their scalability is limited. For those location sensing methods where the sensor must reside in the whole area under surveillance, a technique which allows the use of simple, affordable sensor units is required.

The POISE system (Eyole-Monono, Harle & Hopper, 2006) tries to sense local electrostatic changes on a special floor sensor, allowing the user to be completely unencumbered and sensed only indirectly. The floor is augmented with conductive wires which measure the electrostatic charges produced in insulating material surrounding them.

A standard PVC-sheathed wire has both the wire and the insulator needed. When a person steps on or off the sensor, the triboelectric effect builds a charge in the sheath. The charge is measured through the wire. The wires can be laid unobtrusively beneath a carpet.

The electrostatic sensor is intrinsically scalable and economical, but as a result of its dynamic nature, it does not see an object that is standing still. This property limits its applicability to the elderly care.

Electric NFI systems rely on the fact that the human body has relatively small impedance and thus it is suitable for being sensed by an electrical field (Zimmerman, 1995). This sensing method was used for interfacing with a computer and for navigation in an indoor environment in its first application by Zimmerman.

Capacitive touch sensing is a common way to implement user interfaces in consumer devices. For example, capacitance sensing chips from Analog Devices, Inc. rely on the shunt measurement method. This means that there are a transmitting electrode and a receiving electrode on the surface of the device. The receiving element senses a constant electric field until the finger of the user "steals" a part of it and conducts it to ground (Marsh, 2006). This change is detected as a touch or proximity. The measurement range of touch sensors is usually from zero to tens of picofarads.

There are a couple of commercially available floor based person detection systems using NFI. FutureShape GmbH (Germany) provides Sens-Floor® smart floor system which is implemented using textile laminate sensors. MariMils Oy (Finland) provides Elsi™ underfloor monitoring system with laminated foil sensors. The sensors of both systems allow application of virtually any flooring material.

The ELSI system uses a technique called near-field imaging (NFI) for human tracking. The basic idea is very close to touch sensing, but the

*Figure 1. The operating principle of the NFI floor sensor*

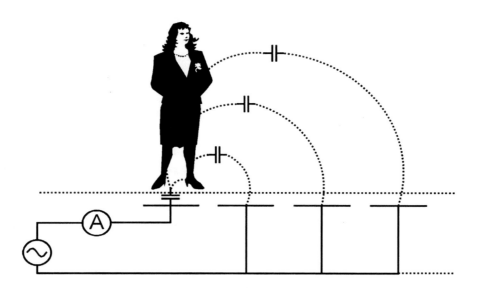

measurement range is different; Elsi is designed to detect the proximity of the whole body of a person. In addition to this, it is designed to withstand much larger bulk capacitances in the sensors. The sensor size is also very different compared to touch sensors; a single element in the sensor array is suitable for detecting the location of one foot of a person, instead of a finger. The size of the whole array is on the scale of a room instead of the scale of a hand-held device.

The ELSI floor sensor system senses the presence of a human body by emitting electric fields and measuring the impedance between conductive elements under the floor covering. The principle of the system is illustrated in Figure 1. This method is not based on weight sensing, but on impedance measurement.

The sensors in the ELSI system are grouped into 0.5-m-wide strips of consecutive sensor elements. At the end of each sensor strip there is a measuring unit, which is fitted to the baseboard. The strips are covered with common floor surfaces, such as plastic membrane or carpet. A schematic illustration of the sensor is in the Figure 2.

The mean positioning accuracy of ELSI is 0.2 m (Rimminen, 2009). This accuracy is approximately nine times better than that of the indoor radio frequency tracking systems found in the literature. These RF systems produce accuracies of approximately 1.8 m (Cho, 2007; Hii, 2005; Hihnel 2004). The accuracy of ELSI is more than enough to determine if a person is standing inside or outside of a door, and enough to separate multiple people from each other in a crowded room. Two people can be separated from each other with a 90% certainty if the gap between them is 0.8 m or more (Rimminen, 2009).

## NFI SYSTEM APPLICATIONS

### Services Utilizing NFI Data

The data obtained from the NFI measurements comprise the signal strengths found in each scanned sensor location. To accomplish useful services, these basic data must be processed to reveal the desired information. In the following,

*Figure 2. The sensor of the ELSI system*

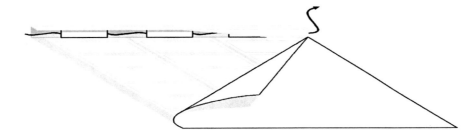

some present and future uses of NFI data are discussed.

## Localization

Localization is a very basic task for NFI. To find out a person's location, one must find out the sensors that are occupied. This is accomplished by comparing the signal to a known empty reference value. Usually at least two sensor cells are occupied by a human target, one cell for each foot. Occasionally there will be even more occupied sensors. When monitoring standing persons, the mean of the occupied sensor coordinates weighted by the observation strengths (i.e. the centroid) is a good approximation of the location.

To localize a walking person is a more complex task. Usually the advancing foot moves high enough to leave the supporting (trailing) foot to contribute to the observations alone. Thus the calculated centroid even shifts backwards a little until it takes a leap forwards when the advancing foot approaches the floor again. The resulting wobbly track easily produces errors in further statistical analysis, not to speak of the odd appearance it produces on the monitoring screen.

Another non-trivial task in human tracking is to distinguish people when there are a number of targets each producing multiple or no observations. One has to decide which of the occupied sensors belong to a particular person. This process is called clustering. The cluster is the group of sensor cells which are estimated to be occupied by the same

*Figure 3. A snapshot of the history playback from room data in the Kustaankartano center for the elderly, Helsinki, Finland. A cluster and one sensor data point are marked*

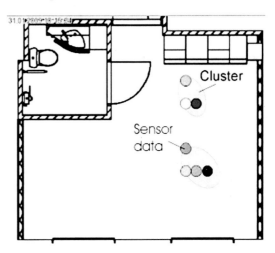

target. By clustering and evaluating the centroid, the person's location can be expressed even more precisely than the size and pitch of the sensors would suggest.

In Figure 3, a typical result of person localization using centroid calculation and clustering can be seen. The signals exceeding the reference values are seen as dots. A darker shade of the dot means a stronger signal.

Using the calculated coordinates of the person, useful services can be provided. In elderly care, information on certain events such as departure from or arrival in a room, visits to the toilet, and getting out of bed can be discerned by the NFI

*Figure 4. A snapshot of the alarm overview of three rooms in the Kustaankartano center for the elderly, Helsinki, Finland*

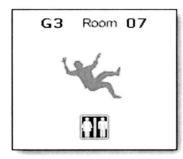 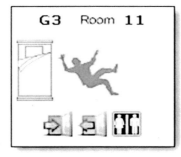 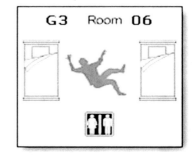

system and the necessary alerts can be forwarded. For example, in Figure 4 there is an overview of three rooms. All the rooms provide an alarm if a person falls or in the event of a visit to the toilet. Room 11 has additional monitoring of arrivals and exits. Rooms 11 and 06 give an alarm when a person leaves their bed. In practice the falling alarm is always active in all premises, while every other alarm setting varies according to the resident's condition.

The localization signal could also be used for other services than monitoring of the elderly. There could be interactive, coordination-intensive games which would be controlled by moving oneself on a room scale. The NFI sensors could be extended to the walls to provide a greater control surface. In the medical field, the room being monitored could be used for the coordination training of stroke patients, brain surgery convalescents, and other neural dysfunction cases. The rehabilitation "games" would be less laborious and of wider effect than normal rehabilitation. There is strong evidence that immediate rehabilitation restores the abilities to a higher level than later intervention.

In Figure 5 there is a schematic presentation of an experimental space where the above-mentioned functions are studied. The space features: floor NFI sensors for location measurements; wall NFI sensors for control and feedback with hand gestures; a highly directive speaker system to produce a sound atmosphere; halogen spots to produce light beams; a video projector to show instructions, and feedback and virtual controllers on the wall. The virtual controls could be a slide fader operated by hand on the NFI sensor.

One application of the localization data could be the use of localization data in planning rescues during fires and other accidents where general confusion easily leads to some people being overlooked. The function could be arranged in such a way that the rescue crew would use the localization information to assess and localize the persons in the danger zone. This would ease the rescue work and lessen the risks in dangerous circumstances.

## Posture

Prompt reaction to fall accidents is the most valued service among professionals in the sphere of elderly care. The NFI data are used to distinguish postures from each other, such as fallen, standing, or crawling. In this section, techniques and problems in posture determination are discussed.

The NFI floor sensor provides impedance values as a function of two dimensional locations. The size of one "pixel" depends on the installation generation, but varies between 0.5 x 0.3 m and 0.5 x 0.25 m. The impedance values of these pixels are approximately 20 ohms when a person is standing with shoes on and approximately 60

*Figure 5. A schematic representation of the proactive space in the University of Art and Design, Helsinki, Finland*

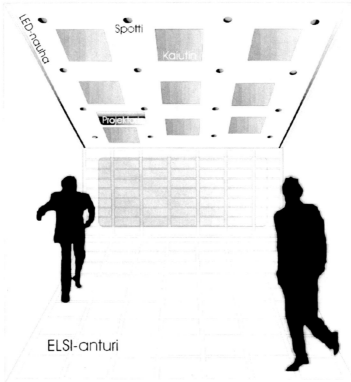

ohms when a person is lying on the floor. Typical observation data can be seen in Figure 6.

The quality of the observation data provides good preconditions for recognizing the characteristics of different postures. The required variety of detected postures determines the sensitivity and specificity of posture recognition.

The most common and the simplest case is where we need to recognize the difference between a standing and a fallen person. The definition of 'fallen' is depicted in Figure 7. The sensitivity and specificity in this case are both 99% when the NFI floor sensor is used.

In the elderly care it is often necessary to distinguish a standing person from a non-standing person. In the non-standing postures we include the following postures: lying supine, lying supine in the form of an X, lying on one's side, lying in a fetal position, crawling, kneeling, and sitting. The 'non-standing' definition is depicted in Figure 7. Preliminary results indicate that for the NFI system the sensitivity is 88% and the specificity 96%.

The results mentioned above were obtained by automatically measuring the longest diagonal length of the observation pattern, such as that shown in Figure 6. The observation pattern includes the cluster of observations that are associated together by a clustering algorithm. The optimum threshold for the diagonal length to indicate a non-standing posture was found to be 0.6 m. The sum of all observations as a detection parameter has also been tried, but with less success.

The results obtained with the NFI method are competitive with other fall detection methods found in the literature. The sensitivities of state-of-the-art methods vary from 77%-100% (Noury, 2007).

*Figure 6. Typical NFI observation data of a supine person*

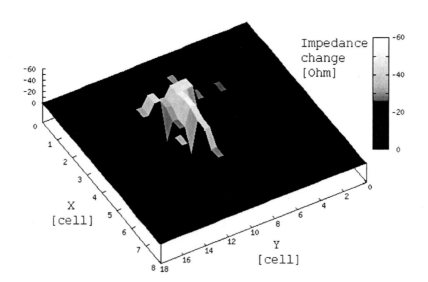

## Identification

One basic property in the NFI system is that it does not distinguish between persons. In some aspects, e.g. privacy, this is an advance, but when providing full functionality to various tracking services, person identification is a must.

The NFI signal alone gives no help to identification. Thus additional techniques must be applied. There are two major techniques available:

- video recognition, where individual characteristics are recognized from a video picture, and
- an identification tag, which communicates with the system and provides identification.

Both systems have their pros and cons. Video recognition techniques require virtually nothing of the recognized object, but the applications are point-based, while in elderly care the recognition should be continuously possible in the entire space. Tag techniques are more versatile, but in elderly care, there is a great obstacle: the

person must carry a tag. A wristband transmitter is feasible if the bearer remembers its purpose and does not try to dispose of it. To gain more reliable identification, one could fit out all other persons than the elderly with identification tags. This has been the solution in the reference sites discussed in this chapter.

There are two major motivations for identifying the caregivers in elderly care. First of all, we need a way to acknowledge alarms that have accumulated in a certain room without adding to the workload by requiring the nurses to press buttons. Buttons can also be mistakenly pressed by the residents themselves, causing the alarms to vanish. RFID tags are therefore an easy, automatic, and safe form of alarm acknowledgement.

The second motivation is related to data logging and to the statistical analysis of the movement of the residents; nurses must not affect the movement statistics of a certain resident. The RFID tags solve this problem too by separating members of staff from the residents.

As previously stated, additional functionalities should be added to the basic NFI system to allow identification. Here the optimum system uses

*Figure 7. The definitions of fallen and non-standing postures*

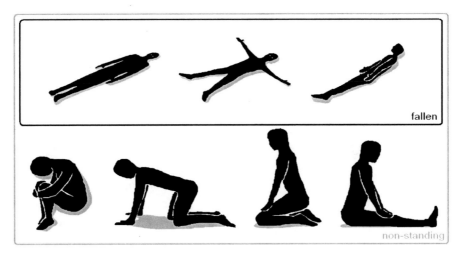

mostly the existing functionalities of the NFI system. We present here two techniques which use the NFI system to different extents.

**NFI Tag**

Because of the short range of the NFI system, a tag which uses NFI technology has to reside practically on the floor. Tags embedded in the soles of the shoes of the care personnel can be used to add a personal code to the NFI signal. The NFI system can then detect the code. The benefit of this technique is that it does not require any further infrastructure beyond the existing NFI floor sensor. The downside is the low read range characteristic of a coactively coupled tag, which limits the placement of the tag; in practice the shoes are the only option. In addition, the functionality of the NFI tag is constrained to one-way communication sending the tag code to the NFI system. In spite of these limitations, the shoe technology is the one most commonly utilized in NFI systems.

**RFID Tag**

If some other infrastructure than NFI is allowed, more functionalities can be added. There are a variety of techniques available, but most of them do not allow the localization accuracy needed in elderly care.

One parallel identification/localization technique has been embedded into the ELSI system (Ropponen, 2009). Its positioning accuracy at best is half the accuracy of NFI. Because of its low frequency, the system is referred as LFID rather than RFID. It utilizes inductive antennas that go around the planar NFI elements forming an array of loops. These loop antennas transmit digital location information with a 125 kHz carrier signal, which is picked up by a mobile device (an active tag) carried by the person, who needs to be identified. The active tag interprets the digital location information from the floor and sends it forward with a ZigBee microwave link. This enables the person not only to be identified but also enables him/her to feed and receive context related information. This technique has a higher read distance than the NFI shoe tag, so the mobile device can be placed more freely.

Typical solution would be to perform only the identification and interfacing by the LFID and utilize the better accuracy of NFI system in the localization.

## Vital Functions Monitoring

The capability of finding out the respiration curve and pulse rate is important when the rescue of a fallen person living independently is being planned. Monitoring of the wellbeing of persons put into segregation is another application. In everyday monitoring the vital functions cannot be measured because the person is in motion.

The vital signs can be recorded when a person stays still on the NFI sensor floor. Weak respiration and pulse signals ride on the basic NFI tracking signal. The strongest vital sign components are found when a person is lying prone. The vital signs are extracted from the tracking signal by amplifying it further by 30 decibels and filtering it. Two types of vital signs can be obtained from this signal: cardiac activity and respiratory activity (Rimminen, 2009). Both of these signal components bear considerable similarities to the same components found in galvanic bioimpedance recording methods. Fine body movements are also clearly visible in the NFI signal.

The vital sign measurement point can be selected freely within the sensor area. This enables the vital sign detection feature to be utilized together with automatic fall detection. When a fall has been detected, the vital data monitoring reveals first whether the person is moving at all. In most cases it is also possible to tell if the person is breathing or if the person has a heartbeat. This information, which is obtained remotely, is crucial in deciding the type of help needed. Elderly people living independently would most probably benefit from this technique. Cell deaths are a problem when people are segregated to avoid criminal or aggressive behavior. The responsible officials are under great pressure to perform checks at short enough intervals. The NFI sensor system can also record vital signs continuously. This kind of monitoring technique is most useful in holding cells for the intoxicated.

## Statistical Analysis of Person Behavior

During its operation, the NFI system constantly logs location data. The logged data are available for various statistical calculations. Below,

some statistical methods applied to the data are presented. The simplest statistical indicator is the distribution of daily locations. Changes in long-term walking speed distributions may also indicate the deterioration of motor functions.

### Data Logging

The logged NFI location data show every activated sensor element at any given time. These data require clustering algorithms for determining the locations of people and separating multiple people from each other. The clustered data are differentiated to get the speed at any given moment and the overall distance walked. The data can also be spatially integrated to get information on the activity distribution in the room.

The speed and distance logging require some special attention concerning the physics of human movement: people tend to shift their weight from one foot to another and otherwise make small movements while standing still. The NFI floor also records this as a propagating movement, which falsely contributes to the momentary speed distribution and distance walked. This is corrected by means of a certain lower threshold to eliminate this "zero-propagating" movement.

### Distribution of Daily Locations

A cumulative activity map is generated by gathering location data over a desired period of time. One map obtained from a home for the elderly can be seen in Figure 8. This map was recorded over a period of twenty days in a two-person room in a ward for the demented. Changes in the distribution of daily locations can reveal changes in overall activity.

### Speed and Length of Daily Walked Path

Differentiated location data reveal momentary walking speeds. The momentary speed distribution gathered can be compared to an earlier data set to detect changes. These changes are thought to be the most promising indicator for deteriorating motor functions. The principle is illustrated in Figure 9.

*Figure 8. Distribution of locations over a twenty-day period. The 20-day data were recorded in a ward for the demented*

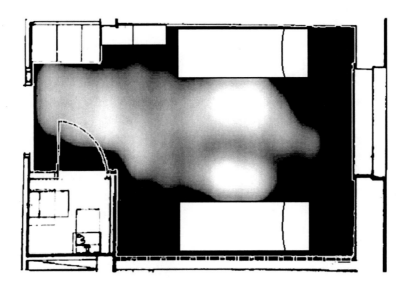

This example shows a diminution in the walking speeds, and some conclusions can be drawn concerning the physical state of the person.

Calculating the overall distance walked over a period of time can also be a very useful indicator in elderly care.

**Behavioral Patterns**

The logged location data can be used to observe walking paths which are typical for a certain starting point in the sensor area. For example, it can be estimated where a person usually aims when he/she gets out of bed in the middle of the night. The estimation is obtained by taking all the walking paths starting from the bedside and forming a spatial distribution of these paths.

The aiming estimation can be used in a similar way to the aforementioned parameters, but also as a building service aid when controlling the lighting or passage automatically.

*Figure 9. Changes in the walking speed distribution can reveal the weakening of motor functions*

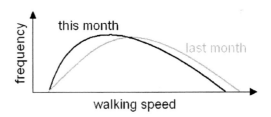

## Practical Software and Hardware Implementation

**Basic Requirements**

The most basic task is the monitoring of the resident's locations. This real-time function is the easiest to realize and most demonstrative to follow, but is of little value in nursing because it requires the attention of a person who probably has a number of other residents to take care of.

Various alarms are the main output of the system. The possibility of relying on alarms has been recognized as the most important factor in making nursing more effective. The residents need different alarm configurations; some of them should never leave their beds unattended and some should be free to move as they wish.

For various advanced services the recording of all tracking is essential. The records provide the possibility of rendering a playback of the events in a room at any selected speed. The playback of the tracking is a useful function. Occasionally a resident is found fallen or injured. To assess the quality of the nursing, the reasons and the events should be sorted out. The playback reveals the exact time and position of the incident, the events leading to it, and also the time when corrective actions were commenced.

## Alarm Configurations

Alarm configuration is performed by care personnel on the basis of the condition of the resident. The person's ability to move and their cognitive state and habits have to be taken into account. The area of the premises is divided into different alarm zones; in Figure 3, typical zones in a room are illustrated. The typical alarms are

- Room exit (leaving the room door zone outwards)
- Room entrance (entering the door zone from outside)
- Toilet entrance (entering the toilet zone)
- Bed entrance (entering the bed zone from the bed)
- Fall

The alarm configurations are made for a certain person. The NFI system, however, does not inherently recognize the person. This creates a problem when there are several persons with different alarm settings.

## Methods of Alarm Forwarding

A number of facilities for the care of the elderly have some kind of emergency call or nurse call system. A basic functionality can be achieved simply by connecting the alarm to it as a closing contact. This approach, however, does not utilize the full capabilities of NFI, although it provides immediate integration with the existing systems of the facility.

Another simple interface which utilizes the existing infrastructure is cellular phone text messaging. The system is equipped with a cellular phone modem which delivers messages to the phones used by care personnel. If multiple phones are used, quite sophisticated alarm forwarding schemes can be applied which relate to time and to persons. Text messaging is a standard 160-character message system which does not allow any alterations to the form or appearance of the message. Its original intended use is person-to-person messaging and both the appearance and handling of messages (retrieving, storing, deleting) are far from optimal.

A better approach is a Java application in a cellular phone which communicates directly with the NFI system. The layout and functions of the interface can be tailored to virtually any need.

However, pilot tests have shown that the cellular phone is not optimal in health care, especially in elderly care. To use the phone takes much attention and the form of a cellular phone is not optimal in nursing work with the elderly. The phone is said to be clumsy.

To optimize the functioning and fulfill most of the requirements, there should be a dedicated multi-function device which could assist the nurse in receiving and acknowledging alarms, automatically retrieving information on the residents and their locations, facilitating passage control, and contributing to other nursing tasks.

This kind of dedicated multi-function device is connected by WLAN to the NFI system. The system follows the location of the user and represents context-sensitive information.

### Methods of Alarm Response

For the evaluation of nursing work, alarms and responses to alarms are important parameters. The nurse should be able to receive and analyze the alarm in as undisrupted a way as possible. The acknowledgement of the alarm should also be smooth and not interfere with the task of rectifying the cause of the alarm.

The most obvious alarm acknowledgement would be to go to the main console of the system, but this is not a viable method. It would be more convenient to use the room buttons of the nurse call system or special room buttons to communicate with the NFI system. However, the resident could also use them and provide false inputs to the system. In addition, a button to be operated in connection with an alarm incident forms an extra memorizing task which stresses the nurse. Moreover, dedicated room buttons are often difficult to provide for economic and technical reasons.

There are, however, solutions to the alarm response problem. First, the NFI locating system can very easily be adapted to read a special NFI tag which sends its code to the floor sensors. Because of the short range of the NFI reading, the tags are incorporated in shoes.

Tagged shoes give the nurse total freedom and facilitate automatic call acknowledgement. The alarm configuration can also be altered upon the identification of a nurse being present. Thus operations in the room (e.g. cleaning and grooming) do not give false alarms.

## Construction Techniques Involved

There are certain requirements for the scheduling of construction work, the durability of sensor components during assembly work, the reliability of electronics, and other matters when planning to realize the NFI measurement system in an apartment.

The planning must first take into account whether the target is a new construction, a renovation, or an add-on object. In a new construction the planner has more influence on the infrastructure that is necessary to support the system. An add-on realization has to use the environment as it is, leading to compromises regarding e.g. the placement of the wiring and components.

The floor area intended for monitoring must be covered with sensors. At the floor edges, there has to be enough unbroken (no doors) wall for continuous baseboards. The sensor foil is less than 1 mm thick so no provisions for floor thickening is needed. The structure and materials of the floor should be checked. The electric field is susceptible to conducting materials such as near by metallic concrete reinforcement. Fortunately a few cm distance is enouch to eliminate the effect.

The arrangements for interfacing the planned system to other services like institution network, nurse call system or patient database prove to be time consuming because of several parties involved. The interfacing planning should be kicked off with no delay.

The assembly of the sensors and the fitting of electronics should be synchronized with the overall contract schedule. One important milestone is the drying of the concrete floors, which enables the sensor assembling. The protection of the already assembled components is an important issue. Although the sensor withstands normal wear extremely well, the construction work includes phases (e.g. wall grouting and painting) which threaten the integrity of the system.

Several factors affect the assessment of the location-sensing system costs in elderly care (Hightower & Borriello, 2001). Time costs include the planning, installation, training and administration. Space costs include the amount of installed infrastructure and the space occupied by hardware. Capital costs include factors such as the price per mobile unit or infrastructure element and the salaries of support personnel.

## CASE STUDIES

### Home for the Elderly

In this case study, an application of the NFI system to a large home for the elderly is presented. The project involves a whole three-story house comprising premises for up to 66 rooms.

The Kustaankartano Center for the Elderly offers retirement home, day activity, and service center services to aged Helsinki residents. Kustaankartano is Finland's second largest retirement home and it takes care of around 600 people. The center is very active in exploring new technical applications in care work which aim to improve safety, promote independent activity, and enhance quality of life. The elderly tracking project at Kustaankartano aimed to give the care personnel a new tool and a way to alter their care work to make it more productive and less stressful. Most of the benefits were expected to be found during the night shift.

The installation of the NFI system was planned to be performed in two stages. The first stage was a two-room pilot installation in building 'A' to map the benefits to the system and to develop the user interface in a small controlled environment. The major installation of building 'G' with 66 rooms was to be installed under a condition that the experiences from building 'A' were positive. The pilot installation in building 'A' was performed by gluing the NFI sensor strips on existing linoleum flooring. This was done to minimize the cost and the time of installation.

The major installation of 66 rooms in building 'G' was scheduled to be simultaneous with a full renovation. This meant that the NFI sensor strips were glued on to bare concrete floors and the data/power cabling were custom made to suit the NFI system. The electronics were installed by automation mechanics and the sensor strips were glued by carpeting professionals. Both of these groups were given special one-day training. The user interface and the operation of the whole system were tuned using the experiences obtained from the pilot in building 'A'. The use of the NFI system in building 'G' was scheduled to start gradually, one floor at a time. At the time of writing two whole floors use the NFI system full time and the last floor is ready for commissioning.

The functionality of the NFI system in building 'G' includes several alarm types, which are configurable for each room, and can be scheduled by a timer. These alarms can result from falling, room exit and bed exit. The alarms are transferred to the cellular phones of the staff (nurses). There are 2-3 cellular phones on a ward, which run a dedicated application for receiving the alarms over a GPRS link.

The nurses have received special training sessions for the use of the NFI system and participate very closely in the further development of the user interface. There have been some problems caused by false NFI observations, failed power supplies and weak sensitivity in few of the rooms. However, the overall user feedback of the NFI system is remarkably good. The system is in everyday use, and has proven its usefulness in institutional elderly care.

The authors have conducted a questionnaire study among the users. The unpublished results reveal that the the system has caused some change in the working methods, especially at nights. The night nurse is feels to have better picture of what happens in the resident´s rooms. The use and functioning were also considered to be easy to understand and no risks to the residents or care was found. Even the traditional phrase "Technology can't replace compassion in health care" (Robinson 2003) turned to be "Technology gives more time to compassion in health care". The time which the nurses had with the residents was considered more relaxing and useful because unnecessary checkings and worrying could be minimized.

## Independent Living

An application of the NFI system in a service house with apartments for assisted independent living is presented in this case study. The project involves 5 apartments equipped with an NFI system. The Harjulan Setlementti non-profit association provides various public services for the local inhabitants in the Päijät-Häme district, Finland. The goal is to support the people – elderly and also others – in having a good life. The association uses a wide palette of means to achieve this goal. One of the activities is to keep up and lease out apartments supporting ambient assisted living. It was decided that a group of apartments to be renovated at Harjulan Settlementti's facilities at Lahti, Finland would be equipped with the NFI system.

The installation of the NFI system followed the renovation schedule of the apartments. The installation was performed sequentially during a period of two years in connection with the general renovation program of the apartments. The planning of the construction schedule was relatively easy because of the modest scale of the project. The sensors were glued on to the old linoleum flooring. Laminate was chosen as the surface material. Most of the electronics and wiring were fitted into a hollow baseboard as usual, so that the system is fully invisible. The toilet was also equipped with sensors. The alarms are forwarded by text messages.

After the renovation and installation of the NFI system the assisted living apartments were put into use. In contrast to institutions for the elderly, the assisted living apartments are inhabited by people with no severe medical issue which would necessitate the services of a professional 24/7 emergency center. Thus the alarms are received by relatives, who decide independently how to respond to the situation.

For this site, there has as yet been no follow-up survey to scientifically assess the functionality and impacts of the NFI system. The characteristics of this installation predict that the alarm rate will be considerably lower than in institutions for the elderly.

One resident commented his experiences about the ELSI system in a newspaper interview (Palokari, 2007). He is generally very happy with the system and the most important thing is the feeling of safety. After a stroke he has become very careful. His adult son receives the alarms to his cell phone and he is also very pleased with the system. In addition to the fall alarms, the system has been set to make an alarm when a long period of inactivity occurs. This has caused some false alarms, when the resident has forgotten to inform his son about a trip away from home. The local project coordinator comments that the system helps the nurses to organize their days better when constant care is not needed. Though, the system will never replace personal contact, he says.

## Vital Signs Monitoring

The police and also some hospitals have holding cells for the intoxicated to avoid criminal or aggressive behavior. In this case study, an application of the NFI system to holding cell for the intoxicated is presented. The project involves one segregation room in one health center in Finland. To avoid cell deaths the NFI sensor system can monitor vital signs continuously when an intoxicated person is placed in segregation. This does not remove the need for frequent check-ups, but only increases the safety of the person. The NFI system is suitable only for an application, where there is no bed in the room. The installation location was chosen because of the lack of bed. The segregation room in this hospital has a covered foam plastic mattress on the floor, which can be moved freely.

The NFI sensor strips were glued on to existing plastic membrane flooring and were covered with another. The electronics were fitted in to a steel housing on the wall to avoid vandalism. A simple indicator of the state of the person was installed in the office of the ward. This indicator has a red and a green light to indicate the following two states: 'no vital signs or movement detected' and 'vital signs or movement is detected'.

At the time of writing the use of the segregation room has not yet been started. There have been some problems with sensing vital signs through the mattress. The mattress will be modified so that the electric field penetrates the foamed plastic. This is done by embedding conductive strips through the mattress to virtually lift the surface of the NFI sensors on top of the mattress. This method allows the mattress to be moved freely inside the room.

## FUTURE RESEARCH DIRECTIONS

As has been seen, there are various methods to gain information on the location of a person. The growing need for location-based services in elderly care will accelerate the development of really scalable (wide area) and affordable systems. An effective care concept requires the integration of several systems, e.g. indoor and outdoor tracking systems, a nurse call system, resident and care personnel databases, and so forth. Thus in the future only those systems which offer integration capabilities such as open code interfaces or internet connectability will survive.

Pervasive integrated systems produce large amounts of data. In the future, new services can be obtained by statistical analysis and data-mining techniques. These new services rely on existing data and no additional infrastructure or measuring systems need to be introduced.

## CONCLUSION

In this chapter, a special emphasis has been on near-field imaging (NFI) technology, which is a special method of gathering both localization and vital functions data of a person. The principle of NFI is simple, but the NFI sensor data can be exploited in various applications such as indoor tracking, automatic fall detection, activity monitoring, bed exit detection, passage control, vital functions monitoring, household automation and other applications

## REFERENCES

Addlesee, M., Jones, A., Livesey, F., & Samaria, F. (1997). The ORL active floor [sensor system]. *IEEE Personal Communications, 4*(5), 35–41. doi:10.1109/98.626980

Alwan, M., Mack, D., Dalal, S., Kell, S., Turner, B., & Felder, R. (2006). Impact of Passive In-Home Health Status Monitoring Technology in Home Health: Outcome Pilot. In 1st Transdisciplinary Conference on Distributed Diagnosis and Home Healthcare (D$_2$H$_2$), 2-4 April 2006 (pp.79-82). Arlington, Virginia.

Bahl, P., & Padmanabhan, V. (2000). RADAR: an in-building RF-based user location and tracking system. In *INFOCOM 2000. Nineteenth Annual Joint Conference of the IEEE Computer and Communications Societies, 26-30 March 2001* (pp. 775-784).Tel Aviv, Israel: IEEE Computer Society.

Celler, B., Earnshaw, W., Ilsar, E., Betbeder-Matibet, L., Harris, M., & Clark, R. (1995). Remote monitoring of health status of the elderly at home. A multidisciplinary project on aging at the University of New South Wales. *International Journal of Bio-Medical Computing, 40*(2), 147–155. doi:10.1016/0020-7101(95)01139-6

Cho, H., Kang, M., Park, J., Park, B., & Kim, H. (2007). Performance analysis of location estimation algorithm in ZigBee networks using received signal strength. In *21st International Conference on Advanced Information Networking and Applications Workshops (AINAW'07), 21-23 May 2007* (pp. 302-306). Niagara Falls, Canada: IEEE Computer Society.

Eyole-Monono, M., Harle, R., & Hopper, A. (2006). POISE: An inexpensive, low-power location sensor based on electrostatics. In *3rd Annual International Conference On Mobile and Ubiquitous Systems: Networks And Services (MobiQuitous 2006), 17 – 21 July 2006* (pp.1-3). San Jose, California: ICST.

Hightower, J., & Borriello, G. (2001). A survey and taxonomy of location systems for ubiquitous computing. *IEEE Computer, 34*(8), 57–66.

Hihnel, D., Burgard, W., Fox, D., Fishkin, K., & Philipose, M. (2004). Mapping and localization with RFID technology. In *IEEE International Conference on Robotics & Automation (ICRA '04), 26 April-1 May 2004*, (pp. 1015-1020). New Orleans, LA: IEEE Robotics and Automation Society.

Hii, P., & Zaslavsky, A. (2005). Improving location accuracy by combining WLAN positioning and sensor technology. In *Workshop on Real-World Wireless Sensor Networks (REALWSN'05)*, 20-21 June 2005. Stockholm, Sweden: Swedish Institute of Computer Science.

Kleinberger, T., Becker, M., Ras, E., Holzinger, A., & Muller, P. (2007). Ambient Intelligence in assisted living: Enable elderly people to handle future interfaces. *Lecture Notes in Computer Science, 4555*, 103–112. doi:10.1007/978-3-540-73281-5_11

Lin, C. C., Chiu, M. J., Hsiao, C. C., Lee, R. G., & Tsai, Y. S. (2006). Wireless health care service system for elderly with dementia. *IEEE Transactions on Information Technology in Biomedicine, 10*(4), 696–704. doi:10.1109/TITB.2006.874196

Marsh, D. (2006). Capacitive touch sensors fulfill early promise. *EDN Europe*. Retrieved April 27, 2009, from http://www.edn.com/contents/images/6339808.pdf

McElligott, L., Dillon, M., Leydon, K., Richardson, B., Fernström, M., & Paradiso, J. (2002). 'ForSe FIElds' - Force sensors for interactive environments. *Lecture Notes in Computer Science, 2498*, 321–328.

Noury, N., Fleury, A., Rumeau, P., Bourke, A. K., Laighin, G. Ó., Rialle, V., et al. (2007). Fall detection –principles and methods. In *Proceedings of the 29th Annual International Conference of the IEEE EMBS*, 23-26 August 2007 (pp. 1663-1666). Lyon, France: IEEE-EMBS.

Palokari, S. (2007, November 5). *Turvana hälyttävä matto*. Helsingin Sanomat, p. D4. (In Finnish)

Perry, M., Dowdall, A., Lines, L., & Hone, K. (2004). Multimodal and ubiquitous computing systems: supporting independent-living older users. *IEEE Transactions on Information Technology in Biomedicine, 8*(3), 258–270. doi:10.1109/TITB.2004.835533

Pollack, M. (2005). Intelligent technology for an aging population: The Use of AI to Assist Elders with Cognitive Impairment. *AI Magazine, 26*(2), 9–24.

Rimminen, H., Lindström, J., & Sepponen, R. (2009). Positioning accuracy and multi-target separation with a human tracking system using near field imaging. *International Journal on Smart Sensing and Intelligent Systems, 2*. Retrieved April 27, 2009, from http://www.s2is.org/Issues/v2/n1/papers/paper9.pdf

Rimminen, H., Linnavuo, M., & Sepponen, R. (2008). Human tracking using near field imaging. In *Second International Conference on Pervasive Computing Technologies for Healthcare (PervasiveHealth 2008), 30 January -1 February 2008* (pp.148-151).Tampere, Finland: ICST.

Rimminen, H., & Sepponen, R. (2009). Biosignals with a floor sensor. In *Second International Conference on Biomedical Electronics and Devices (BIODEVICES 2009), 14-17 January 2009* (pp. 125-130). Porto, Portugal: INSTICC.

Robinson, K. (2003). Technology can't replace compassion in health care. *Critical Care Choices, 34*(1), 1.

Ropponen, A., Linnavuo, M., & Sepponen, R. (2009). LF indoor location and identification system. *International Journal on Smart Sensing and Intelligent Systems,* 2. Retrieved April 27, 2009, from http://www.s2is.org/Issues/v2/n1/papers/paper6.pdf

Varshney, U. (2006). Using wireless technologies in healthcare. *International Journal of Mobile Communications, 4*(3), 354–368.

Zimmerman, T., Smith, J., Paradiso, J., Allport, D., & Gershenfeld, N. (1995). Applying electric field sensing to human computer interfaces. In SIGCHI conference on Human factors in computing systems, May 7-11 1995 (pp. 280–287). Denver, CO: ACM Press.

## KEY TERMS AND DEFINITIONS

**Accuracy:** The degree of closeness of a measured or calculated quantity to its actual value.

**Centroid:** The center of mass of an object. Here the mass means the signal strength.

**GPRS:** A packet oriented mobile data service using GSM or 3G cellular phone systems.

**Near Field Imaging:** A method of localizing a conducting object by measuring the changes in the electrostatic field produced by the sensor near the object..

**Resolution:** The capability of making distinguishable the individual parts of an object.

**Tag:** An object applied to or incorporated into a product, animal, or person for the purpose of identification and tracking using radio waves, ultrasound or other means.

**Triboeletric Effect:** A phenomenon of materials becoming electrically charged when they come into contact with another different material and are then separated.

**Vital Signs:** Body temperature, heart rate, blood pressure and respiratory rate.

**WLAN:** A wireless local area network that links two or more computers or devices to enable communication between devices in a limited area.

# Chapter 5
# SMART:
## Mobile Patient Monitoring in an Emergency Department

**Esteban Pino**
*Universidad de Concepción, Concepción, Chile*

**Dorothy Curtis**
*Massachusetts Institute of Technology, USA*

**Thomas Stair**
*Harvard Medical School, Boston, USA*

**Lucila Ohno-Machado**
*University of California San Diego, USA*

## ABSTRACT

*Patient monitoring is important in many contexts: at mass-casualty disaster sites, in improvised emergency wards, and in emergency room waiting areas. Given the positive history of use of monitoring systems in the hospital during surgery, in the recovery room, or in an intensive care unit, the authors sought to use recent technological advances to enable patient monitoring in more diverse circumstances: at home, while traveling, and in some less well-monitored areas of a hospital. This chapter presents the authors' experiences in designing, implementing and deploying a wireless disaster management system prototype in a real hospital environment. In addition to a review of related systems, the sensors, algorithms and infrastructure used in our implementation are presented. Finally, general guidelines for ubiquitous methodologies and tools are shared based on the lessons learned from the actual implementation.*

## INTRODUCTION

As technology advances, there are more options available for pervasive monitoring. Sensor miniaturization, wireless communication and increasing processing power in smaller packages allow more

efficient, reliable and convenient systems, at least from the end-user perspective. In healthcare, one of the main driving forces behind ubiquitous computing is the increasing need to move patient care from the hospital to non-standard settings such as homes, nursing homes, improvised waiting areas, hazardous locations or the battlefield. For at-risk

DOI: 10.4018/978-1-61520-765-7.ch004

patients, such as those with chronic diseases or the increasingly aging population, being able to live in a familiar and comfortable environment improves quality of life and frees hospital resources. In disaster situations or during seasonal or regional disease outbreaks, response teams move from the hospitals to improvised settings to care for multiple casualties with varying levels of urgency. Firefighters, hazmat teams and soldiers need real-time, ubiquitous monitoring to detect life threatening events. Existing solutions from industry, academia and the military share the same goal of developing unobtrusive, reliable and pervasive monitoring systems.

Powerful, disposable computers, wireless technologies, sensors and energy storage have made possible the development of Body Sensor Networks (BSN) (Aziz et al., 2008). These networks are ubiquitous, allowing patient supervision wherever they may go. Personalized health care is a natural extension of these BSN. Future challenges are user acceptance (from both patients and practitioners), ease of use, and avoiding data flooding with little information.

This chapter presents a particular experience of embedding a pervasive system in a healthcare setting and the steps required in the design and test of such a system in the hospital. We show benefits from fusing information from different sensors, the complications that arise when dealing with untethered subjects and finally the evaluation in a real environment. We also show how the implementation of this system required the skills of a multi-disciplinary team.

## BACKGROUND

### Pervasive Systems in Healthcare

In healthcare, the main technological components in pervasive systems are sensors and network technologies. The most frequently used physiological sensors measure ECG, $SpO_2$, temperature, acceleration, sound, and non-invasive blood pressure (BP). Since most physiologic variables present slow variations, networks are usually low bandwidth, adequate to handle the low data rates. Many of these networks are also characterized by short range transmissions, such as in Body Sensor Networks (BSN) or Personal Area Networks (PAN). These low bandwidth, short range networks are usually implemented using ZigBee or Bluetooth networks (Table 1). As the system aggregates data and forwards it to central servers, higher bandwidth is required. Local Area Networks (LAN) use the widely adopted WiFi networks for their wireless requirements. For larger ranges, cellular networks and WiMAX provide a reasonable solution (Fourty, Val, Fraisse, & Mercier, 2005; Kavas, 2007). Currently, cellular networks are the preferred method to relay data from ambulances and other fast moving patients due to its hand-over capability. WiMAX is being updated to allow roaming but its main strength is its suitability to provide wireless Metropolitan Area Network (MAN) capability to rural, low density areas where cellular networks are not economically viable. Naturally, wired networks provide much better bandwidth and reliability and are used at the earliest opportunity.

Location information is also highly desirable. In a distributed system, finding the patient who has a problem is not easy and a location system should be deployed to solve this problem. Positioning technologies range from GPS or cellular tower referencing used outdoors to RFID, ultrasound or infrared used indoors (Table 2). Sometimes the data network infrastructure acts as a location system by using received signal strength to infer positioning. Some solutions offer a combination of technologies in order to improve their performance.

Korhonen & Bardram (2004) review pervasive healthcare as a multidisciplinary field. It involves hardware, software, sensors, embedded systems, human-computer interfaces, wireless communications and distributed systems among others. In

*Table 1. Wireless technologies for data transmission*

|  | Standard | Max. Bandwidth | Use | Frequency | Range |
|---|---|---|---|---|---|
| *Short range* | | | | | |
| ZigBee | IEEE 802.15.4 | 250 Kbps | PAN | ISM 2.4 GHz | 100 m |
| Bluetooth | IEEE 802.15.1 | 1 Mbps | PAN | ISM 2.4 GHz | 10 m |
| WiFi (b) | IEEE 802.11b | 11 Mbps | LAN | ISM 2.4 GHz | 30 m |
| WiFi (g) | IEEE 802.11g | 54 Mbps | LAN | ISM 2.4 GHz | 100 m |
| WiFi (n) | IEEE 802.11n | 300 Mbps | LAN | ISM 2.4 GHz | 300 m |
| *Long range* | | | | | |
| Cellular (3G) | UMTS | 3 Mbps | MAN | Licensed: 1.95 GHz, 2.14 GHz | ~ 40 km |
| WiMAX | IEEE 802.16 | 70 Mbps | MAN | Licensed: 10-66 GHz Unlicensed: 2-11 GHz | 50 km |

*Table 2. Location technologies*

|  | Use | Advantages | Disadvantages |
|---|---|---|---|
| GPS | Outdoors | Easy to compute position on a map, works anywhere on the planet. | Is obstructed by high buildings, expensive, does not work indoors. |
| Cell tower | Outdoors | Uses existing cell tower network. | Accuracy depends on tower density. |
| RFID | Indoors | Unobstructed by clothing, walls, people. | Requires expensive archway detectors for unattended operation. |
| Ultrasound | Indoors | Excellent room level accuracy, inexpensive. | Tags can be obstructed, low transmission speed limits simultaneous tags in one location. |
| Infrared | Indoors | Excellent room level accuracy. | Easily obstructed by clothing, people. Requires line of sight with detectors. |

healthcare, this multidisciplinary nature is further extended to cope with medical aspects: physiologic sensors, location systems, resource management and intelligent systems. Further, deploying such a system inside a hospital requires collaborating with caregivers, as well as working with the institutional review board, to make sure that patient safety is protected.

Orwat, Graefe, & Faulwasser (2008) present a literature review on pervasive computing in health care. It provides a thorough analysis of 69 articles published from 2002 to 2006. They call for more reports on implementations that evaluate actual acceptance and problems. Privacy concerns are a priority for both patients and caregivers and need to be addressed properly for a wide acceptance

of pervasive monitoring. Saranummi & Wactlar (2008) agree with this view of the current problems in the emerging field of pervasive healthcare. There is a need for more clinical evidence of solution feasibility and user acceptance. Most works are research projects but few present real-world implementation and results.

Regarding networks, Varshney (2003) proposes wireless technology solutions to solve a wide range of challenges in the healthcare industry, including reducing costs, decreasing medical errors and improving service in under-staffed areas. Triantafyllidis, Koutkias, Chouvarda, & Maglaveras, (2008) propose an open and reconfigurable wireless sensor network architecture with emphasis on facilitating the addition of new sensors via a sensor modeling language. Wade & Asada (2007) present a cable-free Body Area Network (BAN) that uses a conductive-fabric garment with both signal and power. It facilitates pervasive monitoring by providing support for multiple sensors per patient.

Commercial monitoring systems range from complete embedded systems that alarm on thresholds and have more than one sensor to a simple $SpO_2$, blood pressure or ECG sensor for occasional self-checking. A few examples are: Welch Allyn Micropaq Monitor (Welch Allyn) provides an ECG and $SpO_2$ patient monitoring solution, Cleveland Medical Devices (CleveMed) provides general acquisition hardware and an assortment of physiological sensors, and Crossbow wireless sensor network (Crossbow), which supplies low level mesh network hardware to support BAN.

The United States military has developed and tested several systems. Originally, they were only used by physicians in the field but later systems recorded soldier data and were able to alert on critical conditions such as low thresholds or soldier unresponsiveness to medics and unit commanders. BMIST-J (now AHLTA-Mobile) (BMIST-J) and the ARTEMIS system (McGrath et al., 2003) are examples of such military systems.

## In the Hospital

Pervasive technologies in a hospital have different requirements than in other settings, such as serving highly mobile personnel, implementing patient-specific management protocols and supporting diverse monitoring goals. Meeting these needs improves monitoring in these complex environments. In 2007, Bardram & Christensen explore Activity-Based Computing (ABC) in hospitals, based on pervasive computing, supporting the naturally collaborative nature of hospital work. Sanchez, Tentori, & Favela (2008) present an activity recognition system for the smart hospital, specific to hospital worker activities. In a different publication, Tentori & Favela (2008) present a set

of tools for activity aware computing in a hospital. Pervasive healthcare systems must be prepared for highly mobile caregivers. This study shows the variety of tasks that are performed during a typical shift. The proposed solution involves a mobile activity monitor that is configured to alert based on patient actions or status. Coronato & Esposito (2008) discuss a localization system that combines two sources of information (RFID and WiFi) to obtain a reliable location in a hospital.

## Mass Casualty Response Systems

Several prototypes of mass casualty response systems, built in academia, are good examples of pervasive systems in healthcare. The basic goal of monitoring a large number of patients with varying degrees of urgency is best served designing a supervisory system that collects physiological data, analyses and provides some decision support to respond to critical patient conditions. In these cases, where patients far outnumber caregivers, a supervisory system that aids in detecting critical patients among many "walking-wounded" is of great value to first responders and caregivers in overcrowded settings.

Lin et al. (2004) implement wireless PDAs to monitor patients during transport. The physiological variables acquired are heart rate (HR), ECG and $SpO_2$. Real-time data transmissions allow a central management unit to supervise patient status and detect deteriorating conditions. A prototype was tested for intra-hospital transport. Lenert, Palmer, Chan, & Rao (2005) propose an "intelligent triage tag" for their Wireless Internet Information System for Medical Response in Disasters (WIISARD) architecture. Location is estimated from received signal strength using the same wireless data network to send data. Only general location is inferred. When the care providers are in the vicinity, the tag can identify itself and stand out among several injured in close proximity. Electronic Tags have bi-directional communication, can display triage status via LEDs and have sensors to determine patient status. Arisoylu, Mishra, Rao, & Lenert (2005) propose a "one switch" wireless access point with access to multiple cellular backhauls for internet connectivity, for use by the WIISARD system. Killeen, Chan, Buono, Griswold, & Lenert (2006) present the caregiver's wireless handheld device for WIISARD. It provides an electronic medical record that replicates the rapidity and ease of use of a standard paper triage tag. Malan, Fulford-Jones, Welsh, & Moulton (2004) present CodeBlue, a sensor network infrastructure to report vital signs and location and seamlessly transmit this data among caregivers. It is meant to enhance responders' ability to triage patients on scene and allocate hospital resources. The network is designed to scale from sparse to very dense deployments, covering a range of settings, from clinics or hospitals to mass casualty response sites. It features encryption, mesh networks, a flexible security model to grants access rights to arriving EMTs and a flexible infrastructure for connecting medical devices and routing physiological data to a central server or hospital information system. In the Advanced Health and Disaster Aid Network (AID-N) project, Massey, Gao, Welsh, Sharp, & Sarrafzadeh (2006) present a low-power electronic triage system with $SpO_2$, blood pressure, ECG and location sensor capability. This work is an extension on the CodeBlue project. Gao, Kim, White, & Alm (2006) present the patient monitoring system for AID-N. The wearable devices use a $SpO_2$ sensor as the primary sensor and implement GPS and MoteTrack location systems for outdoors and indoors positioning respectively. Monitoring is done at a central computer, where location and physiologic data can be seen simultaneously. In the event of requiring assistance, the operator may activate an audible alarm on the patient tag to facilitate aid. Finally, Gao et al. (2007) present the complete AID-N project. In a mass casualty incident a large number of embedded physiologic and location capable electronics report real-time data to a central station where response efforts can be coordinated. Sensor data is transmitted in

three different network layers. A ZigBee-like ad hoc network is used to form a body-area network, connecting each Mote-based embedded system with that patient's $SpO_2$, ECG and/or BP sensors. The ZigBee ad hoc network also provides location data. The second layer connects the embedded system to the Internet backbone. The third layer is the central server at the hospital or with public health authorities. Results from a disaster drill are presented. The large number of small distributed sensors facilitates inferring the actual state of a mass casualty site. Gao, et al. (2008) present the latest version of their original project, this time using miTags with an assortment of possible sensors and a ZigBee based mesh network for data transport. The miTags are based on motes, originally developed at University of California, Berkley and are low power, low bandwidth devices.

All of these pervasive healthcare proposals share some key elements: They implement patient centered, low power, wireless computers (mostly PDAs) to acquire and forward location and physiological data. The most recurring physiological variables monitored are $SpO_2$ and ECG. HR is derived from one or the other of these sensors or is directly reported by one of them. The data are transmitted wirelessly to a central station to supervise patients and coordinate efforts. Data are also transmitted back to caregivers in the field to notify them of events requiring special attention or to provide them with updated patient information. In all proposals, there is an agreement that location and patient status are the basic data required to guide caregiver's efforts.

## SMART

The Scalable Medical Alert and Response Technology (SMART) project is a good example of a pervasive healthcare monitoring system. A prototype was implemented from June 2006 to December 2007 in the waiting area of the Emergency Department at the Brigham and Women's

Hospital in Boston, USA. Originally devised as a disaster management response system, its goal is to monitor, alert and facilitate reprioritization of multiple untethered patients (Waterman et al., 2005; Pino, Ohno-Machado, Wiechmann, & Curtis, 2005; Curtis et al., 2008).

From the point of view of pervasive technology, SMART turns an improvised site or otherwise regular waiting room into an enhanced ambient where subjects can be monitored and located from a central station with low impact in their regular activities. For such a healthcare application, the two main aspects to consider are: (1) physiologic monitoring of key parameters and (2) location of individuals. Such a location system does not need to be of a high precision. Generally, a small room-sized area is enough to select the closest caregivers and to direct them to find the affected patient promptly.

The steps considered in designing SMART were:

1. Selecting physiological sensors and a location technology that can be implemented using low-power and low-cost components
2. Selecting a platform to integrate sensor electronics and wireless data transmission
3. Devising a physical packaging comfortable to the end users
4. Making sure the wireless system can support all the patients
5. Analyzing collected data and presenting aggregated data in a usable way
6. Integrating all components into an easy to set-up, scalable and easy to use system

SMART shares the key elements of other pervasive monitoring systems: distributed patient data collection, location information, central server data aggregation for multiple patient supervision and alarm generation on abnormal conditions. However, SMART incorporates new concepts that allow higher integration into the environment and thus differentiates itself from related projects.

Compared to Lin et al. (2004), SMART uses a similar set of patient sensors, but provides a central management infrastructure to aid in patient categorization and a location system to track patient positions. WIISARD (Lenert, Palmer, Chan, & Rao, 2005) and SMART share a similar architecture, the main difference being the intended use. SMART can be implemented in different settings using commercially available equipment. It is envisioned as a pervasive and ubiquitous system that can be deployed in disaster sites, nursing homes, hospital waiting rooms or even adapted for home use. In an emergency situation, first respondents will be already familiar with the system due to its presence in multiple environments. CodeBlue (Malan, Fulford-Jones, Welsh, & Moulton, 2004) focus more on hardware and network requirements. They propose custom-made, low-power sensors using motes as radio transceivers, while SMART is based on off the shelf equipment and provides a software platform for data analysis, classification and alarm. AID-N (Gao et al, 2007), the follow up project from CodeBlue, is very similar to SMART, both in monitored variables, architecture and intended goal. SMART, however, has several possible deployment scenarios and tries to accommodate patients in a variety of conditions, the most difficult ones being those with higher mobility. Special algorithms that combine sensor information from ECG and $SpO_2$ sources try to minimize false alarms, while keeping the algorithm simple to allow scaling. In sum, SMART is based on three concepts. First, the positioning system can be used for locating patients, caregivers and equipment, thus facilitating resource allocation based on proximity to the point of care. Second, a *Logistics* module is in charge of alarm handling, selecting the closest available caregiver, re-alarming if ignored or escalating the alarm to other caregivers if necessary. Third, a diagnosis suggestion is presented along physiologic data to facilitate supervision of a larger number of patients. The classification algorithm aggregates sensor information to minimize false alarms and allow a

*Figure 1. Patient with location tag and sensor box*

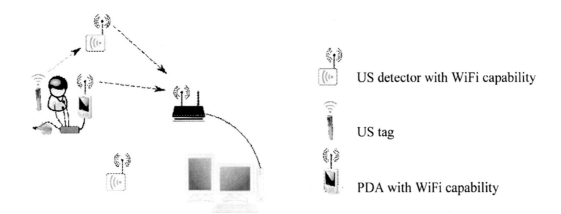

US detector with WiFi capability

US tag

PDA with WiFi capability

supervisor to focus on particular patients. This is a first approximation to automatic triage, which will be critical in a future unattended, fully automatic, triage system for mass casualty incidents.

## System Description

The design considers off-the-shelf parts as primary components. It involves physiologic sensors for patients, a room-level location system, a wireless network infrastructure to cover a waiting area, a central station running software to fuse sensor information and an alarm subsystem for diagnosis support, with the ability to wirelessly notify roaming caregivers.

Figure 1 shows a patient wearing a commercial $SpO_2$ sensor with serial communication and 3 ECG leads (1 signal, monitoring quality). The ECG instrumentation amplifier and serial data board are the only custom made elements in the project. Both data streams are sent to an HP iPaq 5510 PDA running Familiar Linux. A standard 802.11b wireless network (WiFi) carries the data packets to the main server. The location subsystem is implemented via ultrasound (US). An emitter attached to the patient sends its tag number to stationary receivers. The receivers forward the tag id and its signal strength to the main server, where a

simple algorithm associates the tag with the closest detector position. The required bandwidth is less than 50 kbps per patient, considering ECG, $SpO_2$, location and battery data. Power consumption is high due to our requirement for live ECG data that has to be transmitted wirelessly. To this end, an iPaq backpack providing additional battery is used, giving the system 3 to 4 hours of monitoring on a single charge. This autonomy proved enough for our pilot study but has to be addressed in future deployments.

The main server is called SMART Central, a regular commodity PC running Fedora Core Linux. It is wired to a wireless access point that provides 802.11b coverage for the patient and caregiver PDAs and for the US receivers. At SMART Central, the SMART operator is in charge of supervising the system and notifying triage personnel when a patient needs further assistance. The user interface consists of a main display with a patient roster, alarms and real-time physiological data, as shown in Figure 2. A secondary display shows the position of all tagged patients, caregivers and eventually equipment.

The roaming caregiver equipment has the US tag for location purposes and a handheld PDA to receive alarms, review monitored patient information and indicate busy/available status to SMART

*Figure 2. Main user interface and map in SMART central*

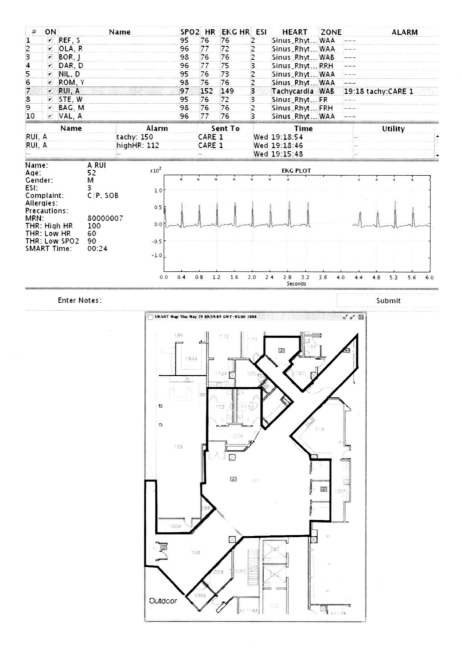

Central. With his (or her) PDA, the caregiver can review clinical data of a patient, real time SpO$_2$ data and ECG tracing. A live ECG and an alarm screen are shown in Figure 3. All communications to and from these PDAs are encrypted because they contain identifiable patient information.

Due to restrictions from the hospital's Institutional Review Board, we could not deploy or test the caregiver subsystem, but a prototype was implemented and used by the SMART operator while away from the main station.

The US location system is shared by all indoor assets that require tracking. Receivers on

*Figure 3. Caregiver view of patient and alarms*

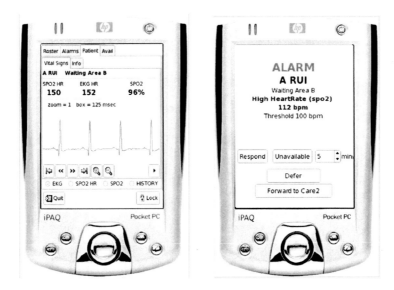

the walls listen to the US tags and report signal strength to determine the closest known location. For SMART, room area accuracy was enough, and allowed caregivers to quickly find a patient or resource when approaching the area. An added benefit of US is that it is blocked by walls, thus getting a wrong location is highly unlikely. Among the alternatives listed in Table 2, US was also the least intrusive in any setting, only requiring affixing detectors in the walls. For outdoor location, such as tracking a patient in an ambulance, a setup with a GPS in lieu of the US for location and the cellular network instead of WiFi for data transmission is used.

## Core Software

All of the software was developed using open source tools, with the goal of producing a flexible system that could accommodate other sensors, subsystems or outputs. Depending on the platform, different programming languages are used, as shown in Figure 4. The PDAs are programmed in Python with GTK. In SMART Central, C and C++ are used in ORNetDB, an engine for stream-

ing databases. The main Graphical User Interface (GUI) is written in Java and the underlying database is implemented in PostgreSQL. Auxiliary GUIs are web–based and implemented as python scripts which have database access.

ORNetDB can accommodate a variable number of connections of various data. Every time a new patient is registered, a new connection is generated for the location, and the ECG and $SpO_2$ data streams. ECG data are fed into a QRS detection node that generates a new stream that contains time-stamped QRS detections in noisy environments. All raw and computed data streams are saved in PostgreSQL databases. The caregiver PDAs have two-way connections to ORNetDB. They receive the patient roster with general information or live streams for a specific patient and send busy/responding notifications when an alarm is issued. SMART Central implements several GUIs, a Decision Support Module and a Logistics Support Module. The SMART Operator interacts with the GUIs to register, monitor and un-register patients. The Decision Module uses real-time information to suggest a classification among 7 medical conditions (bradycardia, sinus

*Figure 4.Component software and data paths in SMART*

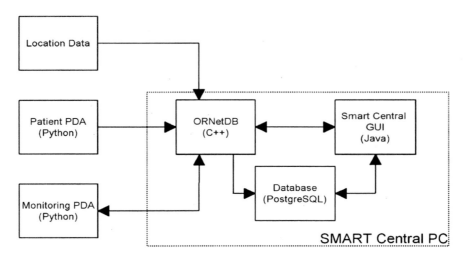

rhythm, tachycardia, ventricular tachycardia, ventricular fibrillation, irregular beats, asystole) and 3 technical conditions (noise, leads off, sensor mismatch). Other straightforward technical alarms are: no ECG signal, no $SpO_2$ signal, no communication from PDA and low battery. When an alarm is due, the Logistics Module is in charge of selecting the closest available caregiver based on the location information, handling re-alarming and escalating alarms to other caregivers if there is no response. As mentioned earlier, administrative restrictions prevented us from fully testing the alarm escalation algorithms, but a prototype showed that it is feasible. This integrated system behavior is possible due to the information fusion from location, physiologic and caregiver status information.

## Results

In general the system performed well. The SMART system was able to monitor multiple roaming patients in the waiting room area for the Emergency Department (ED) at the Brigham and Women's hospital in Boston, MA. The pilot test was conducted from June 2006 to October 2007,

monitoring 145 patients or 6815 minutes of data. Patients with shortness of breath and patients with chest pain were invited to participate in the trial. The system is set up after the patient underwent triage with a nurse. The SMART Operator initiated the process by obtaining consent, handling the hardware pouch, and checking that standard lead II ECG and $SpO_2$ were being recorded. Particular results varied according to the subjects being monitored. In Figure 5, the first patient produced a sinus rhythm alternating only with sinus tachycardia when its HR was consistently over 100 BPM. On the other hand, we also had cases where episodes of highly noisy signals generated false alarms such as ventricular fibrillation or irregular beats. These episodes were always correlated with patient movement, when the beat detection algorithm did not identify the segment as noise and produces false beat annotations. The technical alarms mismatch (when $SpO_2$ HR was normal, but ECG data looked like asystole or ventricular fibrillation) and leads off (when leads act as antennas and ECG data fluctuated among all possible values) were more appropriate, but we had expected more "NOISY" classifications.

*Figure 5. Diagnosis suggestions for two different patients in SMART*

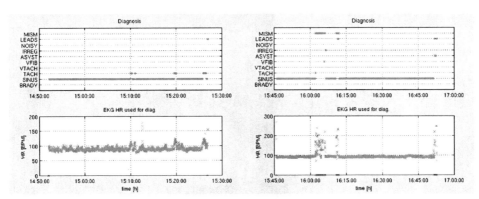

The LEADS (leads off) or ASYST (asystole) diagnoses at the end of the record are generated when the SMART operator removes the equipment from the patient.

The alarms positive predictability fell from over 0.95 in simulated patients to 0.71 in real patients. This decrease was due to inaccurate detection of noise produced by movement and muscle artifacts in the ECG. $SpO_2$ data were used to cross-validate the results and disregard contradictory classifications. Another attempt at improving the noise detection was made using the US tags, but they proved too sensitive to be of practical use. In any case, the incidence of alarms was low, averaging 1 every 12 minutes. During the pilot study, 3 patients were reprioritized and admitted sooner to the ED due to findings while being monitored.

## User Acceptance

A survey conducted for patients who volunteered to participate in the study shows that the system had a very good acceptance. Out of 91 respondents, 87% said that they would probably or likely use such a system again and 68% felt at least a little safer by being monitored. Finally, 38% answered that it improved the care, even though it had been explained to them that it wouldn't.

## FUTURE RESEARCH DIRECTIONS

With increasing miniaturization, improved low-power electronics and further development of algorithms to deal with noisy data, we expect the development and deployment of pervasive health monitoring systems to increase. However, we feel that the first step towards implementing a robust pervasive healthcare system for mass casualty response or for multiple untethered patient monitoring system must be improvement of alarm rates. As the alarms become more trustworthy, it will be possible to augment human resources in a crowded environment with automated supervision. This has to be accomplished by lowering false alarms without sacrificing true alarms. Patient monitoring systems are bound to be biased towards detecting true positives because the cost of missing a real alarm is much higher than the cost of dealing with a false alarm.

From the lessons learned in SMART, the first step to improve alarm generation is enhancing noise detection. In a real environment with ambulatory patients, noise plays a fundamental role in confusing beat detection and diagnosis algorithms that otherwise performs satisfactorily. Movement artifacts and muscle noise, especially when walking, are easily confused with abnormal rhythms. The two possible approaches are via software detection, directly on the noisy signal, or via hardware, incorporating other sensors such

*Figure 6. User acceptance*

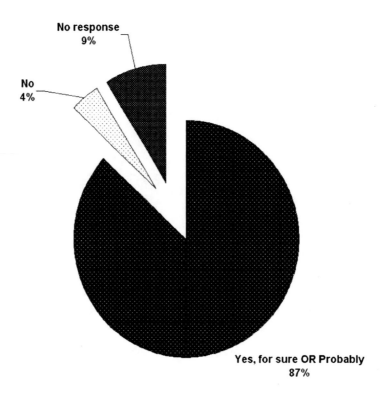

**Would you wear a SMART pouch again?**

**No response**
9%

**No**
4%

**Yes, for sure OR Probably**
87%

as accelerometers, to identify regions of low data quality. SMART's approach is based on software detection, via "leads off", "noisy" and "asystole" classifications. Redmond, Lovell, Basilakis, & Celler (2008) propose an ECG quality measurement based on similar ECG signal characteristics, detecting zones with signal saturation, high frequency noise or lack of signal, and marking unusable ECG with a dilated mask, comparable to SMART's voting mechanism. When the alarm management has matured, we look forward to a future deployment where we can also study the physician acceptance of the system.

Location tracking performed adequately. When patients were transitioning between areas,

we could see that sometimes intermediate areas were not occupied. However, this was not deemed important, as the location system's goal was to inform of patient's last location in order to find and treat him. A future research direction is associating movement with probable noise presence in physiological data.

Power requirements allow 3 to 4 hours monitoring on a single charge. In the future, we will try to lower power consumption in order to increase monitoring length. This can be accomplished by changing to a lower power data transmission such as ZigBee or Bluetooth (Paksuniemi, Sorvoja, Alasaarela, & Myllyla, 2006) and/or by changing the iPaqs as the mobile platform.

*Figure 7. User acceptance. Perceived safety*

**Did the monitoring system make you feel safer?**

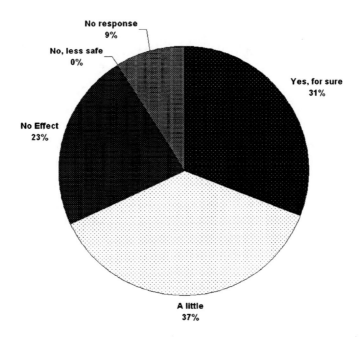

*Figure 8. User acceptance. Perceived effect of monitoring on care*

**Effect of SMART Monitoring on Care**

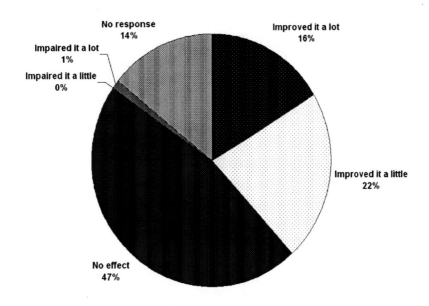

## CONCLUSION

We have presented the SMART system, a pervasive health monitoring system for mass casualty emergencies but also useful in waiting areas of emergency rooms and other ad hoc patient monitoring sites. The system prototype was deployed in a hospital and evaluated over an eighteen month period. Both the implementation and deployment of this system were facilitated by having a multidisciplinary team; computer science researchers and physicians worked together to produce a system that could effectively monitor ambulatory patients awaiting treatment.

From our experience, we conclude that building an acceptable pervasive health monitoring systems requires the interaction of many people: engineers, hospital personnel and patients. Data from real patients allow algorithm designers to produce effective algorithms. While we tested our algorithms on data from various sources, including healthy volunteers and a synthetic patient and web repository of signals, it turned out that data from real patients was qualitatively different, because we monitored them for longer periods of time and even normal patients' ECGs displayed unexpected features. Interacting with hospital personnel makes sure that the system does not adversely affect current standards of patient care. In particular, doctors should not be subjected to excessive false alarms and the nursing staff should not be burdened with additional duties related to prototype systems. The deployment of the networking and location equipment should be done in such a way that the patients are not bothered by it.

Patients in unmonitored areas can benefit from pervasive monitoring systems. These monitoring systems are effective when they do not interfere with patients' normal activities. Systems such as SMART allow a limited number of healthcare personnel to oversee a large number of people with minimal effort. As shown, a wireless system providing simple physiological and location data can be of great help in both improvised and regular settings, and patients evaluate these efforts positively.

## ACKNOWLEDGMENT

We would like to thank the National Library of Medicine for supporting this work through contract number N01LM33509. We would also like to thank our colleagues who provided essential assistance in building the SMART prototype and in deploying and evaluating it: From the Brigham and Women's Hospital Emergency Department: Jacob Bailey, the SMART Operator; from MIT: Jason Waterman, Eugene Shih, and John Guttag; from the Decision Systems Group at Brigham and Women's Hospital: Staal Vinterbo, Rosa Figueroa, and Robert A. Greenes. Terry Aasen and the Sonitor® team provided essential assistance with the deployment of the indoor location system.

## REFERENCES

Arisoylu, M., Mishra, R., Rao, R., & Lenert, L. A. (2005). 802.11 wireless infrastructure to enhance medical response to disasters. In *AMIA Annual Symposium Proceedings*, (pp. 1-5).

Aziz, O., Lo, B., Pansiot, J., Atallah, L., Yang, G.-Z., & Darzi, A. (2008, Oct). From computers to ubiquitous computing by 2010: Health Care. *Philosophical Transactions of the Royal Society A, 366*(1881), 3805-3811.

Bardram, J. E., & Christensen, H. B. (2007, Jan.-March). Pervasive computing support for hospitals: An overview of the activity-based computing project. *IEEE Pervasive Computing / IEEE Computer Society [and] IEEE Communications Society, 6*(1), 44–51. doi:10.1109/MPRV.2007.19

Battlefield Medical Information System Tactical - Joint. (n.d.). *BMIST-J home page.* Retrieved 13 February 2009 from http://www.mc4.army.mil/AHLTA-Mobile_CBT.asp#, CleveMed. Cleveland Medical Devices Inc. (n.d.). home page. Retrieved 13 Feb 2009, from: http://www.clevemed.com/

Coronato, A., & Esposito, M. (2008). Towards an implementation of smart hospital: A localization system for mobile users and devices. In *Proceedings Sixth Annual IEEE International Conference on Pervasive Computing and Communications PERCOM 2008,* (pp. 715-719).

Crossbow. (n.d.). *Home page.* Retrieved 13 Feb 2009 from http://www.xbow.com

Curtis, D. W., Pino, E. J., Bailey, J. M., Shih, E. I., Waterman, J., & Vinterbo, S. A. (2008). SMART - An Integrated Wireless System for Monitoring Unattended Patients. *Journal of the American Medical Informatics Association, 15*(1), 44–53. doi:10.1197/jamia.M2016

Fourty, N., Val, T., Fraisse, P., & Mercier, J.-J. (2005). Comparative analysis of new high data rate wireless communication technologies "from Wi-Fi to WiMAX". In. *Proceedings of the Joint International Conference on Autonomic and Autonomous Systems and International Conference on Networking and Services, ICAS-ICNS, 2005,* 66–71.

Gao, T., Kim, M. I., White, D., & Alm, A. M. (2006). Iterative user-centered design of a next generation patient monitoring system for emergency medical response. In *AMIA Annual Symposium Proceedings,* (pp. 284-288).

Gao, T., Massey, T., Selavo, L., Crawford, D., Chen, B., & Lorincz, K. (2007, Sept.). The advanced health and disaster aid network: A light-weight wireless medical system for triage. *IEEE Transactions on Biomedical Circuits and Systems, 1*(3), 203–216. doi:10.1109/TB-CAS.2007.910901

Gao, T., Pesto, C., Selavo, L., Chen, Y., Ko, J. G., Lim, J. H., et al. (2008) Wireless Medical Sensor Networks in Emergency Response: Implementation and Pilot Results. In *Technologies for Homeland Security, 2008 IEEE Conference on,* (pp. 187-192).

Kavas, A. (2007). Comparative analysis of WLAN, WiMAX and UMTS Technologies. In *Progress In Electromagnetics Research Symposium 2007, Prague, Czech Republic,* (pp. 140-144).

Killeen, J. P., Chan, T. C., Buono, C., Griswold, W. G., & Lenert, L. A. (2006). A wireless first responder handheld device for rapid triage, patient assessment and documentation during mass casualty incidents. In *AMIA Annual Symposium Proceedings,* (pp. 429-433).

Korhonen, I., & Bardram, J. E. (2004). Guest editorial introduction to the special section on pervasive healthcare. *IEEE Transactions on Information Technology in Biomedicine, 8*(3), 229–234. doi:10.1109/TITB.2004.835337

Lenert, L., Palmer, D., Chan, T., & Rao, R. (2005). An intelligent 802.11 triage tag for medical response to disasters. In *AMIA Annual Symposium Proceedings,* (pp. 440-444).

Lin, Y.-H., Jan, I.-C., Ko, P. C.-I., Chen, Y.-Y., Wong, J.-M., & Jan, G.-J. (2004). A wireless PDA-based physiological monitoring system for patient transport. *IEEE Transactions on Information Technology in Biomedicine, 8*(4), 439–447. doi:10.1109/TITB.2004.837829

Malan, D., Fulford-Jones, T., Welsh, M., & Moulton, S. (2004). Codeblue: An ad hoc sensor network infrastructure for emergency medical care. *International Workshop on Wearable and Implantable Body Sensor Networks.*

Massey, T., Gao, T., Welsh, M., Sharp, J. H., & Sarrafzadeh, M. (2006). The design of a decentralized electronic triage system. *AMIA Annual Symposium Proceedings,* (pp. 544-548).

McGrath, S., Grigg, E., Wendelken, S., Blike, G., Rosa, M. D., Fiske, A., et al. (2003, November). *ARTEMIS: A vision for remote triage and emergency management information integration.* Dartmouth University.

Orwat, C., Graefe, A., & Faulwasser, T. (2008). Towards pervasive computing in health care - a literature review. *BMC Medical Informatics and Decision Making, 8,* 26. doi:10.1186/1472-6947-8-26

Paksuniemi, M., Sorvoja, H., Alasaarela, E., & Myllyla, R. (2006). Wireless sensor and data transmission needs and technologies for patient monitoring in the operating room and intensive care unit. In 27th Annual Int. Conf IEEE EMBS05, (pp. 5182-5185).

Pino, E., Ohno-Machado, L., Wiechmann, E., & Curtis, D. (2005). Real-Time ECG Algorithms for Ambulatory Patient Monitoring. In *AMIA Annual Symposium Proceedings*, (pp. 604-608).

Redmond, S. J., Lovell, N. H., Basilakis, J., & Celler, B. G. (2008). ECG Quality measures in telecare monitoring. In *Proc. 30th Annual Int. Conf IEEE EMBC08*, 20th-24th Aug, Vancouver Canada, (pp. 2869-2872).

Sanchez, D., Tentori, M., & Favela, J. (2008, March-April). Activity recognition for the smart hospital. *IEEE Intelligent Systems, 23*(2), 50–57. doi:10.1109/MIS.2008.18

Saranummi, N., & Wactlar, H. (2008). Editorial: Pervasive Healthcare. Selected papers from the pervasive healthcare 2008 conference, Tampere, Finland. *Methods of Information in Medicine, 47*(3), 175–177.

Tentori, M., & Favela, J. (2008, April-June). Activity-aware computing for healthcare. *IEEE Pervasive Computing / IEEE Computer Society [and] IEEE Communications Society, 7*(2), 51–57. doi:10.1109/MPRV.2008.24

Triantafyllidis, A., Koutkias, V., Chouvarda, I., & Maglaveras, N. (2008). An open and reconfigurable wireless sensor network for pervasive health monitoring. In *Proceedings Second International Conference on Pervasive Computing Technologies for Healthcare PervasiveHealth 2008,* (pp. 112-115).

Varshney, U. (2003, Dec.). Pervasive healthcare. *Computer, 36*(12), 138–140. doi:10.1109/MC.2003.1250897

Wade, E., & Asada, H. (2007, Jan.-March). Conductive fabric garment for a cable-free body area network. *IEEE Pervasive Computing / IEEE Computer Society [and] IEEE Communications Society, 6*(1), 52–58. doi:10.1109/MPRV.2007.8

Waterman, J., Curtis, D., Goraczko, M., Shih, E., Sarin, P., Pino, E., et al. (2005). Demonstration of SMART (Scalable Medical Alert Response Technology). *AMIA 2005 Annual Symposium.*

Welch Allyn Micropaq Monitor model Micropaq 404 Monitor (ECG/SpO$_2$). Directions for use. Retrieved February 13, 2009, from http://www.welchallyn.com/documents/Patient%20Monitoring/ Continuous%20Monitoring/Micropaq/user-manual_20070615_402_404_micropaq.pdf

## ADDITIONAL READING

Casas, R., Marco, A., Plaza, I., Garrido, Y., & Falco, J. (2008, February). ZigBee-based alarm system for pervasive healthcare in rural areas. *IET Communications, 2*(2), 208–214. doi:10.1049/iet-com:20060649

Dağtaş, S., Pekhteryev, G., Sahinoğlu, Z., Cam, H., & Challa, N. (2008). Real-time and secure wireless health monitoring. *International Journal of Telemedicine and Applications, 135808,* 1–10. doi:10.1155/2008/135808

Environments, S. M. A. R. T. (Ed.). (2005). *D. Cook. S Das.*

Hayes, T. L., Pavel, M., Larimer, N., Tsay, I. A., Nutt, J., & Adami, A. G. (2007, Jan.-March). Distributed healthcare: Simultaneous assessment of multiple individuals. *IEEE Pervasive Computing / IEEE Computer Society [and] IEEE Communications Society*, *6*(1), 36–43. doi:10.1109/MPRV.2007.9

Orwat, C., Graefe, A., & Faulwasser, T. (2008). Towards pervasive computing in health care - a literature review. *BMC Medical Informatics and Decision Making*, *8*, 26. doi:10.1186/1472-6947-8-26

Proceedings Second International Conference on Pervasive Computing Technologies for Healthcare *PervasiveHealth2008*

## KEY TERMS AND DEFINITIONS

**Pervasive System:** Ubiquitous system with assorted sensors to provide a full picture of monitored subjects at any time and place.

**Patient Monitoring:** Monitoring of patients presenting varying degrees of urgency, to provide better care.

**Ambulatory Monitoring:** Monitoring freely moving patients in non-standard settings such as waiting rooms, home, work, etc.

**Wireless Monitoring:** Wireless transmission of collected data, trying to be as unobtrusive as possible.

**Diagnosis Support System:** System that can provide triage suggestions and alarm generation based on patient monitoring data.

**Mass Casualty Response System:** Patient monitoring system intended for large casualty numbers and high patient to caregiver ratio.

**Disaster Management System:** Mass casualty response system at disaster sites, in non-standard settings.

**Ultrasound Location System:** Location system based on ultrasound signals generated by moving targets and received by detectors to infer location.

*This work was previously published in International Journal of Healthcare Delivery Reform Initiatives, Vol. 1, Issue 4, edited by M. Guah, pp. 1-16, copyright 2010 by IGI Publishing (an imprint of IGI Global).*

# Chapter 6

# An Investigation into the Use of Pervasive Wireless Technologies to Support Diabetes Self–Care

**Nilmini Wickramasinghe**
*RMIT University, Australia*

**Indrit Troshani**
*University of Adelaide Business School, Australia*

**Steve Goldberg**
*INET International Inc., Canada*

## ABSTRACT

*Diabetes is one of the leading chronic diseases affecting Australians and its prevalence continues to rise. The goal of this study is to investigate the application of a pervasive technology solution developed by INET in the form of a wireless enabled mobile phone to facilitate superior diabetes self-care.*

## INTRODUCTION

Diabetes is a chronic disease that occurs when there is too much glucose in the blood because the body is not producing insulin or not using it properly. The total number of diabetes patients worldwide is estimated to rise to 366 million in 2030 from 171 million in 2000 (Wild et al., 2004). With increasingly growing prevalence which includes an estimated 275 Australians developing diabetes daily (Diabe-

tes Australia, 2008), Australia is expected to be a significant contributor to this projected trend.

An estimated 700,000 Australians representing approximately 3.6% of the population were diagnosed with diabetes in 2004-05 and between 1989-90 and 2004-05 the proportion of people diagnosed with this disease more than doubled from 1.3% to 3.3%. Additionally, between 2000-01 and 2004-05, diabetes hospitalisation rates increased by 35% from 1,932 to 2,608 hospitalisations per 100,000 people (AIHW, 2008). Recent statistics also show that for every person diagnosed with diabetes, it is estimated that there is another who has yet to be

DOI: 10.4018/978-1-61520-765-7.ch006

diagnosed which doubles the number of diabetes sufferers (DiabetesAustralia, 2008). Diabetes is, thus, one of the fastest growing chronic diseases in Australia (AIHW, 2008; Chittleborough et al., 2007).

Diabetes can have a major impact on the quality of life of its patients and its long-term effects can evolve into serious complications. For instance, people with diabetes are at greater risk of developing cardiovascular, eye or kidney diseases, lower limb amputation and even reduced life expectancy than people without diabetes (AIHW, 2008; Rasmussen, Wellard, & Nankervis, 2001; Tong & Stevenson, 2007). These complications can lead to death, and currently, diabetes ranks as the sixth leading cause of death in Australia (DiabetesAustralia, 2008)

Evidence also shows that diabetes and its complications incur significant costs for the health system in Australia including costs incurred by carers, government, and the entire health system (DiabCostAustralia, 2002). For instance, in 2004-05 direct healthcare expenditure on diabetes was A\$907 million which constituted approximately 2% of the allocatable recurrent health expenditure in that year (AIHW, 2008). Further costs include societal costs that represent productivity losses for both patients and their carers (DiabCostAustralia, 2002). Diabetes can, therefore, have considerable social, human, and economic impacts and tackling these requires solutions that substantially enhance the existing fragmented and uncoordinated capacity for effective prevention, early detection and management (VictorianGovernment, 2007). Hence, a treatment imperative is to provide patients with appropriate levels of monitoring to ensure containment of the disease and prevention of further complications. Given the exponential growth predicted for patients suffering from this disease coupled with the geographic spread across Australia (AIHW, 2008), a pervasive technology solution would offer the necessary monitoring that is both cost effective, convenient to both

patients and clinicians and least disruptive to patient life style.

Recognizing the need to have a solution that can enable the ubiquitous monitoring of diabetes patients while also continuously educating them, the goal of this chapter is to investigate the application of a pervasive technology solution developed by INET International in the form of a wireless enabled mobile phone to facilitate superior diabetes self-care in the Australian setting. The realization of this goal can contribute by establishing a benchmark for theoretical and empirical testing. To achieve this goal, first, we provide a general background on the Australian health scene and critically review existing research. An elaboration of the proposed pervasive mobile technology solution and of the anticipated barriers and facilitators the Australian setting is then provided. Future trends are subsequently discussed before the chapter is concluded.

## BACKGROUND

### Current Australian Health Scene

Both healthcare professionals and people with diabetes require quality information if disease conditions are to be effectively managed, detected early and/or prevented. Recent research shows that there are several deficiencies and gaps in the information provided by the existing system for monitoring diabetes in Australia (Dixon & Webbie, 2006). First, data collected in hospitals are episode-based rather than patient-based which makes it difficult to determine statistics concerning individual admissions, re-admissions, and treatment patterns. Second, there is lack of data on incidence and prevalence by diabetes type that can help reliably assess the magnitude of the problem. Also, diabetes trend information across the population is sparse. Third, the accuracy of recording data in administrative data sets, such as hospital morbidity, mortality and general practice data is uncertain. Fourth, clinical management information is derived from uncoordinated and fragmented data collections that are not representative of the entire population of diabetes patients which makes comparison, analysis and trend identification difficult. Finally, information is necessary for improving services and maintaining the quality of life of diabetes patients.

These deficiencies are the result of the current health system set up. Based on fee-for-service episodic doctor-patient consultation, the current Australian health system can handle acute short-term illnesses involving a limited range of interventions including their diagnosis and treatment (Hunt, 2007). However, this system is comprised of a mixture of fragmented private and public healthcare subsystems that provide both funding and healthcare delivery. Largely uncoordinated, these subsystems are deemed to be unsuitable for the treatment of long term chronic diseases in general (Dixon & Webbie, 2006). Chronic diseases, such as diabetes, require teams of various health professionals and long term support to help sufferers make effective healthy lifestyle changes and constantly maintain them (Hunt, 2007).

## Current Research

Diabetes management involves a combination of both medical and non-medical approaches with the overall goal for diabetes patients to have a life which is as normal as possible (AIHW, 2008). However, as there is no cure for diabetes, achieving this goal can be challenging because it requires effective lifestyle management and careful and meticulous attention and monitoring by both patients and healthcare professionals (Britt et al., 2007). In particular, to be totally successful, this requires patients to be both informed and active in their treatment regimen. Also known as patient empowerment, this is achieved by effective self-management which is a non-medical approach and which constitutes the focus of this chapter (Mirza et al., 2008).

Self-management is important as it empowers people with diabetes and it acknowledges their central role and responsibility for managing their healthcare (ICIC, 2008). Recent research substantiates the notion that active participation of diabetes patients in self-management is a key strategy for managing their condition (Colagiuri, Colagiuri, & Ward, 1998; Wellard, Rennie, & King, 2008). Therefore, self-management is extremely important in reaching improved treatment outcomes for these patients (Poulton, 1999; Rasmussen et al., 2001).

However, self-management is a constantly time-consuming task that requires significant self-discipline (Russell, Churl Suh, & Safford, 2005) and support strategies that include assessment, goal-setting, action-planning, problem-solving and follow-up (ICIC, 2008). Moreover, because effective self-management may require patient interaction with various healthcare professionals, including general practitioners (GPs), diabetes educators, dieticians, optometrists and community nurses (Knuiman, Welborn, & Bartholomew, 1996), difficulties can arise when people with diabetes encounter problems which range from making appointments to needing to travel to many locations (Van Eyk & Baum, 2002). In particular, in rural and regional areas there can be limited healthcare professionals with diabetes care expertise, thereby, making them difficult and costly to access by diabetes sufferers (Wellard et al., 2008; Zigbor & Songer, 2001).

Given both the importance and complexity of applying self-management effectively for both prevention and early detection of diabetes, there are increasing calls for further research to facilitate self-management (Wellard et al., 2008). A model proposed by Wagner (2008) requires productive interactions between informed and activated patients and prepared and proactive healthcare professionals (ICIC, 2008). One of the most important ways to achieve or at least facilitate this, entails the development of suitable information systems for building patient capacity

Successful web-based projects in healthcare require the consideration of many components. Figure 2 provides an integrative model for all key success factors that we have identified through our research (Goldberg, 2002a, 2002b, 2002c, 2002d, 2002e; Wickramasinghe & Goldberg, 2004; Wickramasinghe & Misra, 2004; Wickramasinghe, Schaffer, & Geisler, 2005). What makes this model unique and most beneficial is its focus on enabling and supporting all areas necessary for the actualization of ICT initiatives in healthcare. By design, the model identifies the inputs necessary to bring an innovative chronic disease management solution to market. These solutions are developed and implemented through a physician-led mobile e-health project. This project is the heart of the model that bridges the needs and requirements of many different players into a final (output) deliverable, a "Wireless Healthcare Program". To accomplish this, the model is continually updated to identify, select and prioritize the ICT project inputs that will:

- Accelerate healthcare system enhancements and achieve rapid healthcare benefits. The model identifies key healthcare system inputs with the four Ps, namely, 1) **People** that deliver healthcare, 2) **Process** to define the current healthcare delivery tasks, 3) **Platform** used in the healthcare technology infrastructure, and 4) **Protection** of patient data.
- Close the timing gaps between information research studies and their application in healthcare operational settings.
- Shorten the time cycle to fund an ICT project and receive an adequate return on the investment.

*Table.1 Components of chronic care model (Rachlis, 2006)*

| Component | Description |
|---|---|
| Organisation of Health System | • Leadership in chronic disease management (CDM)<br>• Goals for CDM<br>• Improvement strategy for CDM<br>• Incentives and regulations for CDM<br>• Benefits |
| Self-management support | • Assessment and documentation of needs and activities<br>• Addressing concerns of patients<br>• Effective behaviour change interventions |
| Decision Support | • Evidence-based guidelines<br>• Involvement of specialists in improving primary care<br>• Providing education for CDM<br>• Informing patients about guidelines |
| Delivery System design | • Practice team functioning<br>• Practice team leadership<br>• Appointment system<br>• Follow-up<br>• Planned visits for CDM<br>• Continuity of Care |
| Clinical Information Systems | • Registry<br>• Reminders to providers<br>• Feedback<br>• Information about relevant subgroups of patients needing services<br>• Patient treatment plans |
| Community | • Linkages for patients to resources<br>• Partnerships with community organizations<br>• Policy and plan development |

*Figure 2. INET-web-based-business model*

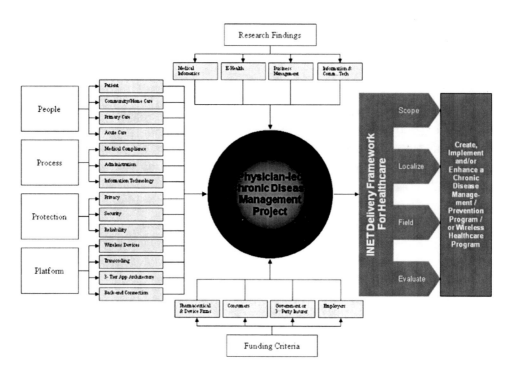

Together the components of the model will help in actualizing physician-led solution for the management of chronic diseases in general and of diabetes in particular. The delivery framework activities (Figure 1a and 2) are ongoing and represent a continuous improvement cyclical approach towards a given wireless healthcare program. These activities however require the relevant and complete inputs from the healthcare system if they are to be carried out successfully. With the refocused SDLC in constructing mobile e-health solutions, both the healthcare inputs (i.e. the four Ps) and the delivery framework may require funding from various sources in return for healthcare improvements and the building up of intelligence in terms of relevant research findings.

To successfully implement the business model described above it was, however, necessary to have an appropriate methodology. Based on this need the adaptive mapping to realization methodology (AMR) was developed (figure 3). The idea of the methodology was to apply a systematic rigorous set of predetermined protocols to each business case and then map the post-prior results back to the model. In this way, it was possible to compare and contrast both *a priori* and *post priori* findings. From such a comparison a diagnosis of the current state was made and then prescriptions were derived for the next business case. Hence, each pilot study incorporated the lessons learnt from the previous one and the model was adapted in real time.

By applying the tools and techniques of today's knowledge economy as presented in the intelligence continuum (IC) it is possible to make the AMR methodology into a very powerful knowledge-based systems development model (figure 4). The IC was developed by Wickramasinghe and Schaffer (2006) to enable the application of tools and technologies of the knowledge economy to be applied to healthcare processes in a systematic and rigorous fashion and thereby ensure superior healthcare delivery. The collection of key tools, techniques and processes

*Table 2. INET practice framework – Compressing the SDLC*

| SDLC (waterfall) | INET Mobile e-Health Project | | | |
| --- | --- | --- | --- | --- |
| | Scope | Localize | Field | Evaluate |
| I.T. Role & Responsibility | Project Management Business Analysis | Data Analysis Technical Tools Expert Programmer Data Administrator Network Architect Database Administrator Network Administrator | Technical Support | Account Manager |
| Investigation | Problem Definition Feasibility Study – can objectives be met at a reasonable cost. Project Definition | | | Document Solution, Data analysis of outcomes, benefits and Next Steps |
| Analysis (Logical Design) | | Define what the IS must do to fix the problem Less temptation to follow existing practices which may not be best Define the user's requirements and priorities Analyze existing system Develop logical design for the new system | | |
| Design (Physical Design) | | Define how the new system will work Detail Schedule and budget Produce a physical design showing system inputs, outputs, user interfaces. | | |
| Implementation | | Research technology Product Acquisitions Test programs, sub-systems and systems acquire or develop software Code programs Software developer manual System operators manual Purchase and Install hardware and software package | User's Manual People Changeover Tasks Data Conversion. Technical Changeover Tasks | |
| Maintenance | | Fix Problem/Solution Determination | Fix Database, Network and 3rd Party Products Fix security and access problems Fix learning curve time disruptions Fix collaboration problems | |

that make up the IC include but are not limited to data mining, business intelligence/analytics and knowledge management (Wickramasinghe & Schaffer, 2006). Taken together, they represent a very powerful system for refining the raw data stored in data marts and/or data warehouses and

*Figure 3. AMR methodology*

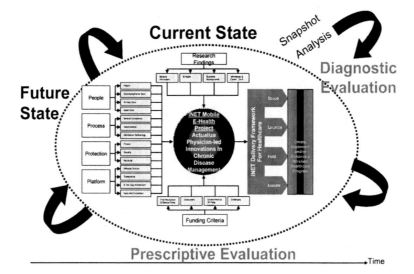

thereby maximizing the value and utility of these data assets for any organization. To maximize the value of the data generated through specific healthcare processes and then use this to improve processes, IC techniques and tools must be applied in a systematic manner. Once applied, the results become part of the data set that are subsequently reintroduced into the system and combined with other inputs of people, processes, and technology to develop an improvement continuum. Thus, the IC includes the generation of data, the analysis of these data to provide a "diagnosis", and their reintroduction into the cycle as a "prescriptive" solution. In this way, the IC is well suited to the dynamic and complex nature of healthcare environments and ensures that the future state is always built upon the extant knowledge-base of the preceding state. Through the incorporation of the IC with the AMR methodology we then have a knowledge-based systems development model that can be applied to any setting, not necessarily to chronic disease management. The power of this model is that it brings best practices and the best available germane knowledge to each iteration and is both flexible and robust.

The preceding discussion has outlined a pervasive ICT enabled solution which while not exorbitantly expensive, it facilitates the superior monitoring of diabetes (figure 5). The proposed solution enables patient empowerment by way of enhancing self-management. This is a desirable objective because it allows patients to become equal partners with their clinicians in the management of their own healthcare (Opie, 1998; Radin, 2006) by enhancing the traditional clinical-patient interactions (Mirza, Norris, & Stockdale, 2008). However, because most work has focused on specific applications and proof-of-concept studies, this chapter would be incomplete without considering the critical success factors, including facilitators and barriers, that are expected to affect the ubiquitous adoption of the proposed solution in the Australian setting (Mirza et al., 2008).

## ANTICIPATED BARRIERS AND FACILITATORS IN AUSTRALIA

In order to move smoothly from idea to realisation we identify and discuss seven factors that may impede or facilitate the success of the proposed

*Figure 4. Knowledge-based systems development model*

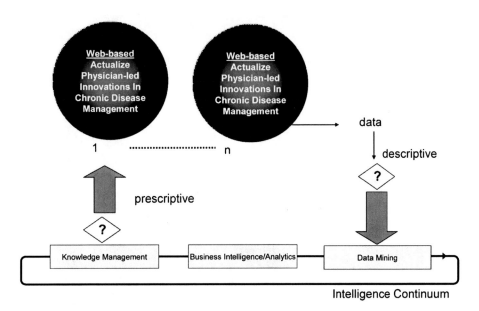

solution in the Australian setting. First, our solution has the potential to reduce face-to-face interaction between patients and their clinicians. While this may be favourable for some patients, it may impact on the social needs of others for human interaction. This may lead to resistance or even rejection for adopting the proposed solution at both conscious and subconscious levels (Vanjara, 2006). However, our solution incorporates mobile phones which are perceived to confer a social status amongst some segments of society which may well become an adoption facilitator. Furthermore, usage of mobile phones may also help eliminate the social stigma that can occur with alternative obvious devices that are used for monitoring chronic diseases (Mirza et al., 2008).

Second, mobile phones are location-independent which makes healthcare monitoring both flexible and ubiquitous, that is, not confined to specific settings, such as hospitals (Istepanian & Lacal, 2003). While also generating potentially significant cost savings (e.g. by reducing false positive or non serious hospitalisations) for managing the care of non-critical diabetes sufferers our solution will also improve their quality of life

(Istepanian, Jovanov, & Zhang, 2004; Mirza et al., 2008; Norris, 2002). This may, thus, facilitate adoption of the proposed solution.

Third, the ageing population in Australia combined with the fragmented nature of the Australian healthcare system that is designed to treat episodic conditions, and the generally poor awareness of life style implications will increase the pressure on this system for better chronic disease treatment standards over longer periods (ABS, 2003; Rowland, 2003). The pervasive nature of our solution combined with its ability to offer targeted and tailored health messages can contribute to ease that pressure, and consequently, become a facilitator for its adoption in Australia (Neville et al., 2002).

Fourth, there is evidence suggesting that to date, some sectors of the healthcare system in Australia have not been convinced of the benefits of ICT in general and pervasive mobile solutions in particular (Yu, Li, & Gagnon, 2008). At least partially, this is due clinicians' preference and bias towards traditional face-to-face forms of interactions with their patients (Skulimowski, 2006). Furthermore, in a recent study, Australian nurses and clinicians

*Figure 5. ICT support for diabetes*

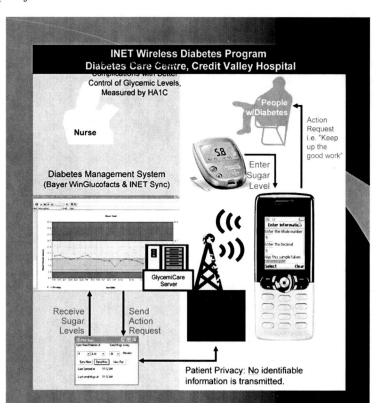

considered that the vast majority of employers did not encourage ICT training, and for those for whom training was available, heavy workloads were considered to be major barriers for training uptake (Eley et al., 2008). Taken together, these factors are expected to become barriers for the adoption of the proposed solution. Organisational changes, including establishment or awareness and training are, thus, required for extended adoption and diffusion (Mirza et al., 2008).

Fifth, our proposed solution is expected to be highly cost-effective for people with diabetes. For example, costs to patients are estimated to be confined to data transfer charges which include the systematic texting (e.g. by SMS) of glycemic levels (measured by HA1C readings). With increasing competition amongst Australian operators, data transfer charges are expected to decrease in the future (Troshani & Rao, 2007a).

Another possible cost to patients may include mobile handset acquisition. However, with a very high mobile penetration rate in Australia, diabetes patients are likely to already be in possession of mobile phones (Rao & Troshani, 2007a, 2007b). Nevertheless, our proposed solution may require investment outlays from health providers. Initial setup, operational, and supporting infrastructure costs may be barriers for the smooth adoption of our solution in Australia (Khambati et al., 2008).

Sixth, perceptions of security and privacy are likely to have a strong bearing on the successful adoption of the proposed solution. Although the proposed model accounts for protection of patient information in terms of privacy, security, and reliability, both individual and organisational adopters are expected to require solid guarantees that continuous security improvements will reliably safeguard the privacy of patient data. Nevertheless, extant research shows that these concerns may dissipate over time as mobile technology matures and benefits and convenience begin to be experienced on a wide scale (Mirza et al., 2008).

Finally, other factors that, in various forms, may become barriers for the adoption or our solution in Australia include existing disparate legacy systems and possible integration costs, lack of standards and limited bandwidth (Mirza et al., 2008).

## FUTURE RESEARCH DIRECTIONS

Given the general global consensus that effective and efficient healthcare delivery will only occur through the judicious application of ICTs (Lacroix, 1999; Frost and Sullivan, 2004; Porter and Tiesberg, 2006; Kulkarni and Nathanson, 2005; Wickramasinghe et al., 2007), it is inevitable that, as we move into the second decade of the 21st century, the prevalence of ICTs to facilitate the delivery of value driven healthcare will increase. We believe in such a climate our proposed solution will be even more appropriate not only because it utilises ICTs to provide superior healthcare delivery in the case of diabetic patients but it is also simple to implement and use and cost effective both at the micro and macro levels. These levels include both individual patients and clinicians and organisations including public and private healthcare providers.

Nevertheless, it is anticipated that increased adoption and diffusion of chronic disease mobile self-care solutions may depend increasingly less on technology and increasingly more on acceptability by both patients and clinicians on the one hand and on organisational healthcare providers on the other. Clearly, these mobile solutions need to suit and be consistent with both patient lifestyles and work practices undertaken by clinicians within healthcare provider organisations. This may be indicative that education programs and promotional campaigns may need to be undertaken for enhancing awareness and incentivising adoption. Tested processes and procedures will result that greatly facilitate the creation of personal medical records and effective and efficient forms of interaction with patients who suffer from a very debilitating chronic disease such as diabetes.

We also believe that this model can be extended and adapted to provide the necessary monitoring and self-care to other chronic diseases including but not limited to hypertension, cardiac conditions and obesity. Diseases of this nature require daily tests and continuous monitoring which are typically essential to recommended treatment. However, widespread adoption and diffusion of mobile self-care solutions for chronic disease management also implies that practical steps may need to be undertaken in the future concerning the development, implementation, and evaluation of information standards as well as subsequent integration with healthcare legacy systems.

## CONCLUSION

We set out to present a case for the need to embrace a pervasive technology solution for the superior monitoring of diabetes self-care for patients in Australia. We proffered the INET wireless solution as a suitable solution, for many reasons including that it is equally successful in controlling both type I and type II diabetes, is as effective irrespective of patient's age, socio economic standing or location and has minimal risks and a very slight learning curve (if at all). We contend that if such a model were to be incorporated into the Australian context the growing segment of the population suffering from diabetes would have a convenient, cost effective and superior means of monitoring and thereby controlling their diabetes while in turn enjoying a better quality of life.

The INET wireless diabetes solution facilitates governments, associations, pharmaceutical firms, researchers, healthcare professionals and other healthcare stakeholders that are looking for improved and measurable outcomes among patients suffering from diabetes. Specific benefits ranges from decreasing diabetes related complications to reducing the economic burden on the health system.

We realise that further research is required to test the proposed solution in the Australian healthcare setting including testing of aspects, such as perceived ease of use, perceived usefulness, etc., however, we close by warning that if a pervasive technology solution is not sought for the monitoring and support of diabetes self-care not only will this chronic disease become a silent epidemic but it will also be a very costly burden for both the healthcare sector and the community at large.

# REFERENCES

ABS. (2003). *Population Projections, Australia, 2002-2101, Cat. No. 3222.0.* Canberra, Australia: Australian Bureau of Statistics.

AIHW. (2008). *Diabetes: Australian Facts 2008.* Canberra, Australia: Australian Institute of Health and Welfare.

Balas, E. A., Krishna, S., Kretschmer, R. A., Cheek, T. R., Lobach, D. F., & Boren, S. A. (2004). Computerized knowledge management in diabetes care. *Medical Care, 42*(6), 610–621. doi:10.1097/01.mlr.0000128008.12117.f8

Bodenheimer, T., Lorig, K., Holman, H., & Grumbach, K. (2002). Patient self-management of chronic disease in primary care. [JAMA]. *Journal of the American Medical Association, 288*(19), 2469–2475. doi:10.1001/jama.288.19.2469

Britt, H., Miller, G. C., Charles, J., Pan, Y., Valenti, L., & Henderson, J. (2007). *General Practice Activity in Australia 2005-06, Cat. no. GEP 16.* Canberra, Australia: AIHW.

Chau, S., & Turner, P. (2006). Utilisation of mobile handheld devices for care management at an Australian aged care facility. *Electronic Commerce Research and Applications, 5,* 305–312. doi:10.1016/j.elerap.2006.04.005

Chittleborough, C. R., Grant, J. F., Phillips, P. J., & Taylor, A. W. (2007). The increasing prevalence of diabetes in South Australia: the relationship with population ageing and obesity. *Public Health, 121,* 92–99. doi:10.1016/j.puhe.2006.09.017

Colagiuri, S., Colagiuri, R., & Ward, J. (1998). *National Diabetes Strategy and Implementation Plan.* Canberra, Australia: Diabetes Australia.

DiabCostAustralia. (2002). *Assessing the Burden of Type 2 Diabetes in Australia.* Adelaide, Australia: DiabCost Australia.

DiabetesAustralia. (2008). Diabetes in Australia. *Journal.* Retrieved from http://www.diabetesaustralia.com.au/Understanding-Diabetes/Diabetes-in-Australia/

Dixon, T., & Webbie, K. (2006). *The National System for Monitoring Diabetes in Australia (AIHW Cat. No. CVD 32).* Canberra, Australia: Australian Institute of Health and Wealfare.

Eley, R., Fallon, T., Soar, J., Buikstra, E., & Hegney, D. (2008). The status of training and education in information and computer technology of Australian nurses: a national survey. *Journal of Clinical Nursing, 17,* 2758–2767. doi:10.1111/j.1365-2702.2008.02285.x

*Frost and Sullivan Country Industry Forecast – European Union Healthcare Industry.* (2004, May 11). Retrieved from http://www.news-medical.net/print_article.asp?id=1405

Goldberg, S. a. (2002a). *Building the Evidence for a standardized Mobile Internet (wireless) Environment in Ontario, Canada, January Update, Internal INET Documentation.* Ontario, Canada: INET.

Goldberg, S. a. (2002b). *HTA Presentational Selection and Aggregation Component Summary. Internal INET Documentation.* Ontario, Canada: INET.

Goldberg, S. a. (2002c). *Wireless POC Device Component Summary, Internal INET documentation.* Ontario, Canada: INET.

Goldberg, S. a. (2002d). *HTA Presentation Rendering Component Summary, Internal INET documentation.* Ontario, Canada: INET.

Goldberg, S. a. (2002e). *HTA Quality Assurance Component Summary, Internal INET documentation.* Ontario, Canada: INET.

Hunt, D. (2007). *Urgent health system reform needed to tackle disease epidemic, says head of new University of Melbourne centre.* Retrieved 25 November, 2008, from http://uninews.unimelb.edu.au/view.php?articleID=4615

ICIC. (2008). Improving Chronic Illness Care: The Chronic Care Model. *Journal.* Retrieved from http://www.improvingchroniccare.org/indix.php?p=The_Chronic_Care_Model&s=2

Istepanian, R. S. H., Jovanov, E., & Zhang, Y. T. (2004). Guest Editorial: Introduction to the special section on m-health: beyond seamless mobility and global wireless healthcare connectivity. *IEEE Transactions on Information Technology in Biomedicine, 8*(4), 405–414. doi:10.1109/TITB.2004.840019

Istepanian, R. S. H., & Lacal, J. C. (2003). *Emerging mobile communication technologies for health: some imperative notes on m-health.* Paper presented at the 25th Annual International Conference of the IEEE EMBS, New York.

Joshy, G., & Simmons, D. (2006). Diabetes information systems: a rapidly emerging support for diabetes surveillance and care. *Diabetes Technology & Therapeutics, 8*(5), 587–597. doi:10.1089/dia.2006.8.587

Khambati, A., Warren, J., Grundy, J., & Hosking, J. (2008). *A model driven approach to care planning systems for consumer engagement in chronic disease management.* Paper presented at the HIC 2008 Australia's Health Informatics Conference, Health Informatics Society of Australia Ltd (HISA).

Knuiman, M. W., Welborn, T. A., & Bartholomew, H. C. (1996). Self-reported health and use of health services: a comparison of diabetic and nondiabetic persons from a national sample. *Australian and New Zealand Journal of Public Health, 20*(3), 241–247. doi:10.1111/j.1467-842X.1996.tb01023.x

Kulkarni, R., & Nathanson, L. A. (2005). *Medical Informatics in medicine.* E-Medicine at http://www.emedicine.com/emerg/topic879.htm

Lacroix, A. (1999). International concerted action on collaboration in telemedicine: G8 sub-project 4. *Studies in Health Technology and Informatics, 64,* 12–19.

Mirza, F., Norris, T., & Stockdale, R. (2008). Mobile technologies and the holistic management of chronic diseases. *Health Informatics Journal, 14*(4), 309–321. doi:10.1177/1460458208096559

Neville, G., Greene, A., McLeod, J., & Tracy, A. (2002). Mobile phone text messaging can help young people with asthma. *British Medical Journal, 325,* 600. doi:10.1136/bmj.325.7364.600/a

Norris, A. C. (2002). *Essentials of Telemedicine and Telecare.* Chichester, UK: Wiley.

Opie, A. (1998). Nobody's asked me for my view: users' empowerment by multidisciplinary health teams. *Qualitative Health Research, 18,* 188–206. doi:10.1177/104973239800800204

Porter, M., & Tiesberg, E. (2006). *Re-defining health care delivery.* Boston: Harvard Business Press.

Poulton, B. C. (1999). User involvement in identifying health needs and shaping and evaluating services: is it being raised? *Journal of Advanced Nursing, 30*(6), 1289–1296. doi:10.1046/j.1365-2648.1999.01224.x

Rachlis, M. (2006). *Key to sustainable healthcare system.* Available http://www.improveinchronic-care.org

Radin, P. (2006). To me, it's my life: medical communication, trust, and activism in cyberspace. *Social Science & Medicine, 6,* 591–601. doi:10.1016/j.socscimed.2005.06.022

Rao, S., & Troshani, I. (2007a). AMC-ER Challenges and Rewards: Experiences of Australian Content Exporters. Adelaide, South Australia: Australian Mobile Content – Export Research Initiative, m.Net Corporation Ltd.

Rao, S., & Troshani, I. (2007b). AMC-ER Initial Selection of Content, Markets, and Distribution Channels for the Australian Mobile Content – Export Research Initiative. Adelaide, Australia: m.Net Corporation Ltd.

Rasmussen, B., Wellard, S., & Nankervis, A. (2001). Consumer issues in navigating health care services for type I diabetes. *Journal of Clinical Nursing, 10,* 628–634. doi:10.1046/j.1365-2702.2001.00550.x

Reach, G., Zerrouki, D., Leclercq, D., & d'Ivernois, J. F. (2005). Adjusting insulin doses: from knowledge to decision. *Patient Education and Counseling, 56*(1), 98–103. doi:10.1016/j.pec.2004.01.001

Rowland, D. (2003). An ageing population: emergence of a new stage of life? In Khoo, S., & McDonald, P. (Eds.), *The Transformation of Australia's Population: 1970-2030* (pp. 239–265). Sydney: UNSW Press.

Rudi, R., & Celler, B. G. (2006). *Design and implementation of expert-telemedicine system for diabetes management at home.* Paper presented at the International Conference on Biomedical and Pharmaceutical Enginering 2006 (ICBPE2006), IEEE, 11-14 December 2006, Singapore.

Russell, L. B., Churl Suh, D., & Safford, M. M. (2005). Time requirements for diabetes management: too much for many? *The Journal of Family Practice, 54*(1), 52–56.

Skulimowski, A. M. (2006). *The Challenges to the Medical Decision Making System posed by mHealth.* Kraków, Poland: Centre for Decision Sciences and Forecasting, Progress & Business Foundation, Institute for Prospective Technological Studies (IPTS). Available http://ipts.jrc.ec.europa.eu/home/report/english/articles/vol81/ICT1E816.htm

Tong, B., & Stevenson, C. (2007). *Comorbidity of cardiovascular disease, diabetes and chronic kidney disease in Australia, AIHW cat. no. CVD 37.* Canberra, Australia: AIHW.

Troshani, I., & Rao, S. (2007a). The diffusion of mobile services in Australia: an evaluation using stakeholder and transaction cost economics theories. *IADIS International Journal of WWW/Internet, 5*(2), 40-57.

Van Eyk, H., & Baum, F. (2002). Learning about interagency collaboration: Trialling collaborative projects between hospitals and community health services. *Health & Social Care in the Community, 10*(4), 262–269. doi:10.1046/j.1365-2524.2002.00369.x

Vanjara, P. (2006). Application of mobile technologies in healthcare diagnostics and administration. In Lazakidou, A. (Ed.), *Handbook of Research on Informatics in Healthcare and Medicine* (pp. 113–130). Hershey, PA: Idea Group.

Victorian Government. (2007). *Diabetes Prevention and Management: A Strategic Framework for Victoria 1007-2010.* Melbourne, Australia: Victorian Government, Department of Human Services.

Wellard, S. J., Rennie, S., & King, R. (2008). Perceptions of people with type 2 diabetes about self-management and the efficiency of community based services. *Contemporary Nurse, 29*(2), 218–226.

Wickramasinghe, N., & Goldberg, S. (2003). *The wireless panacea for healthcare.* Paper presented at the 36th Hawaii International Conference on System Sciences, Hawaii, 6-10 January, IEEE.

Wickramasinghe, N., & Goldberg, S. (2004). How M=EC2 in healthcare. *International Journal of Mobile Communications, 2*(2), 140–156. doi:10.1504/IJMC.2004.004664

Wickramasinghe, N., Goldberg, S., & Bali, R. (2007). Enabling Superior M-health Project Success: A tri-Country Validation. *Intl. J. Services and Standards, 4*(1), 97–117. doi:10.1504/IJSS.2008.016087

Wickramasinghe, N., & Misra, S. (2004). A wireless trust model for healthcare. *International Journal of e-Health, 1*, 60-77.

Wickramasinghe, N., & Schaffer, J. (2006). Creating knowledge driven healthcare processes with the intelligence continuum. *International Journal of Electronic Healthcare, 2*(2), 164–174.

Wickramasinghe, N., Schaffer, J., & Geisler, E. (2005). Assessing e-health. In Spil, T., & Schuring, R. (Eds.), *E-Health Systems Diffusion and Use: The Innovation, The User, and The User IT Model.* Hershey, PA: Idea Group.

Wild, S., Roglic, G., Green, A., Sicree, R., & King, H. (2004). Global prevalence of diabetes: estimates for the year 2000 and projections for 2030. *Diabetes Care, 27*, 1047–1053. doi:10.2337/diacare.27.5.1047

Yu, P., Li, H., & Gagnon, M.-P. (2008). Health IT acceptance factors in long-term care facilities: a cross-sectional survey. *International Journal of Health Informatics.* doi:10.1016/j.ijmedinf.2008.07.006.

Zigbor, J. C., & Songer, T. J. (2001). External barriers to diabetes care: addressing personal and health systems issues. *Diabetes Spectrum, 14*, 23–28. doi:10.2337/diaspect.14.1.23

## ADDITIONAL READING

Al HArkim. L 2007 Web Mobile-Based Applications for Healthcare Management IGI, Hershey

Spil, T., & Schuring, R. (2006). *E-Health Systems Diffusion and Use.* IGI Hershey.

Wickramasinghe, N. (2009). *Healthcare Knowledge Management Primer.* New York: Routledge.

*A previous version of this chapter was originally published in International Journal of Healthcare Delivery Reform Initiatives, Vol. 1, Issue 4, edited by M. Guah, copyright 2010 by IGI Publishing (an imprint of IGI Global).*

# Chapter 7
# Pervasive Process–Based Healthcare Systems on a Grid Environment

**Vassiliki Koufi**
*University of Piraeus, Greece*

**Flora Malamateniou**
*University of Piraeus, Greece*

**George Vassilacopoulos**
*University of Piraeus, Greece*

## ABSTRACT

*Healthcare is an increasingly collaborative enterprise involving many individuals and organizations that coordinate their efforts toward promoting quality and efficient delivery of healthcare through the use of pervasive healthcare information systems. The latter can provide seamless access to well-informed, high-quality healthcare services anywhere, anytime by removing temporal, spatial and other constraints imposed by the technological heterogeneity of existing healthcare information systems. In such environments, concerns over the privacy and security of health information arise. Hence, it is essential to provide an effective access control mechanism that meets the requirements imposed by the least privilege principle by adjusting user permissions continuously in order to adapt to the current situation. This chapter presents a pervasive grid-based healthcare information system architecture that facilitates authorized access to healthcare processes via wireless devices. Context-aware technologies are used to both automate healthcare processes and regulate access to services and data via a fine-grained access control mechanism.*

## INTRODUCTION

Healthcare delivery is a highly complex process involving a broad range of healthcare services (e.g.

in-patient, out-patient, emergency), typically performed by a number of geographically distributed and organizationally disparate healthcare providers requiring increased collaboration and coordination of their activities in order to provide shared and integrated care when and where needed (Koufi &

DOI: 10.4018/978-1-61520-765-7.ch007

Vassilacopoulos, 2008). As healthcare providers are mostly hosting diverse information systems, promoting quality and efficient delivery of healthcare, requires the use of interoperable healthcare information systems (HIS). With the advent of pervasive and ubiquitous computing technologies, the requirements for information technology to healthcare process alignment can be met with the least possible intervention from the participating parties. For example, an HIS architecture that places emphasis on supporting collaboration and coordination among various healthcare services can also fulfill the requirements to support mobility of healthcare professionals that may lead to a pervasive computing infrastructure. Thus, patient information which is scattered around disparate and geographically dispersed systems can be readily accessed in a pervasive manner by authorized users at the point of care.

This chapter will present a grid-enabled HIS architecture that facilitates seamless and pervasive access to integrated healthcare services by utilizing both wireless and agent technologies. This architecture utilizes the Business Process Execution Language (BPEL) for modeling healthcare processes, Grid middleware technology for resolving data integration issues and Radio Frequency Identification (RFID) technology for user identification. Thus, healthcare processes performed within the boundaries of a health district are modeled as flows of Grid database services which provide an integrated or even derived view of data retrieved by multiple distributed data resources, such as relational and XML databases (Open Grid Services Architecture - Data Access and Integration, n.d.). In addition, agent technology is used for implementing a context-aware authorization mechanism to conveniently and effectively regulate user access to patient information while providing confidence that security policies are faithfully and consistently enforced. The system functionality is delivered to the healthcare professionals' personal digital assistants (PDAs) via a customized Grid portal application that complies with the restrictions imposed by PDA technology (e.g. limited display size).

One important consideration in the development of such an HIS is to secure personal information against unauthorized access, collection, use, disclosure or disposal by ensuring a tight matching of permissions to actual usage and need. To this end, the least privilege principle should be enforced which, in turn, requires continuous adjustments of the sets of user permissions to ensure that, at any time, users assume the minimum sets of permissions required for the execution of each task of a healthcare process. The system architecture presented here implements a dynamic, context-aware access control mechanism that incorporates the advantages of broad, role-based permission assignment and administration across object types, as in role-based access control (RBAC) (National Institute of Standards and Technology (NIST), n.d.), and yet provides the flexibility for adjusting role permissions on individual objects during a BPEL process enactment according to the current context. During the execution of a process instance, changes in contextual information are sensed to adapt user permissions to the minimum required for completing a job. Relevant access control policies are enforced at both the BPEL task level and the Grid database service level.

## BACKGROUND

Currently, healthcare providers often have trouble sharing information because of discrepancies between data storage platforms. Thus, a need arises for a more integrated and interoperable health information space. Grid systems may provide a means to manage the increasing volumes of patient data since they can serve as an integration infrastructure for shared and coordinated use of diverse data resources in virtual healthcare organizations comprised of geographically distributed and organizationally disparate healthcare providers (Pereira, Muppavarapu & Chung, 2006; Malamateniou & Vassilacopoulos, 2003). Moreover, service orientation of the Grid makes it a promising platform for seamless and dynamic development, integration and deployment of service-oriented healthcare information systems using business process technologies and Grid database services (Koufi, Papakonstantinou & Vassilacopoulos, 2006). BPEL is one of the strongest business process technologies (Pasley, 2005). It provides a standard, XML-based platform that expresses a business process's event sequence and collaboration logic, whereas the underlying grid database services provide the process functionality. These services can be created by using middleware products such as Open Grid Services Architecture - Data Access and Integration (OGSA – DAI) (Open Grid Services Architecture - Data Access and Integration, n.d.), which is part of the Globus Toolkit (The Globus Alliance, n.d.).

Grid database services are built as an extension to Web services and deliver added-value, high level data management functionality. As the existing Grid middleware, including the Globus Toolkit, does not support mobility in the Grid nodes and is generally suitable only for high-profile service providers and clients (Khatua, Dasgupta & Mukherjee, 2006), system functionality can be delivered to healthcare professionals at the point of care by providing access to the Grid services in a ubiquitous and pervasive manner (i.e. via mobile and wireless clients).

Since their introduction in the early 1990s, Personal Digital Assistants (PDAs) have become increasingly popular for a large variety of applications in the healthcare domain (Grabowski, Lewandowski & Russell, 2004). Several facilities have integrated the use of wireless network enabled PDAs into their practice sites as they consider that it better meets a healthcare professional's needs. This is due to the fact that they provide a considerably larger screen than mobile phones and, as opposed to portable PCs and netbooks, they can slide smoothly in the professional's gown pocket. Thus, PDAs are used as extensions of an integrated office-based computer system and can provide online access to different information services (Bergeron BP, 2002; Muller, Frankewitsch, Ganslandt, Burkle & Prokosch, 2004). Due to the limitations imposed by PDA technology (e.g. operating system restrictions), these services are mostly web-based.

A Grid portal, being a secure and highly customizable online environment for gathering information about Grid services and resources, can deliver complex Grid solutions to users through a web browser without requiring either download and install specialized software or set up networks, firewalls and port policies, accordingly (Thomas, Burruss, Cinquini, Fox, Gannon & Gilbert, 2005). Hence, Grid-enabled portals have been proven to provide effective mechanisms for exposing distributed systems to general user communities without forcing them to deal with the complexities of the underlying systems (Thomas, Burruss, Cinquini, Fox, Gannon & Gilbert, 2005). On these grounds, a Grid portal application that complies with the restrictions imposed by PDA technology seems an ideal solution for the provision of pervasive access to Grid healthcare processes.

One major concern when developing healthcare applications is related to inaccurate patient identification as it may compromise patient safety (e.g. misidentification of a patient may lead to a healthcare professional obtaining an incomplete or incorrect medical history) (BASEscan, n.d.). Automatic patient identification can provide a means to eliminate identification-related medical errors while increasing work efficiency of healthcare professionals. Nowadays, there are two automatic identification technologies vying for acceptance in the healthcare field. These are barcoding and radio frequency identification (RFID). Both perform similar functions but in significantly different ways. However, RFID tends to be preferred over barcoding as there are a few cases where it can prove to be more beneficial. For example, in the case that a patient is in isolation due to an infection, RFID enables identification from just outside the room or contaminated area, eliminating the need to cleanse or sterilize the device (Inglesby & Inglesby, 2005). In RFID, identification and other data are stored in small devices named RFID tags, which can be either active or passive. Active RFID tags have a built-in power supply, such as a battery, as well as electronics that perform specialized tasks (American Barcode and RFID, n.d.). By contrast, passive RFID tags do not have a power supply and must rely on the power emitted by an RFID reader to transmit data (American Barcode and RFID, n.d.). Thus, a passive tag cannot communicate any data if a reader is not present, whereas an active tag can communicate data in the absence of a reader.

## RELATED WORK

During the last few years, there has been a trend towards the development of applications to assist healthcare professionals. Moreover, research efforts regarding the advancement of pervasiveness of existing healthcare information systems have been on the rise (DOCMEM, 2003; MOBI-DEV, 2005; IHE, 2005; C-CARE, 2005; DOC@HAND, 2006, Akogrimo, 2007, TrustCare, 2008).

DOCMEM (DOCMEM, 2003) proposes an advanced interactive environment for getting a ubiquitous, permanent and intelligent access to patients' medical files stored on a secured server in their hospital. In addition, the proposed environment enables ambulatory and in-hospital medical doctors to communicate patient's information with other independent healthcare professionals or with a hospital. Similar functionality is provided by MOBI-DEV (MOBI-DEV, 2005) which provides a new generation of mobile devices for healthcare professionals working in and outside of hospitals. MOBI-DEV enables access to the hospital information system at any time from anywhere. Security is assured via suitable mechanisms for data transmission and management as well as authentication and certification of users.

IHE (IHE, 2005) defines a common framework to deliver the basic interoperability needed for local, regional and nationwide health information networks. C-CARE (C-CARE, 2005) improves access to essential personal clinical data at any time by authorized healthcare professionals. Finally, DOC@HAND (DOC@HAND, 2006) provides healthcare professionals with an integrated environment which helps them to collect the information and knowledge required for a more informed decision making on diagnoses, therapies and protocols. This environment is accessible from portable platforms such as table PCs.

The aforementioned studies involve the provision of pervasive and ubiquitous access to patient medical data through the use of wireless and mobile devices. However, they don't handle data management and access control in the context of a Grid-based, process-oriented healthcare environment. Moreover, both DOCMEM and MOBI-DEV provide access to patient information stored at a specific healthcare organization. IHE initiative profiles enable sharing of patient information in support of optimal patient care but arise new problems due to lack of flexibility for adoption to different organizational conditions and lack of security integration in the different profiles (Wozak, Ammenwerth, Hoerbst, Soegner, Mair & Schabetsberger, 2008). Finally, both C-CARE and DOC@HAND support ubiquitous access to a collection of essential, relevant and up-to-date patient information but the access control mechanisms employed for ensuring patient privacy are static as they lack context-awareness features.

Akogrimo (Akogrimo, 2007) is a research effort concerned with the development of a Grid-based healthcare information system intended for use by both citizens and healthcare providers. In particular, Akogrimo aims at providing pervasive healthcare services by means of dynamic personalized workflows. However, when it comes to security issues it lacks an efficient, context-aware authorization mechanism capable of safeguarding patient privacy.

A combination of pervasive computing and workflow systems technology has been proposed by (Bundgaard Hildebrandt and Hojsgaard, 2008) who initiated research project on Trustworthy Pervasive Healthcare Services (TrustCare). The aim of the project is to contribute to the foundations of IT-systems able to support trustworthy pervasive workflows and services within the healthcare sector.

In this chapter an HIS architecture is proposed that combines BPEL and Grid technologies in an attempt to orchestrate geographically dispersed Grid database services concerned with healthcare delivery within and across healthcare organizations (Ranganathan & McFaddin, 2004). Thus, healthcare processes are modelled using BPEL and Grid database services are created using OGSA-DAI middleware to provide integrated access to healthcare databases irrespective of the network location they reside. Moreover, the system provides pervasive and authorized access both to BPEL tasks and to Grid database services. Security is enforced by a context-aware, certificate-based access control mechanism that mediates between subjects (healthcare professionals) and objects (BPEL tasks and Grid database services) and decides whether access of a given subject to a given object should be permitted or denied. Thus, the risk of compromising patient privacy is reduced.

## METHODOLOGIES AND TOOLS FOR THE DEVELOPMENT OF PERVASIVE HEALTHCARE APPLICATIONS

Healthcare technologies are increasingly pervasive, moving into the working environment of health care professionals and homes of the patients, presenting new challenges to design of pervasive healthcare applications. Experience has shown that designing such pervasive systems is extremely difficult and approaches used for this purpose tend to be subjective, piecemeal or both

(Neely, Stevenson, Kray, Mulder, Connelly & Siek, 2008).

One approach to the design of pervasive healthcare systems is based on the combined use of Unified Modeling Language (UML) and Colored Petri Nets (CPN) language (Jorgensen, 2002). UML models are suitable particularly for modeling the behavior of static aspects of the system while Colored Petri Nets (CPN) language is believed to be suitable for modeling the behavior of the dynamic aspects of the system. This approach, based on the aforementioned models, enables the evaluation and comparison of the behavioral consequences of alternative design proposals prior to implementation.

For the development of pervasive healthcare applications, a model-driven prototyping approach has been proposed according to which a number of tools like graphical editors and generators can be used to simplify the development of pervasive health application prototypes that typically span multiple platforms (Kurschl, Mitsch & Schoenboeck, 2008).

Pervasive applications are distributed, mobile, adaptive and consider context as a first-order concept. Thus, a major challenge that needs to be faced when developing such applications is the implementation of adaptive behavior which is not easy due to its ad hoc specific nature (Augustin, Yamin, Da Silva, Real, Frainer & Geyer, 2006). Suggestions for context-aware infrastructures and applications are numerous in Pervasive and Ubiquitous Computing research, including suggestions for the use of context-aware technologies in a hospital setting. For example, the 'Intelligent Hospital' application (Mitchell, Spiteri, Bates & Coulouris, 2000) uses location awareness to enable video communication to follow clinicians around inside a hospital, and others have been adding context-awareness to the use of mobile technologies in hospitals (Kjeldskov, J. & Skov, M., 2004; Munoz, Rodriguez, Favela, Martinez-Garcia & Gonzalez, 2003).

Among the main approaches that appear in the literature with regard to context-awareness are Agent-Centered Context-Awareness (ACCA), where context revolves around the perception an agent has of its environment, and User-Centered Context-Awareness (UCCA), where context is the global, emergent picture that devices help build of an individual in its environment (Roy, Abdulrazak & Belala, 2008). Under both approaches, agents have to be in a continual state of re-evaluation with respect to available context sources, potential partner nodes to share processing and trade information, failure of shared and ongoing transactions, etc. (Roy, Abdulrazak & Belala, 2008). UCCA strives for at least one globally agreed-upon state, profile, while ACCA accepts local, distinct perceptions of context for each agent (Roy, Abdulrazak & Belala, 2008).

## A HEALTHCARE DELIVERY SCENARIO

The basic motivation for this research stems from our involvement in a recent project concerned with defining and automating cross-organizational healthcare processes spanning a health district in order to implement a district-wide, process-oriented healthcare information system. The interoperability requirements and the stringent security needs of the system, where sensitive patient information is used, motivated this work and provided some of the background supportive information for developing the prototype presented in this chapter.

Typically, a health district consists of one district general hospital (DGH) and a number of peripheral hospitals and health centers. As patient information is scattered around disparate and geographically dispersed systems and patient referrals are usually made among various healthcare providers within a district (e.g. for hospitalization, for outpatient consultation or for performing spe-

cialized medical procedures), there is a need to ensure that an interoperable environment is created and that authorized access to healthcare process tasks and to patient information required through the execution of these tasks is provided.

Suppose a healthcare process which is concerned with the medical activities that may be performed during a physician's clinical ward round. Among others, this process involves assessing patient's condition, accessing the patient's medical record and issuing medical orders. As an example, consider the case where a patient's physician wishes to issue a radiological request for one of his/her patients. The request is sent to the radiology department of the hospital which schedules the radiological procedure requested and sends a message to the requesting physician notifying him/her on the date and time scheduled. After performing the radiological procedure requested, the radiologist accesses the relevant part of the patient record, writes a radiological report and sends it to the requesting physician.

Figure 1 shows a high-level view of the healthcare sub-process concerned with radiology orders using the IBM WebSphere Workflow build-time tool (IBM Corporation, 2005). In this business process two organizational units of the hospital are involved: the clinical department and the radiology department of a hospital. Two of the roles participating in the healthcare process are: clinical physician (physician) and radiologist (radiologist). Table 1 shows an extract of authorization requirements regarding task execution and related data access privileges assigned to these roles, respectively. Similar requirements exist in many healthcare application fields where request-service situations occur (Poulymenopoulou, Malamateniou & Vassilacopoulos, 2005).

From an authorization perspective, the healthcare process of Figure 1 surfaces several requirements with regard to task execution and Grid database services invocation. These requirements include the following:

*Figure 1. A high level view of a radiological request process model using IBM WebSphere Workflow build-time*

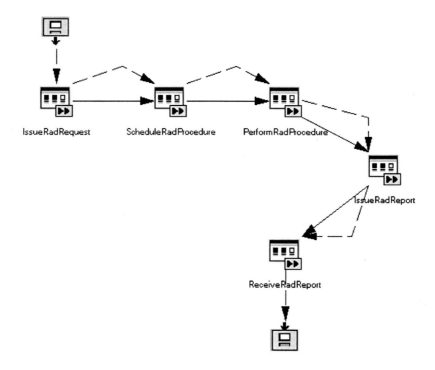

*Table 1. Extract of authorization requirements for the healthcare process of Figure 1 (Task execution and data access permissions)*

| 1. | Physicians may issue requests for radiological procedures on patients while on duty and within the hospital premises (IssueRadRequest). |
|---|---|
| 1.1 | Physicians may write radiological requests for their current patients. |
| 1.2 | Physicians may edit radiological requests for their current patients before sent. |
| 1.3 | Physicians may send radiological requests for their current patients. |
| 1.4 | Physicians may cancel radiological requests for their current patients after sent. |
| 1.5 | Physicians may read patient records of their current patients. |
| 2. | Radiologists holding a specific sub-specialty may perform only relevant radiological procedures on patients (RerformRadProcedure) |
| 3. | Radiologists may issue patient-oriented radiological reports on request by physicians (IssueRadReport). |
| 3.1 | Radiologists may read patient record data before sending their radiological reports. |
| 3.2 | Radiologists may write patient-oriented radiological reports for their current patients. |
| 3.3 | Radiologists may edit patient-oriented radiological reports for their current patients before sent. |
| 3.4 | Radiologists may send patient-oriented radiological requests for their current patients |
| 3.5 | Radiologists may cancel patient-oriented radiological reports after sent. |
| 3.6 | Radiologists may read past patient radiological reports prepared by them. |
| 4. | Physicians may receive patient radiological reports issued by radiologists only if requested by them (ReceiveRadReport). |
| 4.1 | Physicians may read the requested radiological reports on their patients. |
| 4.2 | Physicians may read patient records of their patients. |

- *Task execution:* In certain circumstances the candidates for a task instance execution should be dynamically determined and be either a sub-group of the authorized users or only one, specific authorized user. For example, the request for a radiological report (issued by a physician) should be routed only to the sub-group of radiologists who hold the relevant sub-specialty (e.g. CT or MRI) and the radiological report (issued by a radiologist) should be routed only to the requesting physician.

- *Data access:* Given that a role holder can execute a specific task, he/she should be allowed to exercise a dynamically determined set of permissions on certain data objects only. For example, during the execution of the "IssueRadRequest" task, a physician is allowed to read patient record data and to issue (write, edit and send) radiological requests only for his/her patients while on duty and within the hospital premises.

- *Permission propagation:* Some role holders should receive additional permissions on certain data objects in order to effectively execute a task but these permissions should be revoked upon successful execution of the task. For example, for an effective execution of the "IssueRadReport" task with regard to a patient, in response to a request submitted by a physician, a radiologist should receive the permission to read the patient's record but he/she should not be allowed to retain this permission after successful task execution.

The above requirements suggest that certain data access permissions of the healthcare process participants depend on the process execution context. In particular, contextual information available at access time, such as user-to-patient proximity, location of attempted access and time of attempted access, can influence the authorization decision regarding task execution and, given this permis-

sion, associated Grid database service invocation to access the relevant data objects. This enables a more flexible and precise access control policy specification that satisfies the least privilege principle by incorporating the advantages of having broad, role-based permissions across BPEL tasks and data object types, like RBAC, yet enhanced with the ability to simultaneously support the following features: (a) predicate-based access control, limiting user access to specific data objects, (b) a permission propagation function from one role holder to another in certain circumstances, and (c) determining qualified task performers during a process instance based not only on the role-to-task permission policy, specified at process build time, but also on application data processed during the process instance. In addition, the model should not incur any significant administrative overhead and should be self-administering to a great extent.

## HEALTHCARE INFORMATION SYSTEM ARCHITECTURE

The proposed system architecture facilitates pervasive access to healthcare processes which, in turn, provide access to integrated patient information through the use of a Grid-based integration and interoperability infrastructure. Figure 2 shows a high-level view of the system architecture, which is described by a three-tier model, comprising of the viewer's site, the server site of the DGH and the Grid.

The first tier essentially refers to the PDA carried by a physician on a ward round. A RFID reader is adapted to the PDA which reads the passive RFID tags placed on wristbands worn by patients. RFID tags contain only the patient's identification number which is the patient's social security number in a machine readable form. Thus, privacy concerns imposed by the use of RFID technology are considerably limited. The PDA contains both RFID software, which is responsible for collect-

*Figure 2. System architecture*

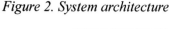

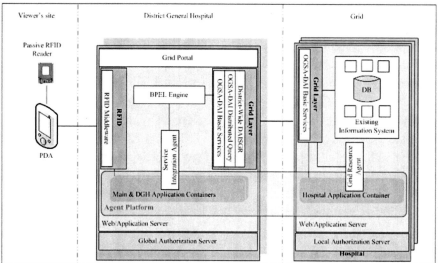

ing raw RFID data, filtering them and submitting them to the RFID middleware installed on a server at the DGH site, and an HTTP(S)-based client, which is the PDA's web browser and provides user interaction with the system.

The second tier is the server site of the DGH and consists of the following components:

- *OGSA-DAI Middleware*: It is the middleware product that addresses the issues related to interoperability of the database management systems residing at each healthcare setting within a health district. In particular, it is used for the generation of the specific Grid database services that manage access to medical data stored in the database of each single healthcare setting. These services can be created by using OGSA-DAI Basic Services and can be combined to provide higher-level web services that support data federation and distributed query processing. The latter are implemented using OGSA-DAI Distributed Query and provide access to district-wide consolidated patient information. A district-wide registry, DAISGR, is

used for discovery of the database services required for a task. WSDL provides the description of these services and how they can be accessed.

- *BPEL Engine*: It handles the execution of BPEL-based healthcare processes provided in the healthcare settings within a health district. The BPEL engine, given a BPEL process definition and a set of inputs, executes the process by invoking the various Grid database services in the right sequence. While executing the process, it controls the data flow between the tasks comprising it and performs monitoring activities.
- *Agent Platform*: It is the software used for the development and deployment of the agents that realize both automated execution of BPEL-based healthcare processes on occurrence of certain events and continuous adjustments of user permissions on BPEL tasks in order to adapt to the current situation. Thus, tight matching of permissions to actual usage and need is ensured.
- *RFID Middleware*: It is the product that mediates between the RFID software

installed on the PDA and the software applications using the information captured by the RFID reader. This middleware applies formatting or logic to tag data captured by the RFID reader in order to convert it to a form that can be processed by any software application. Whenever an event occurs (i.e. a patient's RFID tag is captured) this is communicated along with the processed RFID tag data to the relevant agent which in turn initiates the execution of the relevant process.

- *Grid Portal*: It provides a web-based front end to the system. It consists of a JSR-168 (Java Community Press, n.d.) compliant portlet container that hosts and manages the main portlet of the system, as well as the portlets of the process (BPEL) applications. A portlet is a java web component that generates dynamic content in response to processed requests (Del Vecchio, Hazlewood & Humphrey, 2006). The main portlet of the system provides the Web browser-based portal user interface to the BPEL Engine where all healthcare processes are deployed. In order to provide the required functionality to the users, the portlet uses the engine's web service. Thus interaction with the corresponding processes is enabled. This interaction is performed through certain portlets developed to facilitate the physicians' interaction with the relevant tasks of the process. In particular, a physician accesses the main portlet to instantiate a BPEL process and to execute the tasks he/she is authorized to access. On task execution, the associated Grid database services are located and invoked to retrieve district-wide consolidated patient information.
- *Web/Application Server*: It provides the hosting environment to the aforementioned components.

The third tier is the Grid which comprises of remote data resources where medical data are stored. These are heterogeneous and reside in geographically distributed and organizationally disparate healthcare providers within a health district. The structure of each one of the Grid nodes residing at a healthcare setting is illustrated in Figure 2. Each data resource used for the storing patient information in a healthcare setting is Grid-enabled and the database services exposing it to the Grid are deployed in the web server of the organization and registered with the district-wide DAISGR. The agent platform is used for implementing the agents that perform continuous adjustments of user permissions on Grid database services in order to adapt to the current situation.

## ACCESS CONTROL FRAMEWORK

The movement towards pervasive HIS that meet interoperability requirements has created new challenges for the sharing of health information in a private and secure manner. In particular, when interoperability is realized through the use of a Grid infrastructure on top of which pervasive process-based healthcare systems are built, effort should be put in the development and enforcement of privacy and security policies governing access to both healthcare process tasks and data being accessed through them. Hence, in an interoperable environment like the one illustrated in Figure 2, a robust security framework must be in place in order to ensure that health information follow patients throughout their care in a secure manner.

In this environment, healthcare processes are modeled using BPEL. Access control is one of the aspects of business processes explicitly mentioned to be outside the scope of BPEL (Mendling, Strembeck, Stermsek & Neumann, 2004). Thus, a BPEL process can be executed by everybody who is able to support the relevant partner link types (Mendling, Strembeck, Stermsek & Neu-

*Figure 3. Security architecture*

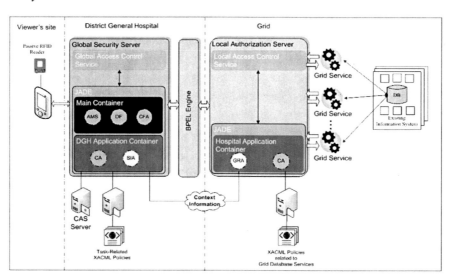

mann, 2004). However, this is inappropriate in the healthcare domain due to the strict security requirements on medical data managed by the Grid database services incorporated into the BPEL process tasks. In addition, integrated access to healthcare information scattered around disparate and geographically dispersed systems is provided by means of Grid database services generated by OGSA-DAI. Access control within the OGSA-DAI framework is currently enforced through the use of local Access Control Lists (ACLs). Such an authorization mechanism is not suitable in the healthcare domain where frequent changes of users' privileges are required, fact that causes waste of valuable time and great administrative overhead.

The number, type and sophistication of tools that protect information in interoperable environments are growing at an ever-increasing rate and provide the opportunity to offer health privacy protections beyond those in the paper environment. In many cases, the utilization of role-based access controls is considered as an effective means of limiting access to a patient's information to only those individuals who need the information for treatment.

In the proposed system architecture, a dynamic access control mechanism is incorporated which is based on the role-based access control (RBAC) paradigm and is provided at two levels: the BPEL task level and the Grid database service level (Koufi & Vassilacopoulos, 2008). As illustrated in Figure 3, this is described by a two-tier model consisted of a global access control service, residing on a server at the DGH site, and one local access control service, residing at each healthcare organization within the health district.

The access control mechanism developed is middleware-based and context-aware as it is employed to mediate between subjects (healthcare professionals) and objects (BPEL tasks and Grid database services) and to decide whether access of a given subject to given object should be permitted or denied by taking into account the current context. In particular, the Java Authentication and Authorization Service (JAAS) (Java Authentication and Authorization Service (JAAS) Reference Guide, n.d) was used for the development of:

- An, external to the BPEL engine, access control service that regulates user access to tasks, and

- An, external to OGSA-DAI, access control service that regulates access to Grid database services. This service essentially enhances OGSA-DAI's mechanism by adding context-awareness features.

In addition, the developed mechanism is certificate-based as it relies on Community Authorization Service (CAS) certificates for user-to-role assignments while role-to-permission assignments are specified by means of access control policies and are subject to constraints holding at the time of the attempted access. These policies are expressed by using the Core and Hierarchical RBAC profile of eXtensible Access Control Markup Language (XACML) (Organization for the Advancement of Structured Information Standards (OASIS), n.d.).

## CAS CERTIFICATES FOR USER TO ROLE ASSIGNMENTS

A health district is a distributed community of resource providers (healthcare providers) and resource consumers (patients). In this community complex and dynamic policies govern who can use which resources for which purpose. In order to facilitate scalability in the specification and enforcement of these policies in our environment, part of the authority for maintaining fine-grained access control policies has been delegated to the community, namely the DGH. In particular, a server at the DGH site hosts Community Authorization Service (CAS) which provides healthcare professionals with the relevant credentials referred to as CAS credentials.

The CAS architecture builds on the public key authentication and delegation mechanisms provided by the Grid Security Infrastructure (GSI) (The Globus Alliance, n.d.). The CAS server uses a backend database to store information regarding users, the groups users belong to as well as policy statements that specify who (which user or group) has the permission, which resource or resource group the permission is granted on, and what permission is granted (The Globus Alliance, n.d.). The permission is denoted by a service type and an action. The action describes the operation (e.g. read, write, or execute program) and the service type defines the namespace in which the action is defined (e.g. file).

In the prototype system, CAS is used for specifying user-to-role assignments in the form of security assertions, expressed in Security Assertion Markup Language (SAML) (Pearlman, Welch, Foster, Kesselman & Tuecke, 2002). In particular, user groups stored to the CAS database correspond to the roles of the parties involved in healthcare delivery situations. Users are made members of these roles by being assigned to the appropriate user group in the CAS database. The assignment of fine-grained privileges to each role/user group and the specification of constraints on it is a responsibility undertaken by each resource provider.

Prior to requesting access to any resource, a user needs to obtain a proxy certificate which is a temporary certificate stored in a server called MyProxy server. The latter is hosted at the DGH site. MyProxy is open source software for managing X.509 Public Key Infrastructure (PKI) security credentials (certificates and private keys) (MyProxy Credential Management Service, n.d.). It combines an online credential repository with an online certificate authority to allow users to securely obtain proxy credentials when and where needed, without worrying about managing private key and certificate files (MyProxy Credential Management Service, n.d.).

Whenever a user needs to gain access to a resource, he presents his proxy credential, which he obtained upon login, to the CAS server which returns a new credential, known as a CAS proxy credential. This credential contains the CAS policy assertions representing the user's roles. The roles used in the certificates are functional and, hence, they remain unchanged until the certificate expires as they are independent of the constraints held at the time of attempted access. The CAS proxy credential is then presented to the resource provider.

In the prototype system, there are two kinds of resources on which access is controlled, namely BPEL processes (in particular, the tasks comprising them) and the underlying Grid database services used for information retrieval. Hence, CAS certificates accompany every request (either for task execution or Grid database service invocation) issued through the portal. The validity of the CAS proxy credential is being verified at the site (DHG or other healthcare organization) hosting the target object (task or Grid database service). After the credential has been verified, the CAS policy assertions are parsed in order to obtain the roles assigned to the healthcare professional owning the credential. Subsequently, these roles are translated in the relevant permissions on the target resource as specified in the relevant policy repository.

The value of this approach stems from the fact that resource providers still maintain ultimate control over their resources.

## XACML POLICIES FOR ROLE TO PERMISSION ASSIGNMENTS

In the prototype system, the mapping of roles to the relevant permissions is performed by means of access control policies expressed by using the Core and Hierarchical RBAC profile of eXtensible Access Control Markup Language (XACML) (Organization for the Advancement of Structured Information Standards (OASIS), n.d.). These policies are expressed in the form of roles, role hierarchies, privileges and constraints. XACML is an OASIS standard for describing access control policies uniformly across different security domains (Organization for the Advancement of Structured Information Standards (OASIS), n.d.).

Due to strict security requirements on medical data, managed by healthcare processes, the specification of access control policies not for the entire resource (e.g. process, database) but for its components (e.g. task, table) is of utmost importance. Since both processes and databases constitute resources which are organized as a hierarchy, when specifying policies on them the hierarchical resource profile of XACML(Organization for the Advancement of Structured Information Standards (OASIS), n.d.) can be used for the representation of these components. This profile specifies how XACML provides access control for resources that are organized as a hierarchy, such as file systems, XML documents and databases. We consider this profile suitable for specifying access control policies on BPEL process tasks as well. According to this profile, non-XML data can be represented by a URI of the following form:

```
<scheme>://<authority>/<pathname>
```

- <scheme> identifies the namespace of the URI and can be either a protocol (e.g. "ftp", "http", "https") or a file system resource declared as "file".
- <authority> is typically defined by an Internet-based server or a scheme-specific registry of naming authorities, such as DNS, and
- <pathname> is of the form <root name>{/<node name>}. The sequence of <root name> and <node name> values should correspond to the components in a hierarchical resource.

Suppose that the process illustrated in Figure 1 is named "RadProcProcess". Then the task "IssueRadRequest" of this process would be represented as follows:

```
"https://localhost:8443/active-
bpel/services/RadProcProcess/Is-
sueRadRequest"
```

*Figure 4. RPS of the role "physician"*

*Figure 4. RPS of the role "physician"*

```
1    <Subject>
2      <SubjectMatch MatchId="&function;anyURI-equal">
3        <AttributeValue DataType="&xml;anyURI"
           Scope="Attiki.DGH">&roles;physician</AttributeValue>
4        <SubjectAttributeDesignator AttributeId="&role;" DataType="&xml;anyURI"/>
5      </SubjectMatch>
6    </Subject>
```

In a similar fashion,

```
"https://localhost:8443/ogsadai/
DataService/Patient"
```

indicates the table "Patient" in the database represented by the specified URI. As retrieval of a patient's medical record involves data retrieval from more that one table, granting access to a patient's medical record would require granting access to each one of these tables. This would cause policies to grow extremely complex to manage. To address this issue, each healthcare provider implements the patient medical record as a view on his database. Hence, granting access to a patient's medical record requires granting access to this view. In OGSA-DAI a view can be realized by means of an activity. The latter is a feature of OGSA-DAI whereby the functionality provided by simple Grid database services can be extended.

An excerpt of the RPS for the role "physician" of the case scenario of Section 3 is illustrated in Figure 4. As opposed to PPS, the form of the RPS is the same regardless of the resource to which access is attempted.

As mentioned above, a resource (target object) may be either a task or a Grid database service invoked on execution of a task. Hence, two kinds of policies need to be specified, each residing at the site where the target object resides. These policies are:

- *Task-related policies*: They reside on the same server of the DGH site with the BPEL engine and assist in the derivation of the exact permissions a subject should acquire for performing a task. For example, a PPS for role "physician" is shown in Figure 5. This constitutes a realization of authorization requirement (1) listed in Table 1. It specifies that the physician has the permission to perform the operation "execute" (specified within <Action>) on the resource identified by the URI "http://localhost/active-bpel/services/RadProcProcess/IssueRadRequest" (specified within <Resource>) only when he is on duty and within hospital premises (specified within <Condition>).

- *Policies related to Grid database services*: They reside on a server at each healthcare organization (i.e. Grid node) and assist in the derivation of the exact permissions a subject should acquire for retrieving the portion of medical information needed. For example, regarding access to the database view mentioned above, namely "PatientMedRecord", the PPS for role "physician" would have the same form as the one illustrated in Figure 5 with the following two differences:

```
DataType of Resource (line
6) would be "https://local-
```

*Figure 5. BPEL task-related PPS of the role "physician"*

```
4    <Resource>
5     <ResourceMatch MatchId="&function;string-equal">
6      <AttributeValue
          DataType="&xml;string">http://localhost/active-bpel/services/RadProcProcess/IssueRadRequest
         </AttributeValue>
7      <ResourceAttributeDesignator AttributeId="&resource;resource-id" DataType="&xml;string"/>
8     </ResourceMatch>
9    </Resource>
10   ...
12    <Action>
13    <ActionMatch MatchId="&function;string-equal">
14     <AttributeValue DataType="&xml;string">execute</AttributeValue>
15     <ActionAttributeDesignator AttributeId="&action;action-id" DataType="&xml;string"/>
16    </ActionMatch>
17    </Action>
18    ...
20   <Condition>
21   <Apply FunctionId="&function;and">
22   <Apply FunctionId="&function;string-equal">
23    <EnvironmentAttributeDesignator
         AttributeId="urn:oasis:names:tc:xacml:2.0:environment:userPatientRelationship"
         DataType="&xml;string"/>
24    <AttributeValue DataType="&xml;string">currentPatient</AttributeValue>
25    </Apply>
26   <Apply FunctionId="&function;string-equal">
27    <EnvironmentAttributeDesignator
         AttributeId=" urn:oasis:names:tc:xacml:2.0:environment:status" DataType="&xml;string"/>
28    <AttributeValue DataType="&xml;yes">onDuty</AttributeValue>
29    </Apply>
30   <Apply FunctionId="&function;string-equal">
31    <EnvironmentAttributeDesignator
         AttributeId="urn:oasis:names:tc:xacml:2.0:environment:location" DataType="&xml;string"/>
32    <AttributeValue DataType="&xml;string">inPremises</AttributeValue>
33    </Apply>
34   </Apply>
35   </Condition>
```

```
host:8443/ogsadai/DataService/
PatientMedRecord"
```

The DataType of Action (line 14) would be "select"

Permissions on both BPEL tasks and Grid database services are dynamically adapted to the constraints imposed by the current context.

## CONTEXT INFORMATION MANAGEMENT

In the prototype system, the management of context information influencing authorization decisions is performed by a Context Manager. Both the context information model and the Context Manager are described below.

### 1.1.1. Context Information Model

Context information is determined by a pre-defined set of attributes related to:

- The user (e.g. user certificate, user/patient relationship),
- The environment (e.g. client location and time of attempted access) and
- The data resource provider, namely to the healthcare organization (e.g. local security policy).

For example, the permissions of a physician accessing the system via his/her PDA, are adapted depending on his/her identity (included in the CAS certificate), location and time of access as well as the security policy of each healthcare organization where a portion of the requested information is stored.

### 1.1.2. Context Manager

Context information is collected by a Context Manager which is realized as a multi-agent system composed of several containers that run on different hosts. In particular, each one of these hosts resides at a healthcare setting within the health district. There is one main container which is deployed in a server at the DGH site and a number of peripheral containers deployed in servers residing at the healthcare organizations of the health district. The main container is the first one to start and all other containers register to it at bootstrap time.

The Main Container holds two special agents, the Agent Management System (AMS) and the Directory Facilitator (DF). The AMS (Agent Management System) that represents the authority in the platform, i.e. it is the only agent that can activate platform management actions such as creating/killing other agents, killing containers and shutting down the platform (Java Agent Development Framework, n.d.). The DF (Directory Facilitator)

that implements the yellow pages service by means of which other agents advertise their services and find other agents offering services they need (Java Agent Development Framework, n.d.).

Peripheral containers hold two kinds of agents:

- *Service Integration Agent (SIA)*: It is held in a container deployed on a server at the DGH site and manages user permissions on BPEL tasks.
- *Grid Resource Agent (GRA)*: It is held in a container on a server at the site of each healthcare organization participating in a healthcare process and manages user permissions on Grid database services.

Each agent uses middleware context collection services to monitor context. At the time of an attempted access (either to a task or to a Grid database service), the relevant agent acquires the context holding and passes it to the relevant access control service which uses it in conjunction with the relevant XACML policies to derive the exact permissions of the requesting party. Changes in user and environment context are sensed by both agents, whereas changes in resource context are sensed and dealt with by the Grid resource agent lying at each Grid node.

## PROTOTYPE IMPLEMENTATION

To illustrate the functionality of the proposed architecture, we describe a prototype system which is based on the case scenario of Section 3.

The prototype system and the underlying security services have been developed on a local Grid. The software tools used are Apache/Tomcat as Web/Application Server and Globus Toolkit (GT4) for the provision of Grid middleware services. OGSA-DAI and its extension, OGSA-DQP, are used for the generation of the Grid database services using the geographically dispersed data resources. In our implementation, a PostGres SQL relational database and a MySQL database are used as data resources. The port types and descriptions of the Grid database services are described by generated WSDL, which also indicates the way these can be accessed. The BPEL engine used for the execution of BPEL healthcare processes is ActiveBPEL (Active Endpoints, n.d.), an open source BPEL Engine (Emmerich, Butchart, Chen, Wassermann & Price, 2006). The portal that provides access to the system is based upon GridSphere portal framework (Gridsphere Portal Framework, n.d.). The GridSphere Portal is a Java Servlets/JSP based framework that builds upon the Java CoG Kit (Java CoG Kit, n.d.), Globus Toolkit (The Globus Alliance, n.d.) and MyProxy (MyProxy Credential Management Service, n.d.) to support such features as single sign-on, job submission and data movement. The GridSphere portal framework is based upon the Java Portlet model (Grabowski, Lewandowski & Russell, 2004). The portlet concept is a Java standard (JSR-168) (Java Community Press, n.d.). Agents are developed using the Java Agent Development Framework Jade) (Java Agent Development Framework, n.d.).

A high-level view of the prototype system functionality is illustrated in Figure 6. At the beginning of a shift, a physician, using his/her X.509 personal certificate and its private key, creates the proxy certificate which is stored on the MyProxy server and is valid for the duration of his/her shift. This certificate provides him/her access to the Grid portal and, consequently, to all the healthcare processes he/she is authorized to access.

While a physician makes a ward round, he/she logs in the portal using his/her Myproxy password. The portal contacts the MyProxy Server and requests the physician's proxy certificate from the MyProxy online credential repository. Hence, the physician's temporary credentials are retrieved, and passed on to the CAS server, which returns a new credential, known as a CAS proxy

credential that contains the CAS policy assertions representing the physician's capabilities (in the form of roles) (Pereira, Muppavarapu & Chung, 2006). When the physician approaches a patient in a ward, the patient's RFID tag is read by the reader attached to the physician's PDA. This generates an event captured by RFID middleware which processes the data received, formats them accordingly and communicates them to the agent that is responsible for initiating the relevant BPEL process that will display the patient medical record on the PDA screen. Before an interaction with the BPEL engine is initiated, the role-based access control mechanism described above is invoked, whereby permission or denial of access to the BPEL task "IssueRadRequest" is determined in accordance to the policy assertions contained in the physician's CAS proxy credential, the XACML security policies and the context holding at the time of attempted access. In particular, on issuing a request for task execution, the roles contained in the CAS certificate accompanying the request are extracted and their relevant permissions regarding access to BPEL tasks are specified using the file storing the XACML policies (Organization for the Advancement of Structured Information Standards (OASIS), n.d.). These permissions are further refined according to the context holding at the time of the attempted access.

Suppose that a physician is permitted to execute the task "IssueRadRequest". As this task involves retrieval of the patient's medical record, it may involve data retrieval using a number of remote Grid database services that access the relevant data resources of the various healthcare settings where the patient has received care. For each remote data resource involved, a request for invocation of the relevant Grid database service is issued which is accompanied by the same CAS certificate. By using this certificate, the portlet authenticates itself (achieving single sign-on through its delegated proxy certificate) and receives the authorized privileges in order to execute the relevant Grid database service on behalf of the physician. To

*Figure 6. System functionality*

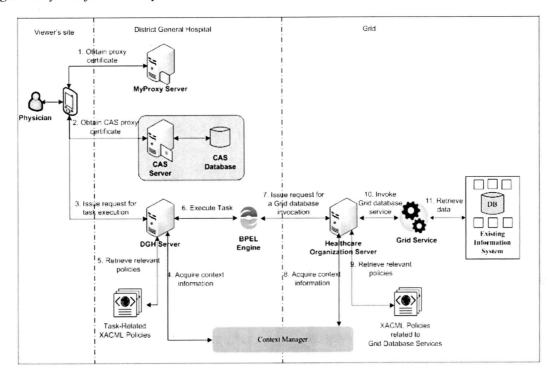

this end, the roles extracted from the extension of the CAS proxy certificate are used in conjunction with the XACML policies stored in one file at each Grid node (i.e. healthcare organization) providing the portion of medical information requested. In this way, the permissions of the physician on Grid database services are derived. As is the case for BPEL tasks, permissions on Grid database services are dynamically adapted by the constraints imposed by the current context.

If the physician has the required privileges, the service is executed and the output, which is in XML format, is transformed in HTML format and rendered back into the physician's web browser. This transformation is supported within the OGSA-DAI framework through XSL Transform.

After reviewing the patient's medical record, the physician may issue a request for a radiological procedure.

## FUTURE RESEARCH DIRECTIONS

The integration of RFID technology with process-based healthcare information systems entails technical as well as privacy and ethical problems with the latter being of utmost importance. Securing RFID-based healthcare information systems constitutes a major challenge to be addressed, thus suggesting directions for future work. In particular, specific security risks that need to be addressed are:

- The contents of an RFID tag can be read by any RFID scanner as RFID tags can't differentiate between readers.
- RFID tags can be read without the patient's knowledge as they don't need to be swiped or obviously scanned (as is the case with magnetic strips or barcodes).
- RFID tags can be read at greater distances with a high-gain antenna.

- Patient RFID tags contain a unique identification number which, if not protected from unauthorized access, may be used for unauthorized access, collection, use, disclosure or disposal of the patient's medical data.

## CONCLUSION

Process-based systems built on a Grid infrastructure can offer great benefits in the development of healthcare information systems. However, for these systems to reach their full potential in providing quality and effective healthcare services, pervasive access to healthcare processes as well as to updated patient medical records anytime, anywhere must be provided to healthcare professionals. This can be achieved by incorporating mobile and wireless devices as clients to these systems and also by utilizing context-aware technologies for automating healthcare process execution. In this chapter, an HIS architecture was presented that facilitates seamless and pervasive access to integrated healthcare services by utilizing both wireless and agent technologies. In such a pervasive environment, security risks arise especially with regard to authorization and access control. Hence, relevant mechanisms must be in place that can conveniently regulate user access to information while providing confidence that security policies are faithfully and consistently enforced within and across organizations residing in a health district. In particular, when adherence to the least privilege principle is considered a prominent feature of a system, the incorporated access control mechanism should provide tight, just-in-time permissions so that authorized users get access to specific objects subject to the current context. The access control mechanism presented in this chapter meets the aforementioned requirements and is embedded in the prototype system. In particular, the mechanism ensures authorized execution of BPEL tasks and invocation of relevant Grid database services in accordance with the current context. Thus, a tight matching of permissions to actual usage and need is ensured.

## REFERENCES

Active Endpoints. (n.d). *ActiveBPEL Open Source Engine Project.* Retrieved August 18, 2007, from http://www.activebpel.org/

*Akogrimo (Access to Knowledge through the Grid in a Mobile World).* (2007). Retrieved April 25, 2009, from http://www.akogrimo.org/modules.php?op=modload&name=AddFile&file=addfile&par=1& datei=scen_ehealth

American Barcode and RFID. (n.d.). *Passive RFID Tags vs. Active RFID Tags.* Retrieved April 15, 2009, from http://www.abrfid.com/rfid/articles/passive-active-tags.aspx

Augustin, I., Yamin, A. C., Da Silva, L. C., Real, R. A., Frainer, G., & Geyer, C. F. R. (2006). ISAMadapt: abstractions and tools for designing general-purpose pervasive applications. *Software, Practice & Experience, 36,* 1231–1256. doi:10.1002/spe.756

Bardram, J. E., Mihailidis, A., & Wan, D. (Eds.). (2007). *Pervasive Computing in Healthcare.* Boca Raton, FL: CRC Press.

BASEscan. (n.d). *Accurate Patient Identification Using Encoded Driver License Information.* Retrieved May 12, 2009, from http://www.medibase.com/pdf/basescan.pdf

Bergeron, B. P. (2002). Enterprise digital assistants: the progression of wireless clinical computing. *The Journal of Medical Practice Management, 17,* 229–233.

Bundgaard, M., Hildebrandt, T., & Hojgaard, E. (2008, June). *Seamlessly Distributed & Mobile Workflow or: The right processes at the right places.* Paper presented at Programming Language Approaches to Concurrency and Communication-cEntric Software (PLACES), Oslo, Norway.

Continuous Care (C-CARE). (2005). Retrieved December 15, 2008, from http://cordis.europa.eu/data/PROJ_FP5/ACTIONeqDndSESSIONeq112422005919ndDOCeq513ndTBLeqEN_PROJ.htm

IBM Corporation. (2005). *IBM Websphere Workflow – Getting Started with Buildtime V. 3.6.*

Del Vecchio, D., Hazlewood, V., & Humphrey, M. (2006, November). *Evaluating Grid portal security.* Paper presented at Supercomputing, Tampa, FL. DOC@HAND, 2006. Retrieved December 15, 2008, from http://services.txt.it/docathand/.

Emmerich, W., Butchart, B., Chen, L., Wassermann, B., & Price, S. L. (2006). Grid service orchestration using the Business Process Execution Language (BPEL). *Journal of Grid Computing, 3,* 283–304. doi:10.1007/s10723-005-9015-3

Grabowski, P., Lewandowski, B., & Russell, M. (2004). *Access from J2ME-enabled mobile devices to Grid services* (White Paper). Poznan University of Technology, Poland.

*Gridsphere Portal Framework.* (n.d.). Retrieved August 18, 2007, from http://www.gridsphere.org/gridsphere/gridsphere

Inglesby, J., & Inglesby, T. (2005, September). Retrieved April 25, 2009, from http://www.psqh.com/sepoct05/barcodingrfid2.html

Integrating the Healthcare Enterprise (IHE). (2005). Retrieved December 15, 2008, from http://www.ihe.net/

Java Agent Development Framework. (n.d.). Retrieved May 15, 2008, from http://jade.tilab.com/

*Java Authentication and Authorization Service (JAAS) Reference Guide for the Java SE Development Kit 6.* (n.d.). Retrieved May 12, 2008, from http://java.sun.com/javase/6/docs/technotes/guides/security/jaas/JAASRefGuide.html

*Java CoG Kit.* (n.d.). Retrieved May 12, 2008, from http://www-unix.globus.org/cog/

Java Community Press. (n.d.). *JSR-168 Portlet Specification.* Retrieved August 18, 2007, from http://www.jcp.org/aboutJava/communityprocess/final/jsr168/

Jorgensen, J. B. (2002, August). *Coloured Petri Nets in UML-Based Software Development – Designing Middleware for Pervasive Healthcare.* Paper presented at the Fourth International Workshop on Practical Use of Coloured Petri Nets and the CPN Tools. Aarhus, Denmark.

Khatua, S., Dasgupta, S., & Mukherjee, N. (2006, June). *Pervasive access to the Data Grid.* Paper presented at the International Conference on Grid Computing and Applications, Las Vegas, NV.

Kjeldskov, J., & Skov, M. (2004, June). *Supporting work activities in healthcare by mobile electronic patient records.* Paper presented at the 6th Asia-Pacific Conference on Human-Computer Interaction, Rotorua, New Zealand.

Koufi, V., Papakonstantinou, D., & Vassilacopoulos, G. (2006, June). *Virtual patient record security on a Grid infrastructure.* Paper presented at the International Conference on Information Communication Technologies in Health (ICICTH'06), Samos, Greece.

Koufi, V., & Vassilacopoulos, G. (2008, January). *HDGPortal: A Grid Portal Application for Pervasive Access to Process-Based Healthcare Systems.* Paper presented at the 2nd International Conference in Pervasive Computing Technologies in Healthcare, Tampere, Finland.

Kurschl, W., Mitsch, S., & Schoenboeck, J. (2008, November). *Model-Driven Prototyping Support for Pervasive Health Care Applications*. Paper presented at the Software Engineering and Applications Conference, Orlando, Florida, USA.

Malamateniou, F., & Vassilacopoulos, G. (2003). Developing a virtual patient record using XML and web-based workflow technologies. *International Journal of Medical Informatics, 70*(2-3), 131–139. doi:10.1016/S1386-5056(03)00039-X

Mendling, J., Strembeck, M., Stermsek, G., & Neumann, G. (2004, June). *An Approach to Extract RBAC Models for BPEL4WS Processes*. Paper presented at the 13th IEEE Int. Workshops on Enabling Technologies: Infrastructure for Collaborative Enterprises, Modena, Italy.

Mitchell, S., Spiteri, M. D., Bates, J., & Coulouris, G. (2000). *Context-Aware Multimedia Computing in the Intelligent Hospital*. Paper presented at the 9th European Workshop on ACM SIGOPS, New York.

Mobile Devices For Healthcare Applications (MOBI-DEV). (2005). Retrieved December 15, 2008, from http://www.mobi-dev.arakne.it/

Muller, M., Frankewitsch, T., Ganslandt, T., Burkle, T., & Prokosch, H. U. (2004). The Clinical Document Architecture (CDA) enables Electronic Medical Records to wireless mobile computing. [Amsterdam: IOS Press.]. *Medinfo, 107*, 1448–1452.

Munoz, M., Rodriguez, M., Favela, J., Martinez-Garcia, A., & Gonzalez, V. (2003). Context-Aware Mobile Communication in Hospitals. *IEEE Computer, 36*(9), 38–46.

MyProxy Credential Management Service. (n.d.). Retrieved October 16, 2007, from http://grid.ncsa.uiuc.edu/myproxy/

National Institute of Standards and Technology (NIST). *Role Based Access Control (RBAC) and Role Based Security*. (n.d.). Retrieved October 16, 2007, from http://csrc.nist.gov/groups/SNS/rbac/

Neely, S., Stevenson, G., Kray, C., Mulder, I., Connelly, K., & Siek, K. A. (2008). Evaluating Pervasive and Ubiquitous Systems. *IEEE Pervasive Computing / IEEE Computer Society [and] IEEE Communications Society, 7*(3), 85–88. doi:10.1109/MPRV.2008.47

Open Grid Services Architecture - Data Access and Integration (OGSA-DAI). (n.d.). Retrieved October 12, 2007, from http://www.ogsadai.org.uk/

Organization for the Advancement of Structured Information Standards (OASIS). (n.d.) *eXtensible Access Control Markup Language (XACML) TC*. Retrieved October 15, 2007, from http://www.oasis-open.org/committees/xacml/

Organization for the Advancement of Structured Information Standards (OASIS). *Core and Hierarchical Role Based Access Control (RBAC) Profile of XACML v2.0*. (n.d.). Retrieved May 12, 2008, from http://docs.oasis-open.org/xacml/2.0/access_control-xacml-2.0-rbac-profile1-spec-os.pdf

Organization for the Advancement of Structured Information Standards (OASIS). *Hierarchical Resource Profile of XACML v2.0*. (n.d.). Retrieved May 12, 2008, from http://docs.oasis-open.org/xacml/2.0/access_control-xacml-2.0-hier-profile-spec-os.pdf

Pasley, J. (2005). How BPEL and SOA are changing web services development. *IEEE Internet Computing, 9*(3), 60–67. doi:10.1109/MIC.2005.56

Pearlman, L., Welch, V., Foster, I., Kesselman, C., & Tuecke, S. (2002, June). *A Community Authorization Service for Group Collaboration*. Paper presented at the 3rd IEEE International Workshop on Policies for Distributed Systems and Networks, Monterey, California, USA.

Pereira, A. L., Muppavarapu, V., & Chung, S. M. (2006). Role-Based Access Control for Grid database services using the community authorization service. *IEEE Transactions on Dependable and Secure Computing, 3*(2), 156–166. doi:10.1109/TDSC.2006.26

Poulymenopoulou, M., Malamateniou, F., & Vassilacopoulos, G. (2005). Emergency Healthcare Process Automation using Workflow Technology and Web Services. *International Journal of Medical Informatics, 28*(3), 195–207.

Ranganathan, A., & McFaddin, S. (2004, June). *Using processes to coordinate web services in pervasive computing environments*. Paper presented at the IEEE International Conference on Web Services (ICWS'04), San Diego, CA.

The Globus Alliance. (n.d.). *The Globus Toolkit*. Retrieved December 12, 2008, from http://www.globus.org/

Thomas, M. P., Burruss, J., Cinquini, L., Fox, G., Gannon, D., & Gilbert, L. (2005). Grid portal architectures for scientific applications. *Journal of Physics: Conference Series, 16*, 596–600. doi:10.1088/1742-6596/16/1/083

*Ubiquitous, Permanent and Intelligent Access to Patients' Medical Files (DOCMEM)*. (2003). Retrieved December 15, 2008, from http://cordis.europa.eu/data/PROJ_FP5/ACTIONeqDndSESSIONeq112422005919ndDOCeq2361ndTBLeqEN_PROJ.htm

Wozak, F., Ammenwerth, E., Hoerbst, A., Soegner, P., Mair, R., & Schabetsberger, T. (2008, May). *IHE Based Interoperability – Benefits and Challenges*. Paper presented at the 21st International Congress of the European Federation for Medical Informatics (MIE), Göteborg, Sweden.

## ADDITIONAL READING

Adamski, M., Kulczewski, M., Kurowski, K., Nabrzyski, J., & Hume, A. (2007). Security and Performance Enhancements to OGSA-DAI for Grid Data Virtualization. *Concurrency and Computation, 19*(16), 2171–2182. doi:10.1002/cpe.1165

Al Kukhun, D., & Sedes, F. (2008). Adaptive Solutions for Access Control within Pervasive Healthcare Systems. In Smart Homes and Health Telematics: Vol. 5120. Lecture Notes in Computer Science (pp. 155-160). Springer Berlin / Heidelberg.

Antonioletti, M., Hong, N. C., Hume, A., Jackson, M., Krause, A., & Nowell, J. (2003, October). *Experiences designing and implementing Grid database services in the OGSA-DAI project*. Designing and Building Grid Services Workshop, GGF9, Chicago IL, USA.

Bertino, E., Crampton, J., & Paci, F. (2006, September). *Access Control and Authorization Constraints for WS-BPEL*. Paper presented at the IEEE International Conference on Web Services, Chicago, USA.

Brennan, P. F., & Hawkins, R. P. (Eds.). (2007). *Gustafson. H.* Investing in E-Health. Springer-Verlag New York Inc.

Da Silveira, M., Guelfi, N., Baldacchino, J.-D., Plumer, P., Seil, M., & Wienecke, A. (2008, January). *A Survey of Interoperability in E-Health Systems: the European Approach.* Poster presented in the 1st International Conference in Health Informatics, Madeira, Portugal.

Dou, W., Cheung, S. C., Chen, G., & Cai, S. (2005). Certificate-Driven Grid Workflow Paradigm Based on Service Computing. In Grid and Cooperative Computing - GCC 2005: Vol. 3795. Lecture Notes in Computer Science (pp. 155-160). Springer Berlin / Heidelberg.

Fischer, S., Stewart, T. E., Mehta, S., Wax, R., & Lapinsky, S. E. (2003). Handheld computing in medicine. *Journal of the American Medical Informatics Association, 10*(2), 139–149. doi:10.1197/jamia.M1180

Hewlett Packard. (2008). *RFID and Privacy.* Guidance for Healthcare Professionals.

Hussain, S., Yang, L. T., Laforest, F., & Verdier, C. (2008). Pervasive Health Care Services and Technologies. *International Journal of Telemedicine and Applications, 2008.*

Juan, F., Fox, J., & Pierce, M. (2006, October). *Grid portal system based on GPIR.* Paper presented at the 2nd International Conference on Semantics, Knowledge and Grid, Guilin, China.

Kinetic consulting, Chips with Everything, Is RFID ready for Healthcare? 2008. Retrieved January 14, 2009, from http://www.kineticconsulting.co.uk.

Power, D., Slaymaker, M., Politou, E., & Simpson, A. (2005). A Secure Wrapper for OGSA-DAI. In Advances in Grid Computing - EGC 2005: Vol. 3470. Lecture Notes in Computer Science (pp. 485-494).

RFID in Healthcare. (n.d.). Retrieved December 22, 2008, from http://www.connectingforhealth.nhs.uk/newsroom/worldview/comment14

Stanford, V. (2002). Pervasive Health Care Applications Face Tough Security Challenges. *IEEE Pervasive Computing / IEEE Computer Society [and] IEEE Communications Society, 1*(2), 8–12. doi:10.1109/MPRV.2002.1012332

Tentori, M., Favela, J., & Rodríguez, M. D. (2006). *Privacy-Aware Autonomous Agents for Pervasive Healthcare.* IEEE Computer Society.

Thomas, J., Paci, F., Bertino, E., & Eugster, P. (2007, July). *User Tasks and Access Control over Web Services.* Paper presented at the 15th IEEE International Conference on Web Services, Utah, USA.

Vaidya, S., & Jain, L. C. Yoshida, & H. (Eds.). (2008). Advanced Computational Intelligence Paradigms in Healthcare. Springer-Verlag Berlin and Heidelberg GmbH & Co. KG.

## KEY TERMS AND DEFINITIONS

**Process-Based Healthcare System:** A healthcare system where collaboration of individual caregivers and departments and coordination of their activities is achieved by means of processes.

**Grid Portal Application:** A portal application that provides a web-based interface to Grid services, allowing users to submit compute jobs, transfer files and query Grid information services from a standard web browser.

**Business Process Execution Language:** An emerging standard for specifying business process behavior based on Web Services.

**Role-Based Access Control:** A method of regulating access to resources based on the roles of individual users within an enterprise.

**Open Grid Services Architecture-Data Access and Integration (OGSA-DAI):** A middleware product that allows data resources, such as relational or XML databases, to be accessed via web services.

**Personal Digital Assistant (PDA):** A pocket-sized computing device, typically having a display screen with touch input or a miniature keyboard.

**Radio-Frequency Identification (RFID):** An automatic identification method, relying on storing and remotely retrieving data using devices called RFID tags or transponders.

**Least Privilege Principle:** A principle whereby users are being assigned no more permissions than is necessary to perform their job function.

**Agents:** A complex software entity that is capable of acting with a certain degree of autonomy in order to accomplish tasks on behalf of its user.

# Section 2
# Security, Dependability, and Performability

# Chapter 8
# Sensor Networks Security for Pervasive Healthcare

**Ioannis Krontiris**
*University of Mannheim, Germany*

## ABSTRACT

*Body-worn sensors and wireless interconnection of distributed embedded devices facilitate the use of lightweight systems for monitoring vital health parameters like heart rate, respiration rate and blood pressure. Patients can simply wear monitoring systems without restricting their mobility and everyday life. This is particularly beneficial in the context of world's ageing society with many people suffering chronic ailments. However, wireless transmission of sensitive patient data through distributed embedded devices presents several privacy and security implications. In this book chapter the authors' first highlight the security threats in a biomedical sensor networks and identify the requirements that a security solution has to offer. Then the authors' review some popular architectures proposed in the bibliography over the last few years and they discuss the methods that they employ in order to offer security. Finally the authors' discuss some open research questions that have not been addressed so far and which they believe offer promising directions towards making these kinds of networks more secure.*

## INTRODUCTION

One of the major challenges Information and Communication Technologies (ICT) have to cope with is to deliver healthcare to citizens at high quality and affordable costs. In particular, this challenge has to be considered in the light of prevalent trends in healthcare, such as prolonged medical care for the

ageing population, increasing expenses for managing chronic diseases, and the demand for personal health systems. Research on this challenge aims at the creation of an "intelligent environment" in which the health status of any given individual can be monitored and managed continuously, which will assist health professionals in addressing major health problems.

A promising technology that can enable the above vision is biomedical wireless sensor networks

DOI: 10.4018/978-1-61520-765-7.ch008

(BWSN), which consist of body-worn sensors and wireless interconnection of distributed embedded devices. The emergence of low-power, single-chip radios has allowed the design of small, wearable, truly networked medical sensors. These tiny sensors on each patient can form an ad hoc network, relaying continuous vital sign data to multiple receiving devices, like PDAs carried by physicians, or laptop base stations in ambulances (Shnayder, Chen, Lorincz, Jones, & Welsh, 2005). In this way, we can provide lightweight pervasive health systems for monitoring vital health parameters, like heart rate, respiration rate and blood pressure, and help patients - and their doctors - monitor and manage their health status. According to a report released recently from OnWorld, San Diego, CA, the use of wireless sensor networks is growing within the healthcare industry, and the technology could save the healthcare industry billions of dollars in 2012 by reducing hospitalizations and extending independent living for seniors (Mareca Hatler, 2008).

Several research proposals that have been presented on the application scenarios of wireless sensor networks reveal the benefits of this technology in healthcare. We can classify these benefits according to the following three main categories:

## Patient Monitoring at Home

Biomedical sensor networks allow monitoring of the patient at home, so that the elderly or patients with chronic diseases can enjoy treatment and medical monitoring in their own environment and provide a unique opportunity to shift health care outside a traditional clinical setting to a patient/home-centered setting. By monitoring continuously these people's health over a period of time, physicians can provide more accurate diagnoses and better treatment. For instance, monitoring patient data can help with early detection of conditions like heart disease. Moreover medical

professionals could react to situations such as strokes and asthma attacks more quickly.

## Patient Monitoring in the Hospital

Biomedical sensor networks substantially increase the efficiency of treatments inside the hospital environment. Today biomedical sensors are wired, attaching patients to machines, in order to read different values of vital data. The implementation of a more flexible wireless technology can lead to improved data quality, data resolution and increase of patient's mobility outside the surgery room. This results in enhanced decision making for diagnostics, observation and patient treatment.

Biomedical sensor networks can also be applied to cases prior to surgery. For example, overcrowding occurs in 40% of all Emergency Rooms in the U.S., where patients wait on the average of 3.5 hours before being seen by a doctor. This has caused a number of deaths in waiting rooms of urban hospital emergency rooms. Wireless sensor nodes can be used to monitor the vital signs of patients who are scattered in the waiting rooms and hallways of the ER waiting to be seen by a doctor. Information is transmitted wirelessly to a central monitoring system. If a patient becomes unstable, medical professionals could be alerted more quickly and provide a more immediate response.

## Emergency Response

Disasters present a number of challenges to sensors due to unique patient, user, and environmental needs. Casualties can be distributed over areas well outside the communication range of pre-installed wireless access points. Wireless sensor nodes can be distributed to casualties at a disaster scene and relay sensor data - including vital signs, location, and triage status - over an ad-hoc mesh network to monitoring stations. In this way, members of the distributed response team, such as treatment officers, incident commanders, receiving hospitals and public health officials can have access to real-time patient information. This allows them to maintain an accurate and global situational awareness of the casualties and provide better coordination between the pre-hospital caseload and receiving care facilities.

Despite the increased range of these potential applications, the gap between the security requirements that they pose and the existing WSN security mechanisms remains unresolved. Existing WSN research so far has focused on monitoring the physical environment. However, a biomedical sensor network has distinct features, like mobility of sensors and sensitive nature of data, which aggravate the security challenges. There are a number of security and privacy implications that must be explored in order to promote its adoption by healthcare providers. This is also the conclusion of Lubrin, Lawrence, Navarro, & Zmijewska (2006), who made a study via the use of online survey and showed that wireless sensor networks is a viable technology for health monitoring in healthcare institutions and patient's homes given that strong security solutions are provided.

## BACKGROUND

The architecture and design of biomedical sensor networks depend greatly on the specific application and deployment environment. In this section we review some of the latest developments in such networks, which we will use as examples in the rest of the paper to qualify and compare the security solutions that they offer. But before that, let us first present a generic architecture that most of these proposed systems follow.

As depicted in Figure 1, a patient wears a body sensor network (BSN) composed by wireless sensor devices that provide physiological or activity sensing. Data from the body network is transmitted in a multi-hop fashion through other emplaced sensors to a base station or a personal health system. The role of these emplaced sensors is twofold.

First they sense the environmental conditions of the living space, such as temperature, light, dust, motion, etc. Secondly they enable the mobility of the patient as they maintain their connectivity with the base station. At any time they can route reports, alerts or queries between the base station and the body sensor network.

In the home environment, any legitimate user of the system (doctor, nurses, etc.) can send a query to the base station and retrieve medical data collected by the network. The base station is connected through the internet to a server located at the hospital. From there the information is managed according to the situation: it can be stored at the electronic patient record database or be directly displayed to the PC of a physician or produce an alert and notify an ambulance and the physician in case of emergency.

One of the proposals that follow the above architecture is ALARM-NET (Wood et al., 2006) from the University of Virginia. ALARM-NET is a wireless sensor network that integrates physiological and environmental sensors in a heterogeneous architecture for pervasive, adaptive health care. The system emphasizes on a Circadian Activity Rhythm (CAR) analysis module that monitors the patterns of daily life of the individuals. Data queries at the base station allow real-time collection and processing of sensor data for authorized care providers and analysis programs.

CodeBlue (Lorincz et al., 2004) is a sensor network based medical research project being developed at Harvard. It is intended for deployment for pre-hospital and in-hospital emergency care, disaster response and stroke patient rehabilitation. The sensor nodes collect heart rate (HR), oxygen saturation (SpO2), and ECG data, which then is relayed over a short-range wireless network to any number of receiving devices, including PDAs, laptops, or ambulance-based terminals.

SNAP (Malasri & Wang, 2007) is an architecture for medical sensor networks that focuses on security. Taken this approach, it does not address routing, mobility or congestion issues in the

*Figure 1. General architecture of a patient monitoring system using sensor networks*

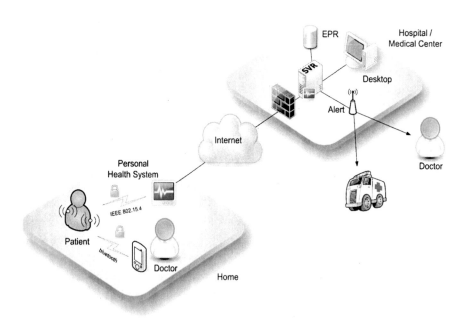

network. In the SNAP architecture, one or more wireless sensors are attached to each patient. The transmitted data are forwarded by a number of wireless relay nodes throughout the hospital area. These nodes are categorized into unlimited-powered and limited powered nodes.

Ayushman is a wireless sensor network based health monitoring infrastructure and testbed being developed at Arizona State University (Venkata-subramanian & Gupta, 2008). The principal component of Ayushman is the Body Area Network (BAN). The BAN is responsible for collecting physiological data from patients. In their current implementation the motes collect three types of physiological data: blood pressure, blood oxygen and acceleration. There are also environmental sensors deployed, which provide the context for the physiological data. All the sensors on a patient send their data at regular intervals to a sink called the *base station*. The sink is responsible for processing the data from the sensors and is much more capable than the sensors (e.g. a PDA). Once the patient data has been processed, the derived

physiological parameters are sent over a Wi-Fi connection to a central server. The central sever stores the data in a database, which is implemented in MS Access, and connects to remote clients over the Internet.

Finally, the WBAN group at the University of Alabama in Huntsville and the Medical Component Design Laboratory at Kansas State University (Warren et al., 2005) are developing wearable health monitoring systems using off-the-shelf ZigBee wireless sensor platforms, custom signal conditioning boards, and the TinyOS software environment, which is an operating system specially designed for wireless sensor networks (Hill et al., 2000). Sensor nodes are strategically placed on the user's body and sample, process, and store information about physiological values.

## SECURITY THREATS

The particular threats that a biomedical sensor network has to face can be categorized into outsider and insider attacks. In an *outsider* attack (intruder node attack), the attacker node is not an authorized participant of the sensor network. Authentication and encryption techniques prevent such an attacker to gain any special access to the sensor network. The intruder node can only be used to launch passive attacks, like the following:

- Passive eavesdropping: the attacker eavesdrops and records encrypted messages, which may then be analyzed in order to discover secret keys or infer information about the network structure.
- Stealth denial of service (DoS) attacks: the attacker can force some nodes to consume all their energy resources. This can be accomplished for example, either by requesting a sensor to continuously transmit data or by continuously route large amount of data through that node.
- Jamming attacks: an adversary attempts to disrupt the networks operation by broadcasting high-energy signals, jamming the communication between legitimate nodes. To realize this attack, attackers can utilize specialized jamming equipment or just normal customized devices to interfere with the medical sensors. In the worst case, this attack can lead to the isolation of certain patients putting their lives at risk.
- Replay attacks: the attacker captures messages exchanged between legitimate nodes and replays them in order to change the aggregation results.

Perhaps more dangerous from a security point of view is an *insider* attack, where an adversary by physically capturing a node and reading its memory, can obtain its key material and forge node messages. Having access to legitimate keys, the attacker can launch several kinds of attacks without easily being detected:

- Unauthorized access to health data.
- False data injection, where the attacker injects false results, which are significantly different from the true health data determined by the biosensors.
- Selective reporting, where the attacker stalls the reports of events by dropping legitimate packets that pass through the compromised node. This requires that the attacker have managed to include her own compromised node into the routing path of the network. This has been proved to be a fairly easy process by launching attacks like the sinkhole attack (Krontiris, Giannetsos & Dimitriou, 2008).
- Alteration of health data of a patient, leading to incorrect diagnosis and treatment.

## SECURITY REQUIREMENTS

Usually in biomedical sensor networks there exist one or more base stations operating as data sinks and often as gateways to IP networks. In general, a base station is considered trustworthy, either because it is physically protected or because it has a tamper-resistant hardware. Concerning the rest of the network, we now discuss the standard security requirements (and eventually behavior) we would like to achieve by making the network secure.

- *Confidentiality*: In order to protect sensed data and communication exchanges between sensors nodes it is important to guarantee the secrecy of messages.
- *Integrity and Authentication*: Integrity and authentication is necessary to enable sensor nodes to detect modified, injected, or replayed packets.
- *Availability*: In many sensor network deployments, keeping the network available for its intended use is essential. Thus, attacks like denial-of-service (DoS) that aim

at bringing down the network itself may have serious consequences to the health and well being of people.

While designing security mechanisms that address the above requirements, one has to keep in mind specific factors that differentiate BSNs from other types of sensor networks. These factors determine some extra requirements, as indicated below:

- Multiple users in different roles must be supported, each with different privacy interests and decision making power.
- Mobility of the patient must be supported, therefore security mechanisms should adapt quickly to dynamic topologies.
- Any security protocol must add a low communication overhead, since throughput is crucial for such networks. Medical data require high data rates, e.g. ECG data are normally sampled at 250 Hz and blood pressure at 100 Hz (Shnayder et al., 2005). If these signals are continuously monitored, the traffic in the network is already dense.
- Any security protocol should take under consideration the strict QoS requirements of a biomedical sensor network. Such networks pose very strict deadlines in reporting the data (e.g. in case of an emergency) and security mechanisms should not hinder QoS. It could be the case that a security protocol could successfully prevent or detect an ongoing attack, at the cost of delaying the reception of a message and causing valuable time for the patient to be lost.
- Many security mechanisms in classical sensor networks take advantage of the large scale of such networks and try to constrain the damage of the attack in a small area. Biomedical sensor networks however, are not usually so large in scale. And most importantly, we do not have the

luxury of tolerating security breaches. The risk of even a single point of failure is simply unacceptable, as it may be enough to compromise the health of the patient.

## UNIQUE CHALLENGES

Addressing the above security requirements becomes very challenging as they must be balanced against the computational, memory, and power constraints of the individual nodes. A wide range of sensor node platforms has emerged over the past five years. So far, for such devices, the trend has been to increase the lifetime of the nodes by decreasing the resources such as memory, CPU, and radio bandwidth. Therefore, motes have tiny resources, on the order of a few kilobytes of RAM and a few megahertz of processor. For example, Table 1 indicates the resources available by some popular mote platforms.

This means that computationally expensive algorithms like asymmetric cryptography cannot be applied here (or should be applied with care). Instead, symmetric encryption/decryption algorithms and hash functions constitute the basic tools for securing sensor network communications. However, symmetric key cryptography is not as versatile as public key cryptography, which complicates the design of secure applications.

Besides resource constraints, one also has to consider the wireless nature of the communication medium as one of the factors that makes securing medical sensor networks even harder. Sensor nodes communicate through wireless communication, which is particularly expensive from an energy point of view (one bit transmitted is equivalent to about a thousand CPU operations (Hill et al., 2000)). Hence one cannot use complicated protocols that involve the exchange of a large number of messages. Additionally, the nature of communication makes it particularly easy to eavesdrop, inject malicious messages into the

*Table 1. Selection of sensor node platforms*

| Platform | MCU | RAM | Program Memory | Radio Chip |
|---|---|---|---|---|
| BTnode3 | ATMega 128 | 64 KB | 128 KB | CC1000/Bluetooth |
| Cricket | ATMega 128 | 4 KB | 128 KB | CC1000 |
| Imote2 | Intel PXA271 | 256 KB | 32 MB | CC2420 |
| Mica2 | ATMega 128 | 4 KB | 128 KB | CC1000 |
| MicaZ | ATMega 128 | 4 KB | 128 KB | CC2420 |
| Tmote Sky | TI MSP 430 | 10 KB | 48 KB | CC2420 |
| Shimmer | TI MSP 430 | 10 KB | 48 KB | CC1000/Bluetooth |

*Table 2. Security schemes used in healthcare architectures*

| System Architecture | Hardware Platform | Security Scheme |
|---|---|---|
| CodeBlue | Mica2 | EccM 2.0. & TinySec |
| ALARM-NET | Tmote Sky | Hardware Encryption |
| SNAP | Tmote Sky | TinyECC |
| Ayushman | MicaZ | Physiological Values |
| WBAN | Tmote Sky | Hardware Encryption |

wireless network or even hinder communications entirely using radio jamming.

Moreover, unlike traditional networks, sensor nodes are often accessible by an attacker, presenting the added risk of physical attacks that can expose their cryptographic material or modify their underlying code. This problem is magnified further by the fact that sensor nodes cannot be made tamper-resistant due to increases in hardware cost. Therefore, sensor nodes are more likely to suffer a physical attack, even in a healthcare environment like a hospital, compared to typical PCs, which are located in a secure place and mainly face attacks from a network.

## SECURITY SOLUTIONS

Several security solutions have been proposed in protecting biomedical sensor network's link layer communication, which constitutes the bottom layer of the sensor network protocol stack. More attention has been given to robust and efficient key management schemes, which serve as the fundamental requirement in encryption and authentication. Here, we describe the main approaches followed by the architectures we mentioned in the previous section (see Table 2) and evaluate them on their suitability for biomedical sensor networks.

### TinySec

TinySec (Karlof, Sastry, & Wagner, 2004) is a link-layer security mechanism for wireless sensor networks that is part of the official TinyOS release. It generates secure packets by encrypting data packets using a group key shared among sensor nodes and calculating a MAC for the whole packet including the header. It provides two modes of operation for communication namely, authenticated encryption and authentication only. Authentication only is the default mode of operation, where the payload in the TinyOS packet is not encrypted; each packet is simply enhanced with a MAC. In the authenticated encryption mode the payload is encrypted before the MAC is computed on the packet. The key distribution mechanism was left out and must be implemented as a separate part of the software.

## Encryption and Authentication

TinySec uses a block cipher algorithm for its encryption scheme that is also used for the message authentication code (MAC) resulting in greater code efficiency. In particular it uses the SKIPJACK block cipher in cipher block chaining (CBC) mode for encrypting TinyOS packets. However, instead of a random IV, it uses a counter, which is pre-encrypted. It also uses the cipher stealing technique to ensure the ciphertext is the same length as the underlying plaintext. For the authentication of packets, TinySec uses the same block cipher encryption in CBC-MAC mode to generate a 4 byte Message Authentication Code (MAC) for each message. To provide additional security, it XORs the encryption of the message length with the first plaintext block.

## TinySec Packet Format

The default TinyOS packet contains six fields; destination address, AM type, length, group, data payload and CRC. Since TinySec supports two security modes, it has one packet format for each mode. Figure 2 shows the packet formats for these two modes, authenticated encryption (TinySec-AE) and authentication only (TinySec-Auth). Note that the header fields do not get encrypted, to allow motes quickly determine whether they should reject the packet. The destination address and the AM type are used by the motes for this purpose.

To detect transmission errors, TinyOS motes compute a 16-bit cycle redundancy check (CRC)

over the packet. At the receiver the CRC is re-computed and verified with the CRC field in the packet. If they are equal, the receiver accepts the packet and rejects it otherwise. However, CRCs provide no security against malicious modifications or forgery of packets. TinySec replaces the CRC and the GroupID fields with a 3-byte MAC. The MAC protects the payload as well as the header fields. So, since the MAC can detect any changes in the packet, it can also detect transmission errors, therefore CRC is no longer needed.

In the TinySec-AE mode, the data field (payload) is encrypted by the block cipher in CBC mode. Then the MAC is computed over the encrypted data and the packet header. In order to reduce overhead, TinySec uses an 8 byte IV, which is composed of all the header fields. In this case the overhead is only 4 bytes, i.e. the source address and a 16-bit counter. This raises an issue on the security level due to the repetition of the IV value. Since the counter is 16 bits, a node can send $2^{16}$ packets before IV reuse occurs. However, when this happens, only the length (in blocks) of the longest shared prefix of the two repeated messages will be revealed, since CBC mode is used.

## TinySec Implementation

Due to its simplicity, TinySec performs very well in computation and communication. Malan et. al. (2008) estimated the costs analytically and measured TinySec's performance experimentally using a variety of microbenchmarks and macrobenchmarks. Their results are summarized by Table 3. Of course, TinySec also comes with an additional cost in memory. The implementation of TinySec adds 822 bytes to an application's RAM and 7,076 bytes to ROM.

## TinySec Limitations

TinySec by default relies on a single key manually programmed into the sensor nodes before deployment. This network-wide shared key provides only

*Figure 2. Packet formats for TinySec-Auth and TinSec-AE modes of TinySec*

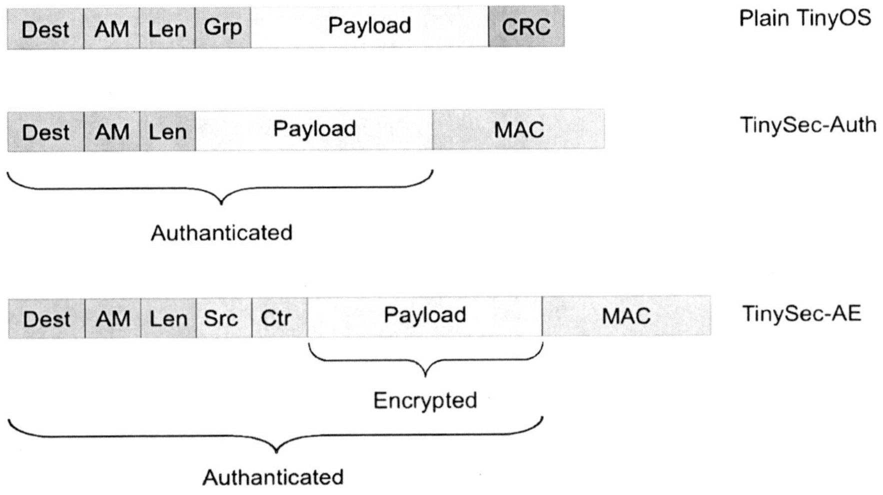

*Table 3. Overhead added by TinySec implementation in TinyOS*

|  | Packet Size Increase | Latency Overhead | Bandwidth Overhead | Energy Overhead | Memory Overhead |
|---|---|---|---|---|---|
| TinySec - Auth | 1.5% | 1.7% | same throughput | 3% | RAM: 20.55% ROM: 5.5% |
| TinySec - AE | 8% | 7.3% | 6% less throughput | 10% | |

a baseline level of security. It cannot protect against node capture attacks. If an adversary compromises a single node or learns the secret key, she can gain access on the information anywhere in the network, as well as inject her own packets. This is probably the weakest point in TinySec, as node capture has been proved to be a fairly easy process (Hartung, Balasalle, & Han, 2005). As we will see in later sections, more recent link-layer security protocols have used stronger keying mechanisms to deal with node capture attacks.

## TinySec Limitations

TinySec by default relies on a single key manually programmed into the sensor nodes before deployment. This network-wide shared key provides only a baseline level of security. It cannot protect against node capture attacks. If an adversary compromises a single node or learns the secret key, she can gain access on the information anywhere in the network, as well as inject her own packets. This is probably the weakest point in TinySec, as node capture has been proved to be a fairly easy process (Hartung, Balasalle, & Han, 2005). As we will see in later sections, more recent link-layer security protocols have used stronger keying mechanisms to deal with node capture attacks.

Another limitation of TinySec is that messages of less than 8 bytes are not addressed efficiently. This is because TinySec uses a $k$-byte block cipher to encrypt the message. For longer messages CBC mode is chosen that encrypts the message block by block. But it is not so unusual for a message (i.e. the payload of the TinyOS packet) to be less than 8 bytes, in which case TinySec will cause a ciphertext expansion, because ciphertext stealing requires at least one block of ciphertext. This kind of ciphertext expansion would cause extra communication power cost when sending data with variable length.

## Elliptic Curve Cryptography

As we said in the previous section, TinySec uses one global key for all the nodes, so compromising one node is equivalent to compromising the whole network. Therefore, a re-keying mechanism is needed. Besides, re-keying is also needed because TinySec's initialization vector (IV) is 4-byte long and therefore, after $2^{32}$ packets, it will be reused. This bound may be insufficient for embedded networks whose lifetime demands long-lasting security.

Obviously, relying on TinySec itself for re-keying would not be a secure solution, since its single secret key may have been compromised. In this case, a public key infrastructure can help our network to securely re-key itself. For example, the CodeBlue architecture employs a form of Diffie-Hellman protocol to address the problem of secret keys' distribution and enable two nodes establish a shared secret key for use as TinySec's key.

Public key algorithms have been widely used for the development of various key establishment protocols. However, until recently they were considered unsuitable for sensor networks because of their large energy demands. Then, Gura et al. (2004) opened the way for the applicability of public key cryptography (PKC) in sensor networks. They ensured that Elliptic Curve Cryptography (ECC) was an appropriate technique for implementing PKC for sensor networks, as it offers a good performance both in computation and memory storage, minimizing energy costs and functional complexity.

The efficiency of ECC resides in the use of much smaller key sizes, compared to that of RSA for the same security level. For example, the strength given by 1024 bit RSA keys is provided by just 163 bit keys in ECC. This results in faster cryptographic operations, like key exchanges or signature generation and verification. Smaller keys

are also more suitable for storage in the limited memory resources of wireless sensor nodes. But except key sizes, ECC is more efficient also in computational requirements and consequently energy consumption. While RSA requires modular exponentiation of the private key, ECC requires scalar point multiplication with selected base point on the elliptic curve.

The exact efficiency of ECC cryptography in wireless sensor networks depends on the choice of elliptic curve parameters and hardware platform. The first implementation of ECC on MICA2 sensor platform by Malan et. al., known as EccM 2.0., used polynomial basis over $F_2^p$ (Malan, Welsh, & Smith, 2004). The time required to compute the public/private key pair was around 34.161 seconds and the time required to calculate the shared secret, given one's private key and another's public key was 34.173 seconds.

Over the last few years there have been several other implementations using ECC optimizations, trying to make this technique attractive for deeply embedded devices. The more applicable implementations are TinyECC (Liu & Ning, 2008) and NanoECC (Szczechowiak, Oliveira, Scott, Collier, & Dahab, 2008). TinyECC is an ECC library that provides elliptic curve arithmetic over various 160-bit prime fields and uses inline assembly code to speed up critical operations on the ATmega128 processor. It requires times of 6.1 seconds and 12.2 seconds for ECDSA signature generation and verification.

Malasri and Wang (2007) also include an ECC-based secure key exchange protocol to set up shared keys between sensor nodes and the base station in their design of wireless medical sensor network. Their implementation is based on TinyECC, but modified to take advantage of the MSP430's hardware multiplier and incorporate a fast modular inversion algorithm with only bit shifts and additions. The resulted code is fairly efficient: it performs a 160-bit scalar point multiplication in 5.3 seconds.

*Table 4. CC2420 security timing examples*

| Mode | Time (μs) |
|------|-----------|
| CCM | 222 |
| CTR | 99 |
| CBC-MAC | 99 |
| Stand-alone | 14 |

## Hardware Encryption

As an alternative to TinySec, one could utilize hardware encryption supported by the ChipCon 2420 ZigBee complaint RF Transceiver, one of the most widely used radio chips in wireless sensor nodes. The CC2420 provides two 128-bit security keys, stored in its RAM, for encryption/decryption. Besides this in-line security, it also provides plain stand-alone security operations with 128-bit plaintext (Healy, Newe, & Lewis, 2007). The plaintext is stored in a buffer located in the RAM and it is overwritten by the cipher-text after encryption.

Based on AES encryption using 128-bit keys, the CC2420 can perform IEEE 802.15.4 MAC security operations, including counter mode encryption (CTR), CBC-MAC (Cipher Block Chaining Message Authentication Code) and CCM, which is the combination of both CTR and CBC-MAC to provide encryption and authentication within an operation and with a single key. To allow real-time data transmission, the encryption and decryption are performed on FIFOs directly. Table 4 shows some examples of the time used by the security module for different operations.

The WBAN group employed this method in their network infrastructure (Warren et al., 2005), where the personal server shares the encryption key with *all* of the sensors in the WBAN during the session initialization. Hardware encryption is also followed by ALARM-NET (Wood et al., 2006). One limitation of the method is that it does not offer AES decryption, so transmitted information cannot be accessed by intermediate nodes if needed (e.g. for aggregation purposes). Any decryption can be performed only at the base station. Another drawback of the method is that it is highly dependent on the specific platform. Other sensor node platforms do not offer hardware encryption support, so a different approach has to be taken in this case.

## Runtime Security Service Composition

In biomedical sensor networks the criticality of data transmitted varies, in contrast with other applications of sensor networks. For example, the monitoring of the physical activities of patients is less critical than the heart rate monitoring. Even more critical is sending an alarm in case the patient is in an emergency. Consequently, the threats are different in each case, requiring different security levels. The provision of such a service from the link-layer security protocol could lead to a better management of the node's resources and extent their lifetime.

ALARM-NET is the only architecture of sensor networks for healthcare that incorporates such a mechanism. In particular, it takes advantage of the fact that hardware-accelerated cryptography in the CC2420 radio chip supports different security modes, as we described in the previous section. It makes those modes selectable for each message, allowing the application to decide which mode to employ, based on message semantics or context. To specify the mode used for each packet, ALARM-NET sacrifices part of the payload, which is used as a bit-field.

We can provide run-time composition of security services *without* removing the AM ID or adding extra fields to support integration of services. We can just use the most significant *three* bits of the data length field in the packet format as an indicator of the security service(s) to be used (from higher order bit to the lower: Replay Attack Protection, Access Control and Integrity, Confidentiality). These three bits are never used by TinyOS, as the maximum data length in TinyOS is chosen to be 29 bytes. Consequently, the provision of this feature comes with no overhead and setting *any* bit means that the related service is provided for that packet (Krontiris, Dimitriou, Soroush, & Salajegheh, 2008).

## Biometric Methods

An emerging key establishment method to secure communications in biomedical sensor networks is biometrics (Cherukuri, Venkatasubramanian, & Gupta, 2003). It advocates the use of the body itself as a means for committing cryptographic keys for symmetric cryptography over an insecure channel. For sensors attached on the same body, if they measure a previously agreed physiological value simultaneously and use this value to generate a pseudo-random number, this number will be the same. Then it can be used to encrypt and decrypt the symmetric key to distribute it securely. Of course, the actual cryptographic key is externally generated, independently from the physiological signals.

The physiological value to be used should be chosen carefully, as it must exhibit proper time variance and randomness. In different case the whole scheme can be vulnerable to brute force attacks. For example, blood glucose, blood pressure or heart rate, are physiological features that are not appropriate. On the other hand, ECG (electrocardiogram) has been found to exhibit desirable characteristics (Bui & Hatzinakos, 2008), since it is time-varying, changing with various physiological activities. Moreover, there exist sensor devices with reasonable costs that can record ECG signals effectively.

Besides randomness, another important requirement is that the generated key should be reproducible with high fidelity at the other sensor nodes on the same body. That translates to recovering identical ECG sequences, which in its turn requires accurate time synchronization, i.e., sensors taking their measurements at the same time produce the same value. To do that, a time synchronization protocol is needed, using reference broadcasts. The nodes listen to an external broadcast command and reinitialize the ECG recording at some scheduled time instant.

Let's assume that the sender and the receiver have measured the physiological values Ks and Kr respectively. If the sender wants to send some confidential data to the receiver, then it generates a random session key $K_{session}$ and transmits the message

$$m = C \parallel \gamma \parallel mac,$$

where $C$ is the encrypted payload,

$$C = E_{Ksession}(\text{Data}),$$

$\gamma$ is an XOR-bound version of the key,

$$\gamma = K_{session} \oplus K_s$$

and *mac* is the message authentication code of the encrypted data with the session key

$$mac = \text{MAC}(K_{session}|C).$$

The receiver, upon receiving the message, uses its own $K_r$ to compute $K_{session}'$ for verifying the MAC. Due to the dynamic nature of the body, $K_s$ and $K_r$ may not be exactly the same, so a *t*-bit error correcting decoder $f(\cdot)$ is used, which can correct errors with a Hamming distance of up to *t*. Therefore,

$$K_{session}' = f(\gamma \oplus Kr) = f(K_{session} + (K_s \oplus K_r)) = f(K_{session} + e).$$

If $K_s$ and $K_r$ are close enough so that $|e| \leq t$, then the key distribution is successful and the receiver will be able to compute the original session key. Then the MAC of the encrypted data is computed as

$$mac' = MAC(K_{session}'|C)$$

and is verified with the MAC from the encrypted data. If the values of *mac'* and *mac* are identical, then the receiver decrypts *C* to obtain the data, otherwise it discards the message received.

There are several disadvantages with solutions using physiological data. First of all they assume the existence of a strict synchronization protocol. Such protocols have been shown to be susceptible to attacks (Manzo, Roosta, & Sastry, 2005) and securing them will require even more of the mote's resources. Moreover, this method assumes that there is a specific pre-defined biometric that all biosensors can measure, which is not necessarily true. In actual systems, when two sensors want to communicate, they must first exchange a list of physiological values that they can measure and use one that they have in common, if this is the case.

Another disadvantage of this method is that only biosensors in and on the body can measure biometrics, so it cannot be applied for securing the communication between other sensor nodes in the general architecture or between biosensors and any on-body local processing unit. Actually, it is hard to be applied for communication between biosensors on the same body, unless they are very close to each other and therefore, the physiological values measured at the two points will vary only slightly. This can allow two biosensors on the same arm to communicate, but the physiological values that they measure will vary significantly with one measured at the leg for instance.

## FUTURE RESEARCH DIRECTIONS

The study of the security problems evolved in biomedical sensor networks are not studies in death so far, and solutions provided by researchers are mainly solutions that try to cover only the basic security requirements. Certainly there is still a long way ahead for the research community to understand the unique characteristics of these systems and provide holistic and trustworthy security solutions. Below we address some of the topics we consider important as future research directions.

### Secure Pairing

Pervasive healthcare systems make extensive use of portable handheld devices that are used by both patients and caregivers. A doctor should be able to directly query the medical sensors of the patient and retrieve real-time data on a mobile device (e.g. smart-phone or PDA). Especially at an emergency situation in the pre-hospital environment, it can be advantageous for the doctor to be able to access medical data independent of the connectivity with the EHR system at the hospital. Unfortunately, all proposed architectures of sensor networks in healthcare so far do not support such operations. They explicitly require that sensor nodes communicate only with the base stations, not with individual medical professional's devices.

Real-time data queries between a hand-held device and a medical sensor node comprise a different communication paradigm than the data collection at the base station through a multi-hop network. Prior work relies on pre-existing associations or secrets to secure such a communication. However, our case is an open-ended scenario, where a-priori planning of access control is frustrated. Therefore, a protocol is necessary to allow access of medical data only when a particular patient and health worker physically meet in a pre-hospital environment.

### Intrusion Detection

Cryptography can provide reasonable defence for outsider attackers, i.e., attackers who have not physically captured a sensor node and compromised its cryptographic primitives and keys. However, cryptography is inefficient in preventing against insider attacks. It remains an open problem for additional research and development. The presence of insiders significantly lessens the effectiveness of link layer security mechanisms. This is because an insider is allowed to participate in the network and have complete access to any messages routed through the network and is free to modify, suppress, or eavesdrop on the contents.

The above problems motivate the need for an intrusion detection system, which can act as a second line of defence: it can *detect* third party break-in attempts, even if this particular attack has not been experienced before. If the intruder is detected soon enough, one can take appropriate measures before any damage is done or any data is compromised. This is a novel research direction for sensor networks and only recently some works started considering intrusion detection as a solution for biomedical sensor networks (Giani, Roosta, & Sastry, 2008; Ng, Sim, & Tan, 2006).

## Privacy

Even though remote patient monitoring through ubiquitous computing systems provide many benefits for health care delivery, yet there are a number of privacy implications that must be explored in order to promote and maintain fundamental medical ethical principles and social expectations. While in this chapter we have focused on the security of the systems, there is also a great need to address the privacy of the individuals. While there are current regulations for medical data, these must be reevaluated and adapted to the new technological changes of health care delivery.

Some of the questions that must be addressed concerning privacy are the following: How owns the medical data collected by the user? How has access to them and under which circumstances? What type of medical data and for how long is stored? Can the patient have full control over how much of the data is sent to the central monitoring station? Guidelines need to be drawn which will regulate what sensor data collection entails and who will have control over it.

## Context Aware Security

In order to address several of the aspect of the privacy concerns addressed in the previous section, a necessary technology is access control. In particular, role-based access control is the dominant model for advanced access control. Healthcare systems have complex access rules because of the many actors in the system and their interlocking access privileges. With context-aware security, the system can dynamically adapt its security policies according to the context and not just the role of the user. For example, a context-aware system can exploit user's location for access control: if the user is within a certain area (e.g. a hospital) it can enforce different authorization rules than in the case where the user is outside the hospital. Other context-aware parameters can be life-threatening situations (e.g. public health emergency) that could alter security restrictions and accommodate emergency access to data. Sensor networks can provide this context awareness as their role is to integrate environmental, physiological and activity information into the same system.

Context information could also be used in order to automatically reconfigure the level of security provided by security mechanisms, optimising the use of resources. Providing a high level of security at all times may render the system unusable and providing no security is equally bad. An intelligent system should make security context aware and adaptive to patient's needs. We believe that providing context aware security will also improve the acceptance of the health monitoring system by healthcare providers. One of the important search needs here is not only to support context awareness, but also to secure the collection of the context itself.

## CONCLUSION

Recent advances in the area of wireless sensor networks have enabled the idea of remote patient monitoring. In this chapter we have discussed the security issues that arise when integrating this new technology into health care systems. The viability and long-term success of biomedical wireless sensor networks depends upon addressing these security threats successfully. We explored some of the existing solutions that have been employed and discussed their pros and cons. Then we identified some areas that are relatively unexplored at the moment and offer some promising research directions. But we should also stress that there is clearly a need for a biomedical sensor network architecture that takes security under consideration from the beginning and not add it as an extra "desirable" feature.

## REFERENCES

Bui, F. M., & Hatzinakos, D. (2008). Biometric methods for secure communications in body sensor networks: resource-efficient key management and signal-level data scrambling. *EURASIP J. Adv. Signal Process, 8*(2), 1–16. doi:10.1155/2008/529879

Cherukuri, S., Venkatasubramanian, K. K., & Gupta, S. K. S. (2003). BioSec: A biometric based approach for securing communication in wireless networks of biosensors implanted in the human body. In *Proceedings of the workshop on wireless security and privacy (wispr), international conference on parallel processing workshops* (pp. 432–439).

Giani, A., Roosta, T., & Sastry, S. (2008, January). Integrity checker for wireless sensor networks in health care applications. In *Proceedings of the 2nd international conference on pervasive computing technologies for healthcare.*

Großschädl, J. (2006). TinySA: A security architecture for wireless sensor networks (extended abstract). In *Proceedings of the 2nd international conference on emerging networking experiments and technologies (conext 2006)*. New York: ACM Press.

Gura, N., Patel, A., Wander, A., Eberle, H., & Shantz, S. C. (2004). Comparing elliptic curve cryptography and RSA on 8-bit CPUs. In *Proceedings of the workshop on cryptography hardware and embedded systems (CHES 2004),* (pp. 119–132).

Hartung, C., Balasalle, J., & Han, R. (2005, January). *Node compromise in sensor networks: The need for secure systems* (Technical Report No. CU-CS-990-05). Department of Computer Science, University of Colorado.

Mareca Hatler, Darryl Gurganious, Charlie Chi. (2008, August). *WSN for healthcare* (Market Report). OnWorld.

Healy, M., Newe, T., & Lewis, E. (2007). Efficiently securing data on a wireless sensor network. *Journal of Physics: Conference Series, 76.*

Hill, J., Szewczyk, R., Woo, A., Hollar, S., Culler, D., & Pister, K. (2000). System architecture directions for networked sensors. *ACM SIGPLAN Notices, 35*(11), 93–104. doi:10.1145/356989.356998

Karlof, C., Sastry, N., & Wagner, D. (2004, November). A link layer security architecture for wireless sensor networks. In Second ACM conference on embedded networked sensor systems (SenSys 2004) (pp. 162–175). TinySec.

Krontiris, I., Dimitriou, T., Soroush, H., & Salajegheh, M. (2008). In Lopez, J., & Zhou, J. (Eds.), *Wireless sensors networks security* (pp. 142–163). Amsterdam: IOS Press.

Krontiris, I., Giannetsos, Th., & Dimitriou, T. (2008). Launching a Sinkhole Attack in Wireless Sensor Networks; the Intruder Side. In *Proceeding of the first international workshop on security and privacy in wireless and mobile computing, networking and communications (SecPriWiMob 2008)*, (pp. 526-531).

Liu, A., & Ning, P. (2008). TinyECC: A configurable library for elliptic curve cryptography in wireless sensor networks. In *Proceedings of the International Conference on Information Processing in Sensor Networks (IPSN 2008), 0*, 245-256.

Lorincz, K., Malan, D. J., Fulford-Jones, T. R. F., Nawoj, A., Clavel, A., & Shnayder, V. (2004). Sensor networks for emergency response: Challenges and opportunities. *IEEE Pervasive Computing / IEEE Computer Society [and] IEEE Communications Society, 3*(4), 16–23. doi:10.1109/MPRV.2004.18

Lorincz, K., Malan, D. J., Fulford-Jones, T. R. F., Nawoj, A., Clavel, A., & Shnayder, V. (2004). Sensor networks for emergency response: Challenges and opportunities. *IEEE Pervasive Computing / IEEE Computer Society [and] IEEE Communications Society, 3*(4), 16–23. doi:10.1109/MPRV.2004.18

Lubrin, E., Lawrence, E., Navarro, K. F., & Zmijewska, A. (2006, July). Awareness of wireless sensor network potential in healthcare industry: A second UTAUT study. In *Proceedings of the IASTED international conference on wireless sensor networks,* Banff, Canada.

Malan, D., Welsh, M., & Smith, M. (2004). A public-key infrastructure for key distribution in TinyOS based on elliptic curve cryptography. In *Proceedings of the first annual IEEE communications society conference on sensor and ad hoc communications and networks (SECON 2004)* (pp. 71-80).

Malan, D. J., Welsh, M., & Smith, M. D. (2008). Implementing public-key infrastructure for sensor networks. *ACM Transactions on Sensor Networks, 4*(4), 1–23. doi:10.1145/1387663.1387668

Malasri, K., & Wang, L. (2007). Addressing security in medical sensor networks. In *Healthnet '07: Proceedings of the 1st ACM SIGMOBILE international workshop on systems and networking support for healthcare and assisted living environments* (pp. 7–12). New York: ACM.

Malasri, K., & Wang, L. (2008). Design and implementation of a secure wireless mote-based medical sensor network. In *Ubicomp '08: Proceedings of the 10th international conference on ubiquitous computing* (pp. 172–181). New York, NY, USA: ACM.

Manzo, M., Roosta, T., & Sastry, S. (2005). Time synchronization attacks in sensor networks. In *SASN '05: Proceedings of the 3rd ACM workshop on security of ad hoc and sensor networks* (pp. 107–116).

Marci Meingast, S. S. Tanya Roosta. (2006, August). Security and privacy issues with health care information technology. In *Embs '06: Proceedings of the 28th annual international conference of the IEEE engineering in medicine and biology society* (pp. 5453–5458).

Messina, M., Lim, Y., Lawrence, E., Martin, D., & Kargl, F. (2008). Implementing and validating an environmental and health monitoring system. In *ITNG '08: Proceedings of the fifth international conference on information technology: New generations* (pp. 994–999).

Ng, H. S., Sim, M. L., & Tan, C. M. (2006). Security issues of wireless sensor networks in healthcare applications. *BT Technology Journal, 24*(2), 138–144. doi:10.1007/s10550-006-0051-8

Shnayder, V., Chen, B., Lorincz, K., Jones, T., & Welsh, M. (2005). Sensor networks for medical care. In *Sensys '05: Proceedings of the 3rd international conference on embedded networked sensor systems.*

Stoa, S., Balasingham, I., & Ramstad, T. A. (2007). Data throughput optimization in the IEEE 802.15.4 medical sensor networks. In IEEE international symposium on circuits and systems (pp. 1361-1364).

Szczechowiak, P., Oliveira, L. B., Scott, M., Collier, M., & Dahab, R. (2008). NanoECC: Testing the limits of elliptic curve cryptography in sensor networks. In *Proceedings of the 5th European conference on wireless sensor networks (EWSN),* (Vol. 4913, p. 305-320). Berlin: Springer.

Tan, C., Wang, H., Zhong, S., & Li, Q. (2008). Body sensor network security: an identity-based cryptography approach. In *WiSec '08: Proceedings of the first ACM conference on wireless network security* (pp. 148–153). New York, NY, USA: ACM.

Uhsadel, L., Poschmann, A., & Paar, C. (2007). Enabling Full-Size Public-Key Algorithms on 8-bit Sensor Nodes. In *Proceedings of european workshop on security in adhoc and sensor networks (ESAS 2007)* (Vol. 4572, pp. 73–86). Berlin: Springer-Verlag.

Venkatasubramanian, K., & Gupta, S. (2007). Security in distributed, grid, mobile, and pervasive computing. In Y. Xiao (Ed.), (p. 443-464). Auerbach Publications, CRC Press. Jih, W., Cheng, S., Hsu, J. Y., & Tsai, T. (2005). Context-aware access control in pervasive healthcare. In EEE '05 workshop: Mobility, agents, and mobile services.

Venkatasubramanian, K., & Gupta, S. (2008). Demo - Ayushman: A secure, usable pervasive health monitoring system. In *Proceedings of the 1st ACM SIGMOBILE international workshop on systems and networking support for healthcare and assisted living environments (Healthnet 2008).*

Warren, S., Lebak, J., Yao, J., Creekmore, J., Milenkovic, A., & Jovanov, E. (2005). Interoperability and security in wireless body area network infrastructures. In *Proceedings of the 27th annual international conference of the IEEE engineering in medicine and biology society,* (pp. 3837–3840).

Washington, DC, USA: IEEE Computer Society. Orwat, C., Graefe, A., & Faulwasser, T. (2008, June). Towards pervasive computing in health care - a literature review. *BMC Medical Informatics and Decision Making, 8,* 26–44. doi:10.1186/1472-6947-8-26

Wood, A., Virone, G., Doan, T., Cao, Q., Selavo, L., Wu, Y., et al. (2006). *ALARM-NET: Wireless sensor networks for assisted-living and residential monitoring* (Tech. Rep. No. CS-2006-1). Department of Computer Science, University of Virginia.

## ADDITIONAL READING

Kargl, F., Lawrence, E., Fischer, M., & Lim, Y. (2008). Security, privacy and legal issues in pervasive e-health monitoring systems. In *ICMB '08: Proceedings of the 2008 7th international conference on mobile business* (pp. 296–304). Washington, DC, USA: IEEE Computer Society.

# Chapter 9
# Trustworthiness of Pervasive Healthcare Folders

**Tristan Allard**
*University of Versailles, France*

**Nicolas Anciaux**
*INRIA Rocquencourt, France*

**Luc Bouganim**
*INRIA Rocquencourt, France*

**Philippe Pucheral**
*University of Versailles, France*

**Romuald Thion**
*INRIA Grenoble, France*

## ABSTRACT

*During the last decade, many countries launched ambitious Electronic Health Record (EHR) programs with the objective to increase the quality of care while decreasing its cost. Pervasive healthcare aims itself at making healthcare information securely available anywhere and anytime, even in disconnected environments (e.g., at patient home). Current server-based EHR solutions badly tackle disconnected situations and fail in providing ultimate security guarantees for the patients. The solution proposed in this chapter capitalizes on a new hardware device combining a secure microcontroller (similar to a smart card chip) with a large external Flash memory on a USB key form factor. Embedding the patient folder as well as a database system and a web server in such a device gives the opportunity to manage securely a healthcare folder in complete autonomy. This chapter proposes also a new way of personalizing access control policies to meet patient's privacy concerns with minimal assistance of practitioners. While both proposals are orthogonal, their integration in the same infrastructure allows building trustworthy pervasive healthcare folders.*

DOI: 10.4018/978-1-61520-765-7.ch009

## INTRODUCTION

Driven by the need to improve the quality of care while decreasing costs, many countries around the world are setting up large scale Electronic Health Record (EHR) systems gathering the medical history of individuals. Interoperability among heterogeneous healthcare information systems and privacy preservation are two main challenges in this context. Pervasive healthcare on its side strive to remove location and time constraints to access patient's healthcare folders. Cares provided at home to elderly or disabled people illustrate well the need for pervasiveness. In this context healthcare data is mainly collected and consulted at home by practitioners having different privileges and acting at different time periods. Healthcare information must be safely exchanged among practitioners to improve care coordination but no connection to the Internet can be always guaranteed. Data can also be issued by institutions external to the care coordination (e.g., a medical lab) and join the patient's folder. Finally, data is sometimes accessed by practitioners outside patient's home (e.g., doctor's office, hospital). In this chapter, we discuss how smart objects can be used to implement healthcare folder pervasiveness efficiently and without privacy breach.

EHR systems aim at answering most of the requirements mentioned above. The objective of centralizing medical information in database systems is manifold[1]: completeness (i.e., to make the information complete and up to date), availability (to make it accessible through the internet 24h-7 days a week), usability (to organize the data and make it easily queryable and interpretable), consistency (to guarantee integrity constraints and enforce atomicity and isolation of updates) and durability (to protect the data against failure). A recent report identified more than 100 EHR running projects worldwide at the scale of a country or regions in 2007 (Door, 2008). Other reports suggest that about 25% of US healthcare practices use EHR systems. Within Europe these figures vary greatly between countries, from 15% in Greece up to 90% in the Netherlands today.

Regarding pervasiveness, healthcare folders can be reached by allowing internet connections to the server(s) through mobile devices (e.g., laptop, PDA, tablet PC). This however requires that every point of the territory be connected through a secure, fast, reliable and cheap network, a situation uncommon in many countries and regions today.

In addition, and despite the unquestionable benefit of EHR systems in terms of quality of care, studies conducted in different countries show that patients are reluctant to use existing EHR systems arguing increasing threats on individual privacy (The Times, 2008; The International Council on Medical & Care Compunetics, 2009). This suspicion is fueled by computer security surveys pointing out the vulnerability of database servers against external and internal attacks (Gordon et al, 2006). Indeed, centralizing and organizing the information make it more valuable, thereby motivating attacks and facilitating abusive usages. Regardless of the legislation protecting the usage of medical data and of the security procedures put in place at the servers, the patient has the sense of losing control over her data.

Hence, implementing pervasiveness of healthcare folders requires addressing accurately the following issues:

1. How to access patient's healthcare folder in a disconnected mode (e.g., at home)?
2. How to access patient's healthcare folder seamlessly in a connected area?
3. How to make the patient trust the EHR security?
4. How to get the patient consent about a pervasive use of her healthcare folder?

As discussed above, existing EHR systems answer well issue 2 but fail in answering issue 1 and issue 3. Therefore, EHR systems fail also in answering issue 4 precisely due to the lack of server trustworthiness.

This chapter suggests a new way of organizing EHR to address issues 1 to 4 all at once. The solution proposed capitalizes on a new hardware device called Secure Portable Token (SPT) hereafter. Roughly speaking, a SPT combines a secure microcontroller (similar to a smart card chip) with a large external Flash memory (Gigabyte sized) on a USB key form factor (Eurosmart, 2008). A SPT can host on-board data and run on-board code with proven security properties. Embedding a database system and a web server in a SPT gives the opportunity to manage securely a healthcare folder in complete autonomy. Accessing the on-board folder at patient's home requires a simple rendering device (e.g., a netbook or PDA) equipped with an USB port and running a web browser. Then issue 1 is tackled by construction. The SPT security properties (tamper-resistant hardware, certified embedded software) answer issue 3 with a much higher confidence than any traditional server can provide.

Issue 2 becomes however more difficult to address. Indeed, the patient folder cannot be accessed without being physically in possession of the patient's SPT. To tackle situations where remote access to the folder is mandatory, the solution proposed is to reintroduce a server in the architecture so that a secure exchange of information can be organized between the patient and a trusted circle of persons. The solution is such that patient's data is never stored in the clear on the server and encryption/decryption keys are known only by the SPT participating to the trusted circle of person defined by the patient. Hence, issue 2 can be tackled in a practical way without compromising issue 3.

One may consider that answering issue 3 leads to answer issue 4 as well. This is unfortunately not true. Trusting the EHR security is a prerequisite for the patient to give her consent about a pervasive use of her medical folder but it is definitely not a sufficient condition. Expressing an enlightened consent means understanding and accepting an access control policy specifying who (individuals or roles) is granted access to which part of her folder. The high number of people interacting with the folder, the diversity of their roles, the complexity of the medical information and the intrinsic difficulty to determine which data (or data association) reveals a given pathology makes this objective highly difficult to reach. This chapter proposes a new and pragmatic alternative to define access control policies manageable by a patient with minimal assistance of practitioners. This solution complements well the SPT-based EHR architecture by answering issue 4. This solution is however orthogonal to the SPT-based architecture and we believe it could apply to many healthcare information systems.

As a conclusion, the objective of this chapter is twofold. First, it discusses to which extent existing EHR architectures can meet the four requirements introduced above (Section 2) and proposes an alternative based on the SPT hardware device (Sections 3 and 4). Second, it discusses whether existing access control policies and confidentiality mechanisms can capture the patient's consent (Section 5) and proposes a solution relying on a new access control model (Section 6). Section 7 relates an experimentation in the field of a pervasive EHR architecture combining both proposals, in the context of home care provided to elderly people.

## BACKGROUND

An Electronic Health Record (EHR) system is a collection of electronic patient folders, each containing the complete medical history of an individual, managed and consulted by authorized health professionals across several organizations (Alliance, 2007). Building an EHR system requires interconnecting various heterogeneous health information systems of disparate organizations in order to aggregate the medical data they maintain separately (e.g., hospitals, practitioners and pharmacists data related to a same individual).

Hence, the first challenge tackled by EHR programs is providing interoperability between heterogeneous systems. As pointed out in the introduction, ensuring data availability even in disconnected environments and enforcing data security are two additional and mandatory challenges. The next subsections present a state of the art on these three challenges.

## EHR Interoperability

Three main approaches can be distinguished according to the level of integration targeted between existing health information systems.

The first approach consists in interconnecting existing autonomous systems in a wider infrastructure with no data centralization and a minimal central control. The Danish Healthcare Data Network (Pedersen, 2006)[2] is representative of this category. It connects the already secure intranets of care organizations via VPNs over the Internet, progressively from organizations to counties, counties to regions, and regions to nation. The Danish EHR effort has mainly consisted in defining a common data model representing clinical data. The USA have adopted a federal approach to build the EHR. At the region scale, Regional Health Information Organizations (RHIOs) are multi-stakeholder organizations that enable the exchange of health information between local health organizations (e.g., CalRHIO for the Californian RHIO). At the nation scale, the Nationwide Health Information Network (NHIN) project, supervised by the Office of the National Coordinator for Health IT (ONC), aims at enabling secure health information exchange across the USA by using RHIOs as regional building blocks. The NHIN will be a "network of networks" built over the Internet.

The second approach strengthens the integration thanks to centralized indexes and/or data summaries. The National Health Society in the United Kingdom has launched the Care Record Service (CRS) project. First, CRS aims at linking together the existing EMRs (Electronic Medical Record) of an individual, thus constituting a virtual unique health folder. Navigating between the EMRs of an individual and gathering detailed data will be easier; furthermore, by sharing data across EMRs, duplication of - e.g., administrative - data will be useless. Second, CRS aims at storing summaries of detailed data on the "Spine", an already existing central system currently in charge of delivering health related services (e.g., ePresciptions, eReservations). Summarized data will serve to draw reports and analysis about collected care information. With its two-level functional architecture, the Diraya project from Andalusia is similar to the CRS UK project. First, detailed data in EMRs are kept where they are produced (e.g., hospitals) and the central Diraya system indexes them. Second, Diraya centralizes what is called the "main data", that is the data most frequently accessed. In the Netherlands, the National Healthcare Information Hub project (LSP in Dutch), lead by Nictiz is basically a central index storing the location of every individual's EMRs. The Austrian ELGA initiative (Husek, 2008) is similar to the LSP project. The Canadian national program Infoway-Inforoute funds provincial EHR projects, most of these focusing on interoperability between care organizations. For example, the Alberta Netcare EHR centralizes regionally the patients' summary data. The Yukon Telehealth project makes local EMRs accessible to remote specialist practitioners.

The most integrated approach seeks to gather all EMRs related to the same individual into a centralized healthcare folder. In the USA, some private organizations had already felt the need to aggregate all their patients' data in a single folder before the coming of RHIOs. For example, the Veteran Administration Medical Center developed the VistA system (Brown et al, 2003), a Health Information System (HIS) enabling health centers with VistA to share their patients' data. The French national program Dossier Medical Personnel (DMP) aims also at centralizing healthcare folders hosted by selected Database Service Providers. In another spirit, systems like Google Health™ and Microsoft's HealthVault™ propose individuals to centralize their Personal Health Records (PHRs) on their own initiative. Both load medical data directly from the patient's health centers that do agree, offer practical tools for individuals (e.g., drug interactions, hospitals searches), and can provide a controlled access to the PHR to a selected set of persons. Both are free and the users are simply asked to trust their privacy policy.

## EHR Availability

All EHR systems mentioned above provide a 24h/7day a week availability assuming the servers are active and an internet connection can be established to reach them. This is unfortunately not the case in every place and every situation, introducing the need for disconnected accesses to healthcare folders.

In the United Kingdom, the Health eCard is a private initiative that proposes to store encrypted copies of full EMRs in specifically designed smart cards, making patients' health data available in disconnected situations (e.g., emergency situations, home consultation).

The German organization Gematik leads the eGK, an ambitious project mixing a traditional infrastructure with smart cards in order to tackle connected and disconnected situations (Smart Card Alliance-b, 2006). Both patients and professionals are equipped with a smart card, patient smart cards storing EHRs while professional smart cards are being used for strong authentication, digital signature and encryption/decryption of documents. The infrastructure holds a centralized copy of the EHRs, accessible through the internet. This project is still at a preliminary stage.

In the USA, many private initiatives issued by care centers tackle the "disconnected access"

requirement (Smart Card Alliance-a, 2006), e.g., the University of Pittsburgh Medical Center Health Passport Project (HPP), the Florida eLife-Card, Queens Health Network, Mount Sinai Medical Center Personal Health Card. All of them store a copy of critical health information encrypted on a smart card to make it available in case of emergency.

Taiwan has launched in 2001 a project to replace the traditional paper health cards by smart cards (Smart Card Alliance, 2005). Smart cards are used exactly as paper cards were used. They permanently store administrative personal and summary health data, and temporarily store the medical data related to the last six visits. Every six visits, the temporary medical data are uploaded into the Taiwanese health infrastructure. The smart card health project is seamlessly integrated with the previous health infrastructure, providing a strong patient authentication and a paperless data management.

While many initiatives tackle the disconnected access challenge, the low storage capacities of the smart cards used in the aforementioned projects (i.e., at best a few hundreds of Kilo-bytes) severely limit the quantity of on-board data, and then the benefit of the approach.

## EHR Security

Strong authentication is usually required to connect to EHR servers. Health professionals authenticate with a smart-card (e.g., the CRS in UK, the LSP in the Netherlands), as well as patients accessing to their medical folder (e.g., the Diraya initiative in Andalusia). In addition, communication channels can be protected by cryptographic techniques, based on protocols such as TLS (The Transport Layer Security, 2008), enabling entities to securely exchange messages (i.e., encryption, integrity protection, non repudiation of messages), and security measures are implemented on central servers. However, this is not sufficient to put trust in the system.

The suspicion is fueled by computer security surveys pointing out the vulnerability of database servers against external and internal attacks (Gordon et al, 2006). Database systems are identified as the primary target of computer criminality (Gordon et al, 2006), and even the most well defended servers, including those of Pentagon (The Financial Times, 2007; Liebert, 2008), FBI (The Washington Post, 2007) and NASA (Computer World, 2003), have been successfully attacked. In addition, nearly half of the attacks (Gordon et al, 2006) come from the inside (employees) of the companies or organizations. In addition, there are many examples where negligence leads to personal data leakages. To cite a few, thousands of Medicare and Medicaid patients in eight states have been lost in a HCA regional office (FierceHealthIT news, 2006) and Hospitals County published by accident medical records on the web (FierceHealthIT news, 2008; WFTV, 2008) including doctors' notes, diagnoses, medical procedures and possibly names and ages of patients. A recent study shows that 81% of US firms declare loosing employees laptops with sensitive data (Computer World, 2006). Data loss is so frequent that a research project called DataLossDB has been created to report such incidents.

In practice, EHRs are thus very difficult to protect. This legitimates the reserves expressed by both practitioners and patients about EHR programs (The Times, 2008; eHealth Insider, 2008). In the Netherlands, privacy and access concerns are major arguments for the postponement of the national EHR (The International Council on Medical & Care Compunetics, 2009). In particular, the lack of security measures limiting data access for service providers and the loss of control on their own data has been identified as a main reason for citizens to opt-out of the system.

Only EMRs stored in personal and secure hardware such as smart-cards (see Section 2.2) can benefit from true privacy enforcement. However, (1) the storage capacity of the smart-cards used by current projects (e.g., from KB to MB) is too low to store a complete EHR, limiting the data availability in disconnected situations, (2) their low connectivity makes the hosted data seldom available, and (3) their portable nature makes them subjects to losses or destruction. Moreover, to tackle availability, these projects rely on central servers unable to enforce the smart-cards security level (Eurosmart, 2008).

We believe that both data privacy and full availability can be achieved altogether. The solution we propose is centered on a personal smart-card based device storing (the most significant part of) the patient folder and extending the security sphere of its secure hardware to traditional central servers.

## A SECURE, PORTABLE MEDICAL FOLDER

Researches conducted in the PlugDB[3] project led us to design a lightweight Database Management System (DBMS) embedded in a new form of tamper-resistant token, called hereafter Secure Portable Token (SPT). Roughly speaking, a SPT combines a secure microcontroller (similar to a smart card chip) with a large external Flash memory (Gigabyte sized) on a USB key form factor (Eurosmart, 2008). A SPT can host a large volume of on-board data and run on-board code with proven security properties thanks to its tamper-resistant hardware and a certified operating system (Eurosmart, 2008). The main target of the PlugDB technology is the management of secure and portable personal folder. Healthcare folders are very good representative of large personal folders where security and portability are highly required.

Compared to smart cards used in other EHR projects (see Section 2), the storage capacity of a SPT is roughly four orders of magnitude higher. Henceforth, this makes sense to embed the whole patient folder in her SPT and make it available in disconnected mode. In addition to the data, a complete chain of software is embedded in the SPT microcontroller: (1) a Web server, (2) servlets implementing the application, (3) a JDBC bridge, (4) a DBMS engine managing the on-board database and enforcing access control. Hence, the SPT along with its embedded database and software can be seen as a full-fledged server accessible through any web browser running on any device equipped with a USB port (e.g., laptop, tablet-PC, PDA and even cell-phone). Compared to a regular server, the SPT server is personal, pluggable, does not require any network connection and provides unprecedented security guarantees.

The specific hardware architecture of the SPT introduces however many technical challenges. We detail below the most important ones.

## SPT Hardware and Operating System

A SPT combines in the same hardware platform a secure chip and a mass storage NAND FLASH memory (several Gigabytes soon). The secure chip is of the smart card type, with a 32 bit RISC CPU clocked at about 50 MHz, memory modules composed of ROM, tens of KB of static RAM, a small quantity of internal stable storage (NOR FLASH) and security modules. The mass storage NAND FLASH memory is outside the secure chip, connected to it by a bus, and does not benefit from the chip hardware protection.

Gemalto, the smart card world leader has developed an experimental SPT platform. This platform includes a new multi-tasking operating system allowing the development of Web applications based on JAVA and Servlet technology, and thus offering a standardized means to integrate services or embedded Web applications to the SPT. The operating system supports natively: the USB 2.0 protocol and the internet protocol IP for communicating with the external world (Vandewalle, 2004); Multi-threaded Java applications; Cryptographic primitives (some of which implemented in hardware); Memory management and

garbage collection; Servlet management and Web server. For more technical details on the hardware platform and the operating system, we refer the reader to (http://www-smis.inria.fr/~DMSP).

## Embedded Database System

DBMS designers have produced light versions of their systems for personal assistants (e.g. Oracle-lite, DB2 everyplace, SQLServer for Window CE) but they never addressed the more complex problem of embedding a DBMS in a chip. Initial attempts towards a smart card DBMS was ISOL's SQL Java Machine (Carrasco, 1999), the ISO standard SCQL (ISO/IEC, 1999) and the MasterCard Open Data Storage (MasterCard International, 2002). All these proposals concerned traditional smart cards with few resources and therefore proposed basic data management functionalities (close to sequential files). Managing embedded medical folders requires much more powerful storage, indexation, access control and query capabilities. PicoDBMS was the first full fledged relational DBMS embedded in a smart card (Pucheral et al, 2001) and was implemented on top of Gemalto's smart card prototypes (Anciaux et al, 2001). PicoDBMS has been designed for managing databases stored in a (Megabyte sized) EEPROM stable memory integrated in the secure chip and protected by the chip tamper-resistance.

The SPT framework introduces important new challenges (Anciaux, Bouganim, et al, 2007):

1. How to support complex queries over a large on-board database (Gigabyte sized) with very little RAM (a few Kilobytes)?
2. How to organize the data storage and the indexes with an acceptable insert/update time considering the peculiarities of NAND Flash memory (fast reads, costly writes, block-erase-before-page-rewrite constraint)?
3. How to protect the on-board database against confidentiality and integrity attacks (the external Flash being not hardware

*Figure 1. Secure portable token*

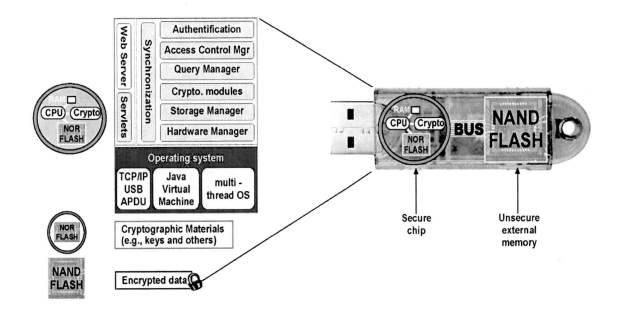

protected) while keeping acceptable query performance?

The SPT architecture and the organization of the embedded software components are illustrated in Figure 1. The on-board code and sensitive data (e.g., cryptographic keys) reside in the secure chip; patient's data reside in the insecure external memory, previously encrypted by the secure execution environment. We detail below the components related to the technical challenges mentioned above.

The Query Manager is in charge of parsing the incoming database queries, building an optimal query execution plan and executing it. This module must consider peculiar execution strategies to answer complex SQL queries over a large quantity of data with little RAM (challenge 1). To tackle this challenge, we designed a massive indexing scheme presented in (Anciaux, Benzine, et al, 2007), which allows processing complex queries while consuming as little RAM as possible and still exhibiting acceptable performance. The idea is to combine in the same indexing model

generalized join indices and multi-table selection indices in such a way that any combination of selection and join predicates can be evaluated by set operations over lists of sorted tuple identifiers. The operator library (algorithms for the operators of the relational algebra, e.g., select, project, join and aggregate) and the execution engine integrate those techniques.

The Storage Manager on which the query manager relies to access the database content (index and tables) is directly concerned with challenge 2. Indeed, the proposed massive indexation scheme causes a difficult problem in terms of Flash updates, due to the severe read/write constraints of NAND Flash (rewriting NAND Flash pages is a very costly operation). Therefore, we designed a structure which manages data and index keys sequentially so that the number of rewrites in Flash is minimized. The use of summarization structures based on bloom filters (Bloom, 1970) and vertical partitioning reduce the cost of index lookups (Yin et al, 2009). These additional structures are also managed in sequence. A first implementation of this principle has been patented jointly by INRIA and Gemalto (Pucheral & Yin, 2007) and is integrated in the current DBMS prototype.

The Hardware Manager embeds the methods for accessing the different memory modules of the SPT. It includes techniques associated with challenge 3 to protect the confidentiality and the integrity of the data, in an efficient way with respect to DBMS access patterns. Indeed, our massive indexation technique leads to numerous, random and fine grain accesses to raw data. We conducted preliminary studies (Anciaux et al, 2006), in which we combine encryption, hashing and timestamping techniques with query execution techniques in order to satisfy three conflicting objectives: efficiency, high security and compliance with the chip hardware resources.

The Access Control Manager is in charge of enforcing the access control policy defined to grant/deny access to pieces of the patient folder to the current user. Privileges can be associated to individual users or roles. To help collecting patients' consent, each patient should be given the chance to personalize a predefined access control policy. Hence, the Access Control Manager plays an important role in answering challenge 4 identified in the introduction. Access control is more deeply discussed in Section 6.

## Data Availability and Security

Any terminal equipped with an USB port and a Web Browser can interact with the SPT and get the data he is granted access to. Hence, when no Internet connection is available (e.g., emergency situations, home intervention, remote server breakdown) SPTs guarantee patients' data availability, thereby achieving challenge 1 identified in the introduction. Furthermore, local connections to SPTs do not suffer from unpredictable performance due to overloaded remote servers or low quality connections: the embedded server is mono-user and USB-2 communication throughput is guaranteed.

In terms of security, patient's data resides in the external NAND Flash memory. As stated in section 3.2, this memory is not hardware protected so that its content must be encrypted to prevent confidentiality attacks and hashed to prevent integrity attacks. The cryptographic keys serving this purpose reside in the NOR Flash memory and are protected by the tamper-resistance of the secure chip. The encryption/decryption/hashing processes physically take place in the secure chip and are similarly hardware protected (i.e., see the red circle of Figure 1). More generally, the complete software chain (web server, servlets, DBMS) runs in the secure chip and benefits from its tamper-resistance. Hence, the authentication, access control, and query steps are all hardware protected. The security of the complete architecture thereby relies on the tamper-resistance of the secure chip. The security of our hardware platform and of the embedded code is under certification with the goal to reach the highest security level (EAL4[+]), usually required for smart card chips used in the medical domain. This makes attacks highly improbable and extremely costly to conduct. Considering that the security of a system lies in the fact that the cost to conduct an attack outweighs its benefit, the security of our architecture is reinforced by the extreme cost of attacks and their small benefit (disclosure of a single patient's folder). Consequently, we argue that our architecture achieves convincingly challenge 4 identified in the introduction.

## A SECURE, PERVASIVE MEDICAL FOLDER

Section 3 tackled challenges 1 and 3; this section focuses on challenge 2: remote accesses to health folders. How can the family doctor express her opinion about an emergency situation without having the patient's SPT? We introduce a central server in the architecture as a mean to obtain data availability, i.e., the ability to readily access data, despite the patient's SPT absence.

This must be achieved without losing the benefits of the SPT in terms of security and control by its owner. This entails never revealing sensitive information to the central server. Two rules arise from this statement: (1) sensitive data must be stored encrypted on the server storage media, and (2) sensitive data must be encrypted and decrypted in a secure execution environment, i.e., a SPT.

To be available to Health professionals, medical folders reside (encrypted) on the central server and can be downloaded to their SPTs on demand. To gain access to the folder, the SPT of the professional must host the cryptographic keys of the patient and hold access privileges on her folder. It is up to the patient to define the trusted circle of professionals holding her key.

To secure the communications, we use protocols such as TLS (Internet Engineering Task Force, 2008). TLS relies on a certificate authority to emit trusted certificates linking an identity to a public key. The Professionals, patients and central server safely communicate after having exchanged and checked their respective certificates. Certificates are inserted in the SPTs' secure internal memory at the beginning of their life cycle, before being delivered to its owner. The server is in charge of securing his own certificate. Note that SPTs are not durable: they may be lost or broken. Hence, to make certificates and pairs of (public key, private key) durable, they must be replicated in a trusted third party (TTP). We do not detail those protocols further in this chapter.

In this section, we first classify data according to their needs in terms of privacy and depict an SPT-centered architecture fulfilling these needs. Second, we focus on synchronization issues between the patient's SPT, the central server, and external entities (e.g., laboratories). Finally, we describe a comprehensive use case of the system.

## A Data Classification Driven by Privacy Concerns

We call *Regular Data* (RD) the pieces of information the patient consent to replicate on a remote server in the clear. Such data is protected by the security policy enforced by the server and can be accessed on line by any practitioner having the required privileges. The access control policy enforced by the server and the SPT is assumed to be identical. However, the server does not benefit from the tamper-resistance of the SPT and Regular Data can be accessed on the server without prior patient knowledge. What is actually considered as Regular Data depends on the patient feeling, e.g., administrative data, non-sensitive medications (e.g., aspirin), non sensitive diagnosis (e.g., flue). Being replicated on the server, Regular Data benefits from the server on-line availability and durability properties.

We call *Secret Data* (SD) the pieces of information the patient considers so sensitive (e.g., psychological analysis) that he cannot accept to delegate their storage to a remote server. Secret data remains confined to the patient's SPT. Hence SD durability is under the patient responsibility and SD availability requires the presence of the patient's SPT.

Finally, we call *Confined Data* (CD) the pieces of information too sensitive to be managed as RD but for which on-line availability and/or durability is mandatory for care practice (e.g., HIV diagnosis, chemotherapy medication, MRI image). CD is replicated encrypted on the server but the encryption keys are never present at the server. Hence CD is protected against server attacks. Encryption keys are stored and managed by SPT devices only. To ensure on-line availability, encryption keys can be shared by the SPTs of a selected set of persons, named hereafter *trusted circle* (e.g., the family doctor and some specialist physicians). Members of the trusted circle can access CD on the server and their SPT can decrypt them. Defining trusted circles is up to the patient.

*Figure 2. Functional architecture*

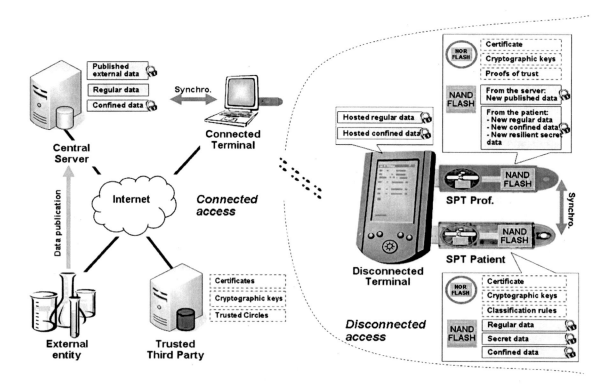

Durability is guaranteed by the server similarly to clear-text data. However, recovering CD entails recovering the related encryption keys. This can be achieved either by a pass phrase or by a trusted third party (TTP) registering encryption keys. Note that Secret Data can be made durable by declaring them as Confined Data, without sharing the encryption keys and assuming the patient trusts the cryptographic protocols.

Data classification is under patient responsibility, possibly with external help (e.g., his family doctor). The patient can change his mind afterwards (e.g., following the advice of his doctor) according to the following hierarchy: secret data → confined data → regular data. Any other change is uncertain, e.g., when changing from regular data to secret data, the clear regular data could have been queried or copied beforehand; the patient cannot be sure of its secrecy.

Figure 2 depicts the global architecture, showing where information resides and whether it is encrypted or not. Data located in dashed rectangles resides in a trusted storage (either the SPT's internal memory or the TTP) contrary to data located in solid rectangles. Data aside yellow locks is encrypted. This architecture provides stronger privacy preservation guarantees than any traditional EHR. Attacks conducted at the server (bypassing the traditional security measures) can only reveal regular data, secret data being absent from the server and confined data being encrypted with keys let under the control of the SPTs and the trusted third party. Attacks conducted over a patient's SPT are made highly difficult by its secure hardware.

## Synchronization

Replicating data on the central server provides availability and durability, but raises a synchronization problem. When a server and a SPT are directly connected with each other, traditional synchronization methods apply. However, a SPT may never connect directly to the central server (e.g. a patient who never leaves home). In this case, SPTs of health professionals must behave as "proxies", carrying encrypted synchronization messages from patients' SPTs to the central server, and vice-versa.

Health professionals carry encrypted synchronization messages from patients' SPTs to the central server when they visit the patients. During the visit, the professional may insert new data in the Patient's SPT. At the end of the visit, newly created regular and confined data (i.e., not present yet in the server) is copied into the professional's SPT. The central server is refreshed every time a professional connects to it. Conversely, the professional SPT carries encrypted data newly created at the server in order to refresh the patient's SPT replica. This situation occurs when external entities produce medical data directly on the central server, e.g., a laboratory producing examination results. However, data cannot be produced in the clear and the data is not yet classified by the patient. To circumvent this problem, external entities must encrypt data with the patient's public key before publishing them on the central server. At synchronization time, the patient will be able to decrypt this data, classify it, and store it according to its privacy class.

## Use Case

Let us illustrate the behavior of the system through a scenario involving four participants: an elderly patient named Patrick, his family doctor David, a nurse Nora, and a spy Sandra. Patrick, David, and Nora have each their own SPT. Several medical examinations are prescribed to Patrick who clas-sifies them as regular, confined, and secret data. Patrick recently went through blood exams into a medical laboratory. The medical lab performing the examination has published the encrypted results on the central server. Results were encrypted with Patrick's public key obtained from the trusted third party.

Nora frequently visits Patrick at home. Patrick has no internet connection and leaves home seldom. Thus, Nora acts as a synchronization means for Patrick's folder (as do any other person visiting Patrick and owning a SPT). Before the visit, Nora downloads from the central server the latest updates performed in Patrick's folder, encrypted with Patrick's public key. This includes the recent examination results. During the visit, Nora's and Patrick's SPTs synchronize: Nora's SPT send to Patrick's SPT the encrypted examination results, Patrick's SPT decrypts them with his private key, classifies and encrypts them accordingly to their classes – lab results are confined data – and sends them back to Nora's SPT which will refresh the central server the next time it connects to it. Nora's SPT also copies the latest updates performed in Patrick's local folder, if any. Nora cannot get access to this data, protected by the tamper resistance of the SPT.

During a previous visit, Patrick asked David to join his trusted circle. Patrick's SPT hashed and signed David's certificate, who uploaded this proof of trust onto the TTP. After Nora's visit, at his office, he can connect to the central server and view Patrick's up-to-date folder, including the results of the recent examinations (classified as confined data) and possible updates carried back by Nora (in the limit of David's access rights). When visiting Patrick at home, David gets the same information by accessing data directly through Patrick's SPT.

One day, Patrick's looses his SPT which is found by Sandra. Missing the PIN code, Sandra cannot authenticate to the SPT. She can open the SPT and snoop at the NAND FLASH memory content but data is encrypted. If she tries to tamper the secure chip to obtain the decryption key, security counter measures will destroy the embedded components. The only attack which could be successfully conducted is against the regular data on the central server. Any sensitive data is stored encrypted (the key being within SPTs or on the trusted third party). A few days after, Patrick receives a new SPT, containing both his keys and his data, and continues to receive visits at home from his health practitioners.

## EXPRESSING PATIENT'S CONSENT

Trusting the EHR security is a prerequisite for the patient to give her consent about a pervasive use of her medical folder but it is definitely not a sufficient condition. Expressing an enlightened consent means understanding and accepting an access control policy specifying who (individuals or roles) is granted access to which part of her folder. This section details the notion of user's privacy and surveys the current models and mechanisms to achieve it.

### Privacy Protection

#### Legal Approach

Roughly, privacy is the protection of Personally Identifiable Information (PII), by means of restricting access, transfer, storage, etc. of PII. The concept of "informed consent" is a cornerstone of most privacy regulations. The consent of use of personal data must be an enlightened, free, univocal and unilateral act. Protecting PII is a prime concern for the deployment of pervasive computing systems such as EHR (Langheinrich, 2005).

The European Union Directive 95/46/EC sets the protection of individuals with regard to the processing of personal data. Article 29 of this directive establishes a set of core principles of privacy, which are quite close to the ten found-

ing principles of Hippocratic database systems (Agrawal et al., 2002):

1. the *purpose limitation principle*: data must be processed for a specific and declared purpose.
2. the *data quality and proportionality principle*: data must be accurate, adequate and relevant wrt the declared purpose.
3. the *transparency principle*: information must be provided as to the purpose of the processing, the identity of the data controller must be ensured.
4. the *security principle*: appropriate security measures must be taken.
5. the *rights of access, rectification and opposition*.
6. *restrictions on onward transfers*.

As stated by the Article 29 Working party (Article 29 Data Protection Working Party, 2007), one of the essential principles concerning EHR is limiting access to a folder to only those healthcare professionals who are involved in the patient's treatment. Data protection could be enhanced by modular access rights: the patient should be given the chance to prevent access to his EHR data if he so chooses. This requires prior information about the possible consequences of not allowing access.

### Privacy Preferences

A lot of attention has been dedicated to expression of privacy preferences, which are consent of use of PII expressed according to the above mentioned principles. The Platform for Privacy Preferences (P3P) defined by the W3C is a machine readable format of privacy preferences. The Platform for Enterprise Privacy Practices (E-P3P) (Karjoth et al., 2002) or EPAL (Ashley et al., 2003) define the enterprise privacy enforcement system for privacy policies internal to the enterprise. P3P is used to state an enterprise's privacy policy when collecting PII from the customers whereas E-P3P is used for internally enforcing the enterprise's policy to control accesses to the collected PII.

As coined by the title of (Massacci & Zannone, 2004) "Privacy Is Linking Permission to Purpose", the purpose (e.g. from P3P: marketing, surveys, payment etc.) is the intended use of the data queried and is the backbone of informed consent. Thus, integrating purpose (and obligations related to these purposes) into control is one of the main challenges and research directions investigated in privacy protection.

## Control Mechanisms for Privacy

### Traditional Access Control

An Access Control (AC) (or authorization) policy is a specialized form of security policy, dedicated to permission management. AC primarily aims at enforcing confidentiality (Samarati & Di Vimercati, 2001). Access control is one of the means to enhance privacy by restricting access to personal data. An AC policy is structured according to a model. The model formally describes the language in which policies are expressed and how to decide whether an access request should be granted or denied.

Traditional AC models are the Mandatory Access Control (MAC) and the Discretionary Access Control (DAC). MAC is a label-based (e.g. Unclassified, Confidential, Secret, Top Secret) AC mechanism. Each user and each data is associated to a unique label. Access on a data is allowed if the user is granted sufficient clearance level. DAC is a decentralized user-based mechanism where the creator of a data defines the set of authorizations.

Intermediate concepts between data and users have been introduced to simplify administration of AC policies. In the Role-Based Access Control (RBAC) models family, roles are assigned to users and permissions are assigned to those roles (Ferraiolo et al., 2003). Thus, an RBAC policy is a set of assignments between users and roles and between roles and permissions. The core rule of RBAC states that an access request is granted iff the issuer endorses a role with this privilege.

From the RBAC initiative, several models have been studied in the literature. These models may either extend RBAC (e.g. with temporal or geographical constraints), or organize policies by mean of additional concepts (e.g. team, task, organization) to enhance their expressive power and flexibility. First-order logic has been advocated as a general framework suitable to formalize AC models and policies (Halpern & Weissman, 2008).

### Access Control for Privacy

Traditional AC models such as RBAC are commonly used to organize access rights. However, they are not adequate to express finer control on data usage. Usage CONtrol model (UCON) is a foundation for next-generation access control models. In this model, a usage control decision is determined by combining authorizations, obligations, and conditions (Zhang et al., 2005). Usage control is a way to implement digital rights management, for instance by providing guarantees of restriction on onward transfers.

In order to guarantee the purpose limitation principle, the notion of purpose should be used for access control. A policy should ensure that data can only be used for its intended purpose, and the access purpose should be compliant with the data's intended purpose. The authors (Yang et al., 2007) have proposed a purpose-based AC model on this basis. (Ni et al., 2007) have bound purposes to RBAC in an integrated model Privacy-Aware RBAC (P-RBAC). This model has been refined to include the definition of conditional obligations. The integration of purpose control and RBAC for privacy protection of relational data has been investigated too (Byun & Li, 2008).

## Specialized Access Control Models for Health Record

Several models have been defined to organize rights on medical data. Alhaqbani and Fidge propose a cascaded AC architecture made of three AC layers (Alhaqbani & Fidge, 2007). First layer is based on DAC, second one on RBAC and last one on MAC. When all the three policies agree, access is granted. The authors of (Røstad & Nytrø, 2008) have more tightly combined DAC and RBAC into the Personally Controlled Health Record (PCHR) AC system. In their approach, two policies are defined: a common one and personalized one. Only the personalized one is defined by EHR's owner. A conflict resolution rule (e.g. deny overrides, permit overrides) is defined, it is used whenever the two policies disagree on the access decision.

The authors of (Alhaqbani & Fidge, 2007) and (Røstad & Nytrø, 2008) concentrate on policies defined by the owner of the EHR, data being centralized and held in a single device. Becker and Sewell focus on high level regulations expressed at national level (Becker & Sewell, 2004). They propose a logical language called Cassandra. This language is based on Datalog with constraints, a fragment of first-order logic studied by the databases community which enjoys good decidability properties.

## Toward a Health Record Masking Model

Researches on usage control, purpose-based AC, privacy preferences and practices provide many valuable results to deal with privacy protection and consent expression. Current researches address a broad scope of privacy issues (e.g., enterprise-wide privacy practices or preference language) able to deal with complex rules (e.g., conditional obligations, time restricted usage, logic rules and constraints). However, access control policies usually defined to regulate accesses to EHR systems are far too complex to expect collecting an enlightened consent of the patients on them, as required by the law. This is due to two main characteristics of these policies:

C1. Huge number of AC rules, due to a high number of people interacting with a folder, combined with a large diversity of roles and privileges.
C2. Complexity of the data to be protected, usually described with a highly specialized terminology, and combined with an intrinsic difficulty to determine which data (or data association) reveals a given pathology.

The default access control policy defined for the future French DMP (Personal Medical Folder) illustrates this complexity quite well. As pictured in Figure 3, this RBAC-based policy is expressed as a matrix Document × Role, where elements of Document are the classes of documents constituting a healthcare folder, elements of Role are the roles which can be played by practitioners and each entry gives the corresponding Read and Write privileges. In its current form, this matrix already contains more than 400 entries while classes of documents are very coarse grain to implement an effective control (e.g., Radiographies may reveal very different pathologies depending on the organ). What is finally revealed remains obscure to the patient.

In the light of this example, default access control policy must be considered as the expression of the need-to-know principle (i.e., a user should be granted access to the information strictly required to accomplish the tasks related to his role) rather than a tool which can be configured by the patient to better protect his own privacy. The right to hide part of his medical history has however been recognized by the law to the patients, with a prior information about the possible consequences of this action. We believe that collecting the enlightened consent of the patient requires providing

*Figure 3. Default matrix of the French DMP (Personal Medical Folder) http://www.d-m-p.org/docs/TabCxPS.pdf*

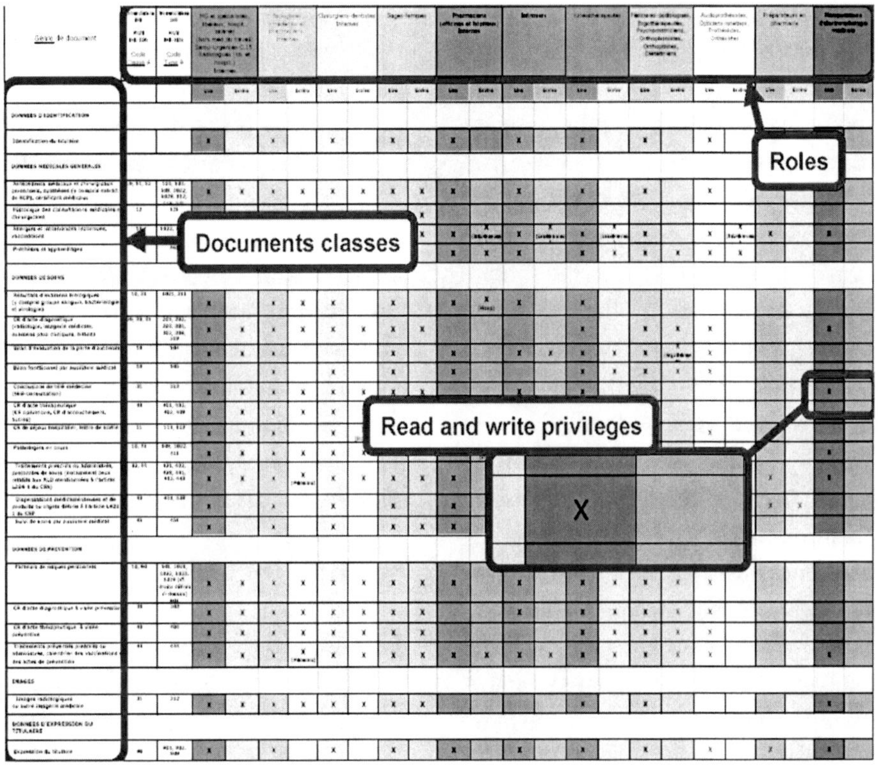

them with effective and comprehensive tools to mask the undesirable information in his folder. To this end, we devised a masking model which consists in defining additional rules, semantically meaningful for each patient (based on self defined terms) and which takes priority over the default access control policy the patient cannot master.

## EBAC: AN EVENT-BASED ACCESS CONTROL MODEL

The Event-Based Access Control model (EBAC) has been designed to help the patient in masking sensitive healthcare records in his folder. Design rational of EBAC is simplicity and accuracy. The model is organized according to the main concepts of events, episodes and relation of confidence.

- *Event*: any document added to a medical folder is associated to an event. Events are endowed with properties, among which the *author* of the document (i.e., a practitioner) and the medical *episode* it belongs to.

- *Episode*: an *episode* is a set of events semantically linked and for which the patients wants to define a common masking policy. For example, the patient may define episodes "MyAbortion2008", "MySecondDepression" and associate incoming events to them, potentially with the help of his family doctor. The patient defines his masking policy on an episode basis by defining who (role or identified users) is granted to participate to this episode.

- *Relation of confidence*: the participation of a practitioner P to an episode is regulated by a relation of confidence with the patient stating (1) which event P can see in this episode and (2) who can see the events produced by P himself in this episode (e.g., Dr Guru can see only the events he produces and nobody else than Guru and the patient can see these same events). In other words, the participants of an episode constitute a trusted circle as defined in Section 4.1 and the relation of confidence defines the scope of their respective actions in this episode. To make the model simple and intuitive, we introduce two scopes for the read the write actions termed *shared* (denoted by S) and *exclusive* (denoted by X). Combining these scopes leads to four possible relations of confidence:

SS: practitioner P can read the shared events in the episode, and produces himself shared events for the episode;

SX: practitioner P can read the shared events in the episode, and produces exclusive events for the episode;

XS: practitioner P can read the exclusive events produced by himself in the episode, and produces shared events for the episode;

XX: practitioner P can read the exclusive events produced by himself in the episode, and produces exclusive events for the episode;

The main ideas of the model are therefore:

- There exists a default (role-based) AC matrix which is defined at the regulation level and that cannot be modified by the owner of the EHR,
- Each healthcare record is associated to an event, itself related to (at most) one episode and the owner defines his masking policy at the episode level,
- Access decision is taken according to the identity of the querier, the author of the event and the episode the event belongs to, with priority given to the masking rule in case of conflict with the AC matrix,
- Only read permission is considered: the aim on the EBAC model is only to prevent from privacy disclosure, other actions are controlled at the regulation level.

The next section formalizes the EBAC model with sets and functions. Note that we do restrict ourselves to information related to AC decision. In a real implementation, basic types would be refined into more complex types. In the definitions, $\nabla$ denotes the absence of value, $A \times B$ is the Cartesian products of sets $A$ and $B$, and $\wp(U)$ denotes the set of all subsets of a set $U$.

## Formal Definitions

Let's introduce basic types:

- *Identifiers*: the set of events' identifiers.
- *Users*: the set of users' identifiers.
- *Form*: the set of documents (or forms) constituting the medical folder.
- *Episodes*: the set of episodes.
- *SS, SX, XS and XX:* four functions that maps each episode to a set of users ($Episodes \rightarrow \wp(Users)$). Moreover $SS(e) \cap SX(e) \cap XS(e) \cap XX(e) = \varnothing$.
- *Events*: the set of events.
- $id : Events \rightarrow Indentifiers$, $form : Events \rightarrow Forms$, $author : Events \rightarrow Users$ and $episode : Events \rightarrow Episodes \cup \{\nabla\}$ :four functions that maps an event to (respectively) an identifier, a form, an author and an episode.

Note that the sets $S_{ep}$ and $S_{\nabla}$ defined respectively as $S_{ep} = \{e \in Events \mid episode(e) = ep\}$ and $S_{\nabla} = \{e \in Events \mid episode(e) = \nabla\}$ define a partition of events according to the (unique) episode they belong:

$$\bigcup_{ep \in Episodes} S_{ep} \cup S_{\nabla} = Events$$

Now we introduce two relations for the default access control matrix. Actually, it is role-based, but on more generic treatment it could be any access control model provided that a function *Users* × *Event* → {*true, false*} exists. The definitions we propose are related to the flat RBAC model but may be easily extended by role hierarchy. Following definitions are from [Ferraiolo et al. 2003]:

- *Roles*: the set of roles
- *URA* ⊆ *Users* × *Roles:* a relation for "user-role assignment"
- *PRA* ⊆ *Roles* × *Forms:* a relation for "permission-role assignment"
- *DefaultMatrix* ⊆ *Users* × *Forms* = {(*u,f*) ∈ *Users* × *Forms* | ∃*r* ∈ *Roles* ∧ (*u, r*) ∈ *URA* ∧ (*r, f*) ∈ *PRA*} the relation defined as the join on roles of *URA* and *PRA* relations.
- *defaultAccess* :: *Users* × *Event* → {*true, false*} a function that determine whether a user's access query on an event is granted. The function is defined as:
  - *defaultAccess*(*u, e*) = *true*, iff *form*(*e*) = *f* and (*u, f*) ∈ *DefaultMatrix*

Now, we define the semantic of the sets of users SS, SX, XS and XX of a given episode e. The idea is to use these sets to define rights based on the identity of the user who try to access and the identity of the user who wrote the event. A user is always able to access an event he wrote himself.

- *perceive* : *Episodes* → ℘(*Users*), *perceive*(*e*) = *SX*(*e*) ∪ *SS*(*e*) is the set of users who may read events related to the episode.
- *hidden* : *Episodes* → (*Users*), *hidden*(*e*) = *XX*(*e*) ∪ *SX*(*e*) is the set of users whose events are hidden to others.
- *access'* : *Episodes* × *Users* × *Users* → {*true, false*} : the function that tell whether access to an episode *e* by a user *u*, on a event written by user *a* is granted. The function is defined as:
  - *access'* (*e, u, a*) = *true* iff (*a* = *u*) ∨ (*u* ∈ *perceive*(*e*) ∧ *a* ∉ *hidden*(*e*))
- *access* : *Users* × *Events* → {*true, false*}: the function that tell whether an access by a user *u* on an event *e* is granted or not. If the event is not related to any episode (∇), access is granted, else, we rely on function *access'*. The function *access* is defined as:
  - *access*(*u, e*) = *true* if *episode*(*e*) = ∇,
  - if *episode*(*e*) = ∇ and *access'*(*episode*(*e*), *u*, *author*(*e*)) = *true*,
  - *access*(*u, e*) = *false* otherwise.

Finally, we combine the access decision based on the default access control model, which express the need to know based on role assignment, and on the episode related to the event. Access is granted iff both access control decisions agree.

- *granted* : *Users* × *Events* → {*true, false*}: the function that combines *defaultAccess* and *access*, it is defined as:
  - *granted*(*u,e*)=*true* iff *defaultAccess*(*u, e*) ∧ *access*(*u, e*)

## Sample Policy

To illustrate the approach, we define a sample EBAC policy. Four professionals named Guru (an adept of alternative medicine), MyPhysician, MyNurse, and AnotherPhysician are acting with the system. The patient we consider has defined two episodes, one for a cancer and another one for an abortion, with the following rules:

- *E1*, "Cancer": *XX(E1)={Guru}, SS(E1)={ MyPhysician, MyNurse }*. This rule states that Guru, MyPhysician and MyNurse constitute the trusted circle for episode E1, in addition to the patient himself. No other user can read events in this episode whatever the default access control policy. MyPhysician and MyNurse share the

*Table 1.*

| | $\nabla$ | | E1 | | E2 | | |
|---|---|---|---|---|---|---|---|
| | *e1* | *e2* | *e3* | *e4* | *e5* | *e6* | *e7* |
| *Guru* | T | T | F | T | F | F | F |
| *MyPhysician* | T | T | T | F | T | T | F |
| *MyNurse* | T | F | T | F | F | F | F |
| *AnotherPhys.* | T | T | F | F | F | F | T |

documents produced in this episode, except those produced by Guru, because the patients wants to hide that he consults Guru for his cancer.

- *E2, "Abortion": SX(E2)={My Physician, AnotherPhysician}, SS(E2)={MyNurse}* MyPhysician, AnotherPhysician and MyNurse constitute the trusted circle of episode E2. MyNurse, who did practice the abortion, produces shared events. MyPhysician and AnotherPhysician share these events but what they produce themselves is kept invisible to each other. Such a rule may be defined by the patient after consulting MyPhysican about a problem following the abortion, and before consulting AnotherPhysician for a second opinion, whether the patient does not fully trust MyPhysician diagnosis.

Let us define a sample flat RBAC:

- *(Guru, Physician)* $\in$ *URA, (MyPhysician, Physician)* $\in$ *URA, (MyNurse, Nurse)* $\in$ *URA*
- *(Physician, General)* $\in$ *PRA, (Physician, Treatment)* $\in$ *PRA, (Nurse, General)* $\in$ *PRA*

The health record is composed of 7 events:

1. *e1 = (General, MyNurse, $\nabla$)*
2. *e2 = (Treatment, MyPhysician, $\nabla$)*

3. *e3 = (General, MyPhysician, E1)*
4. *e4 = (Treatment, Guru, E1)*
5. *e5 = (Treatment, MyPhysician, E2)*
6. *e6 = (General, MyPhysician, E2)*
7. e7 = *(General, AnotherPhysician, E2)*

Using function *granted* the following AC matrix can be computed, where T denotes true and F denotes false:

A proof of concept of the EBAC model has been developed in the Haskell (http://www.haskell.org) functional programming language.

## Implementation Issues

This section sketches how the EBAC model is implemented in the embedded DBMS (see Section 3.2) and how it is used by patients.

A patient can incrementally define episodes (e.g., "Cancer", "Abortion") for his folder. Then, for each event, he chooses:

1. the set of practitioners constituting the trusted circle for this episode;
2. the relation of confidence attached to each.

To implement those access policies in the SPT using the relational model (Codd, 1970), the following relations are added to the database (the view below is simplified for the sake of simplicity):

Event (**Event_id**, *Episode_id, User_id,* Write_ scope, ...)

Episode (**Episode_id**, Label, …)
User (**User_id**, User_name, …)
Privilege (**Privilege_id**, *Episode_id, User_id,* read_scope, write_scope, …)
Notations: attributes in bold are primary keys; attributes in italic are foreign keys.

Relation Event logs the events occurring on the medical folder (e.g., insertion of a document), and refers to relations User and Episode. Relation User stores the set of practitioners interacting with the medical folder, and relation Episode stores the set of episodes defined by the patient. The relations of confidence are stored in the relation Privilege with references to relations Episode and User.

At the time of creation of each event, the reference to the user (User_id) originating the event is specified. The reference to the corresponding episode (Episode_id) is created on demand, i.e., at the time of the insertion or later, and the corresponding write scope (write_scope is set to S or X) is filled at that time by querying the relation Privilege.

For example, at creation of event $e3 = ($*General, MyPhysician, E*1$)$ of the previous example, event e3 in relation Event refers to the practitioner MyPhysician in relation User and is linked to the episode Cancer. Since the write scope of MyPhysician for episode Cancer is S, the attribute value write_scope in Event is set to S.

At execution time, a query Q issued by a practitioner P on the folder is rewritten to integrate access control. Our implementation requires joining each result of Q with relation Event, and projecting the event tuples on attributes Event. write_scope, Event.user_id and Event.episode_id. Before delivering the tuples to P, access control is checked by applying the following filtering condition:

Event.user_id = current_user OR (Event. write_scope = S AND Event.episode_id IN CC), where CC denotes the set of episodes the current user participates in (i.e., is member of the related trusted circle). This condition is checked by a system query on relation Privileges executed and stored at the time of the connection of the practitioner to the SPT.

Each result tuple qualified on this condition satisfies the access control policy defined by the user. Finally, attributes Event.write_scope, Event. user_id and Event.episode_id are removed before delivering the result tuple to P.

## FUTURE WORK

The SPT hardware platform is today operational and the main software components described in the preceding sections have been developed and integrated: central server, embedded web server, embedded DBMS and synchronization protocol. The application itself is being developed and will be experimented in the field by the end of 2009 on a population of about 100 elderly patients and 25 practitioners. The ageing of population makes the health monitoring of elderly people at home crucial. In this context, sensitive data has to be shared between all participants of medical-social networks (doctors, nurses, social workers, home help and family circle) with different access rights. The data must be available at the patient's bedside for a better monitoring of their health cares. For this purpose, the Yvelines District in France has decided to carry out an experimental project of Shared Medical-Social Folder (DMSP in French). In the first step, this project targets elderly people from two gerontology networks. At mid-term, it could be extended to other vulnerable people in unstable or handicapped situation.

ALDS (a home care association) has already carried out a "Common Medical Folder" in paper format, which enables professionals and participants from medical-social sectors to write down crucial facts related to the monitoring of elderly people. While the day-to-day use of this paper folder has proved its efficiency, two burning issues were still unresolved:

- N*o privacy*: all participants (practitioners but also social workers, home help and family circle) can read all records in the patient's folder while some patients are facing complex human situations (diagnosis of terminal illness, addictions, financial difficulties, etc).
- *No remote access to the folder*: consequently, the folder is not updated consistently and timely, leading to a lesser accurate monitoring.

The objective of this experiment in the field is precisely to demonstrate the accuracy of the proposed technology to tackle these two issues. This project involves INRIA (the French National Research Institute in Computer Sciences), University of Versailles, SANTEOS (a French EHR provider), Gemalto (the smart card world leader), ALDS (a home care association) and COGITEY (a clinic for elderly people).

## CONCLUSION

EHR projects are being launched in most developed countries. The benefits provided by centralizing the healthcare information in database servers in terms of information quality, availability and protection against failure are unquestionable. Yet, patients are reluctant to abandon the control over highly sensitive data (e.g., data revealing a severe or shameful disease) to a distant server. In addition, the access to the folder is conditioned by the existence of a high speed and secure internet connection at any place and any time.

This chapter capitalizes on a new hardware portable device, associating the security of a smart card to the storage capacity of a USB key, to give the control back to the patient over his medical history. We have shown how this device can complement a traditional EHR server (1) to protect and share highly sensitive data among trusted parties and (2) to provide a seamless access to the data

even in disconnected mode. From the architectural point of view, the key point is the embedding in a secure chip of the complete software chain usually running on traditional servers: web server, servlets, DBMS and finally the database itself. From the usage point of view, the key point is a new way of personalizing access control policies with minimal assistance of practitioners. While both contributions are orthogonal, their integration in the same infrastructure allows building trustworthy pervasive healthcare folders.

The solution proposed will be experimented in the context of a medical-social network providing medical care and social services at home for elderly people. The expected outcome of this experiment is to demonstrate the effectiveness of the proposed technology with a positive impact on the coordination of medical and social workers and on the acceptance of patients of an electronic usage of their medical history.

## ACKNOWLEDGMENT

This work is partially funded by the Yvelines District Council through the DMSP project and by ANR (the French National Agency for Research) through the PlugDB project. The authors wish to thank Laurent Braconnier and Jean-François Navarre (Yvelines District Council), Philippe Kesmarszky (ALDS), Sophie Lartigue (COGITEY), Morgane Berthelot (SANTEOS), Jean-Jacques Vandewalle (Gemalto) and Karine Zeitouni (University of Versailles) for their active participation in these two projects.

## REFERENCES

Agrawal, R., Kiernan, J., Srikant, R., & Xu, Y. (2002). Hippocratic Databases. *Proceedings of VLDB'02 (pp.* 143-154).

Alhaqbani, B., & Fidge, C. J. (2007). Access Control Requirements for Processing Electronic Health Records Business. In Process Management Workshops, (pp. 371-382).

Anciaux, N., Benzine, M., Bouganim, L., Pucheral, P., & Shasha, D. (2007). GhostDB: querying visible and hidden data without leaks. In *ACM SIGMOD Conference* (pp. 677-688).

Anciaux, N., Bobineau, C., Bouganim, L., Pucheral, P., & Valduriez, P. (2001). PicoDBMS: Validation and Experience. In *International Conference on Very Large Data Bases (VLDB)* (pp. 709-710).

Anciaux, N., Bouganim, L., & Pucheral, P. (2006). Data Confidentiality: to which extent cryptography and secured hardware can help. *Annales des Télécommunications, 61*(3-4), 267–283.

Anciaux, N., Bouganim, L., & Pucheral, P. (2007). Future Trends in Secure Chip Data Management. *IEEE Data Eng. Bull., 30*(3), 49–57.

Ashley, P., Hada, S., Karjoth, G., Powers, C., & Schunter, M. (2003). *Enterprise Privacy Authorization Language (EPAL 1.2). Technical report. IBM Tivoli Software.* IBM Research.

Becker, M. Y., & Sewell, P. (2004). Flexible Trust Management, Applied to Electronic Health Records. In *Computer Security Foundations Workshop* (pp. 139–154). Cassandra.

Bloom, B. (1970). Space/time tradeoffs in hash coding with allowable errors. *Communications of the ACM, 13*(7), 422–426. doi:10.1145/362686.362692

Byun, J., & Li, N. (2008). Purpose based access control for privacy protection in relational database systems. *The VLDB Journal, 17*, 603–619. doi:10.1007/s00778-006-0023-0

Carrasco, L. C. (1999). RDBMS's for Java Cards? What a Senseless Idea! White paper. *ISOL Corp.*

Codd, E. F. (1970). A Relational Model of Data for Large Shared Data Banks. *Communications of the ACM, 13*(6), 377–387. doi:10.1145/362384.362685

Eurosmart. (2008, April). *Smart USB Token.* White Paper. Retrieved February 17, 2009, from http://www.eurosmart.com/images/doc/WorkingGroups/NewFF/Papers/eurosmart_smart_usb_token_wp_april08.pdf

Ferraiolo, D. F., Kuhn, R. D., & Chandramouli, R. (2003). *Role-Based Access Control.* Boston: Artech House Publishers.

Halpern, J. Y., & Weissman, V. (2008). Using First-Order Logic to Reason about Policies. *ACM Transactions on Information and System Security, 11*, 1–41. doi:10.1145/1380564.1380569

Internet Engineering Task Force. (2008). *The Transport Layer Security (TLS) Protocol Version 1.2.* Retrieved February 17, 2009, from http://tools.ietf.org/html/rfc5246

ISO/IEC. Integrated Circuit(s) Cards with Contacts – Part 7: Interindustry Commands for Structured Card Query Language (SCQL). (1999). *Standard ISO/IEC 7816-7.* International Standardization Organization.

Karjoth, G., Schunter, M., & Waidner, M. (2002). *Platform for Enterprise Privacy Practices: Privacy-Enabled Management of Customer Data* (pp. 69–84). Privacy Enhancing Technologies.

Langheinrich, M. (2005). *Personal Privacy in Ubiquitous Computing.* Doctoral dissertation. ETH Zurich.

Liebert, T. (2008, March). Ongoing concern over Pentagon network attack. *IT News Digest.* Retrieved February 17, 2009, from http://blogs.techrepublic.com.com/tech-news/?p=2098.

Massacci, F., & Zannone, N. (2004). *Privacy Is Linking Permission to Purpose* (pp. 179–191). Security Protocols Workshop.

MasterCard International. (2002). *MasterCard Open Data Storage Version 2.0.* Technical Specifications.

Ni, Q., Trombetta, A., Bertino, E., & Lobo, J. (2007).Privacy-aware role based access. In *Proceedings of the 12th ACM symposium on Access control models and technologie,* (pp. 41-50).

Pucheral, P., Bouganim, L., Valduriez, P., & Bobineau, C. (2001). PicoDBMS: Scaling down database techniques for the smartcard. [VLDBJ]. *Very Large Data Bases Journal, 10*(2-3), 120–132.

Pucheral, P., & Yin, S. (2007). System and Method of Managing Indexation of Flash Memory. *European Patent by Gemalto and INRIA,* N° 07290567.2.

Røstad, L., & Nytrø, O. (2008). Personalized access control for a personally controlled health record. In *Proceedings of the 2nd ACM workshop on Computer security architectures* (pp. 9-16).

Samarati, P., & di Vimercati, S. D. C. (2000). Policies, Models, and Mechanisms. In *Foundations of Security Analysis and Design on Foundations of Security Analysis and Design 2000* (pp. 137–196). Access Control.

Vandewalle, J.-J (2004). Smart Card Research Perspectives. *LNCS Construction and Analysis of Safe, Secure and Interoperable Smart devices.*

Yang, N., Barringer, H., & Zhang, N. (2007). A Purpose-Based Access Control Model. In *Symposium in Information Assurance and Security,* (pp. 143-148).

Yin, S., Pucheral, P., & Meng, X. (2009). A Sequential Indexing Scheme for Flash-Based Embedded Systems. In *International Conference on Extending Database Technology (EDBT).*

Zhang, X., Parisi-Presicce, F., Sandhu, R., & Park, J. (2005). Formal model and policy specification of usage control. *ACM Transactions on Information and System Security, 8,* 351–387. doi:10.1145/1108906.1108908

## ADDITIONAL READING

Alliance. (2008, April 28). The National Alliance for Health Information Technology, on Defining Key Health Information Technology Term. Report to the Office of the National Coordinator for Health Information Technology. Retrieved February 17, 2009, from http://www.hhs.gov/healthit/documents/m20080603/10_2_hit_terms.pdf.

Article 29 Data Protection Working Party (2007). *Working Document on the processing of personal data relating to health in electronic health records (EHR).* Technical report 00323/07/EN WP 131. European Commission.

Brown, S. H., Lincoln, M. J., Groen, P. J., & Kolodner, R. M. (2003). VistA, U.S. Department of Veterans Affairs national scale HIS. *International Journal of Medical Informatics, 69,* 135–156. doi:10.1016/S1386-5056(02)00131-4

Computer World. (2003, December). NASA Sites Hacked. Retrieved February 17, 2009, from http://www.computerworld.com/securitytopics/security/cybercrime/story/0,10801,88348,00.html

Computer World. (2006, August). Survey: 81% of U.S. firms lost laptops with sensitive data in the past year. Retrieved February 17, 2009, from http://www.computerworld.com/action/article.do?command=viewArticleBasic&articleId=9002493&source=NLT_PM&nlid=8.

Dahl, M. R. (2006). *Status and perspective of personal health informatics in Denmark.* Denmark: University of Aarhus, Section for Health Informatics, Institute of Public Health. Retrieved February 17, 2009, from http://www.ieee2407. org/files/ws01_mads01.pps.

Door, J.-P. (2008). *Le dossier médical personnel (Information Rep. No. 659).* France: Assemblée Nationale.

eHealth Insider. (2008, January 16). German doctors say no to centrally stored patient records. Retrieved February 17, 2009, from http://www.e-health-insider.com/news/3384/.

FierceHealthIT news. (2006, August 20). Massive data loss at HCA. Retrieved February 17, 2009, from http://www.fiercehealthit.com/story/ massive-data-loss-at-hca/2006-08-21.

FierceHealthIT news. (2008, September). GA hospital health data breach due to outsourcing error. Retrieved February 17, 2009, from http://www. fiercehealthit.com/story/ga-hospital-health-data-breach-due-outsourcing-error/2008-09-28.

Gordon, L. A., Loeb, M. P., Lucyshin, W., & Richardson, R. (2006). 2006 CSI/FBI Computer Crime and Security Survey. *Computer Security Institute.* Retrieved February 17, 2009, from http://i.cmpnet. com/gocsi/db_area/pdfs/fbi/FBI2006.pdf.

Husek, C. (2008, August). ELGA The Electronic Health Record in Austria. *International Conference of Society for Medical Innovation and Technology.* Vienna, Austria.

Pedersen, C. D. (2006, September 8). MedCom - the Danish Healthcare Data Network. *Meeting with AGFA.*

Smart Card Alliance. (2005). The Taiwan Health Care Smart Card Project. Retrieved February 17, 2009, from http://www.smartcardalliance.org/ resources/pdf/Taiwan_Health_Card_Profile.pdf

Smart Card Alliance. (2006-a). Smart Card Applications in the U.S. Healthcare Industry. White Paper N°HC-06001. Retrieved February 17, 2009, from http://www.smartcardalliance.org/ resour ces/hc/Smart_Card_Healthcare_Applications_FINAL.pdf

Smart Card Alliance. (2006-b). German Health Card. Retrieved February 17, 2009, from http://www.smartcardalliance.org/resources/ pdf/German_Health_Card.pdf.

The Financial Times. (2007, September). Chinese military hacked into Pentagon. Retrieved February 17, 2009, from http://www.ft.com/cms/ s/0/9dba9ba2-5a3b-11dc-9bcd-0000779fd2ac. html.

The International Council on Medical & Care Compunetics. (2009, January 23). Dutch nationwide EHR postponed. Are they in good company? Retrieved February 17, 2009, from http://articles. icmcc.org/2009/01/23/dutch-ehr-postponed-are-they-in-good-company/.

The Times. (2008, December 26). Patients avoid NHS database blunders by keeping cards close to their chest. Retrieved February 17, 2009, from http://www.timesonline.co.uk/tol/life_and_sty le/ health/article5397883.ece.

The Washington Post. (2007, July). Consultant Breached FBI's Computers. Retrieved February 17, 2009, from http://www.washington-post.com/wp-dyn/content/article/2006/07/05/ AR2006070 501489_pf.html.

WFTV. (2008, August 14). Medical Center Patient Records Posted On Internet. Retrieved February 17, 2009, from http://www.wftv.com/ news/17188045/detail.html?taf=orlc.

## ENDNOTES

[1]     The term centralization refers to the fact that the data is stored, organized, made available and controlled by database servers, whatever the computer system infrastructure is (either centralized or distributed).

[2]     The term centralization refers to the fact that the data is stored, organized, made available and controlled by database servers, whatever the computer system infrastructure is (either centralized or distributed).

[3]     database servers, whatever the computer system infrastructure is (either centralized or distributed).

*A previous version of this chapter was originally published in International Journal of Healthcare Delivery Reform Initiatives, Vol. 1, Issue 4, edited by M. Guah, copyright 2010 by IGI Publishing (an imprint of IGI Global).*

# Chapter 10
# Communication Issues in Pervasive Healthcare Systems and Applications

**Demosthenes Vouyioukas**
*University of the Aegean, Greece*

**Ilias Maglogiannis**
*University of Central Greece, Greece*

## ABSTRACT

*This book chapter provides a systematic analysis of the communication technologies used in healthcare and homecare, their applications and the utilization of the mobile technologies in the healthcare sector by using in addition case studies to highlight the successes and concerns of homecare projects. There are several software applications, appliances, and communication technologies emerging in the homecare arena, which can be combined in order to create a pervasive mobile health system. This study highlights the key areas of concern and describes various types of applications in terms of communications' performance. A comprehensive overview of some of these homecare, healthcare applications and research are presented. The technologies regarding the provision of these systems are described and categorised in two main groups: synchronous and asynchronous communications' systems and technologies. The recent advances in homecare using wireless body sensors and on/off-body networks technologies are discussed along with the provision of future trends for pervasive healthcare delivery. Finally, this book chapter ends with a brief discussion and concluding remarks in succession to the future trends.*

## INTRODUCTION

The shifting of telemedicine from desktop platforms to wireless and mobile configurations has a significant impact on future healthcare. Obstacles for healthcare services are time and space between the providers and the patients. Wireless technology came to encompass the e-health monitoring everywhere from any given location. The benefits of wireless technology have been illustrated in a number of different examples and applications. Today, patients at rural areas, at accident scenes or even at home are often physically remote to suitable healthcare providers.

Research and development advances in the e-health community include data gathering and

DOI: 10.4018/978-1-61520-765-7.ch010

transfer of vital information, integration of human machine interface technology into handheld devices, data interoperability and integration with hospital legacy systems and electronic patient records. However, several major challenges still need to be clarified so as to expand the implementation and use of mobile health devices and services and reinforce the market development.

In recent years, there has been increased research on commercial mobile health systems based on WLAN (Wireless Local Area Networks), GPRS (General Packet Radio Service) and 3G UMTS (3rd Generation Universal Mobile Telecommunications System) networking technologies. These technologies have been utilized in the deployment of emerging healthcare and homecare systems. The introduction of high speed data rate, wide bandwidth, digital and encrypted communication technology, makes possible the delivery of audio, video and waveform data to wherever and whenever needed. It is hoped that the current deployment of 3G based systems with global operational morphologies will improve some of the limitations of the existing wireless technologies and will provide a well-organized platform for homecare services.

Mobile and wireless concepts in healthcare are typically related to bio-monitoring and home monitoring. Bio-monitoring using mobile networks includes physiological monitoring of parameters such as heart rate, electrocardiogram (ECG), electroencephalogram, (EEG) monitoring, blood pressure, blood oximetry, and other physiological signals. Alternative uses include physical activity monitoring of parameters such as movement, gastrointestinal telemetry fall detection, and location tracking. Using mobile technology, patient records can be accessed by healthcare professionals from any given location by connection to the institution's internal network. Physicians now have ubiquitous access to patient history, laboratory results, pharmaceutical data, insurance information, and medical resources. Handheld devices can also be used in home

healthcare, for example, to fight diabetes through effective monitoring.

The mission of this book chapter is to provide a detailed analysis of the pervasive healthcare technology, applications and uses of mobile technologies in the health sector by using in addition case studies to highlight the successes and concerns of relevant projects. There are a variety of applications, devices, and communication technologies emerging in the electronic healthcare arena, which can be combined to create a pervasive mobile health system. This book chapter will highlight the key areas of concern and describe the various types of applications. A comprehensive overview of some of these electronic health applications and research will be presented. Meanwhile, the technologies regarding the provision of the pervasive health systems will be described and categorised in two main groups: synchronous and asynchronous communications' systems and technologies. Correspondingly, the classification of the wireless technologies will also be categorized according to their total throughput into small and high data rates within the relevant applications following the end-users view. The recent advances in mobile health (m-health) systems using wireless body sensors and on/off-body networks technologies will be discussed along with the provision of future trends for pervasive healthcare delivery.

In addition, the pervasive healthcare systems operating in patient's homes define the field of the so called homecare systems. These systems will be presented in a different section of this chapter issue, since the delimitations of the home environment dictates special technical objectives and introduces important problems and obstacles. However, the use of this wireless sensor technology in medical practice not only allows a supreme level of complexity in patient monitoring with regards to existing parameters (such as vital signs), but also offers the prospect of identifying new ways of diagnosing and preventing disease. The book chapter will end with a description of various applied pervasive health platforms along with their applications and services. A comparison of these platforms will be prepared in conjunction with some results and suggestive extensions. A brief discussion, concluding remarks and additional reading will also be given in succession to the future trends.

## BACKGROUND

### Patient Biosignals and Acquisition Methods - Biosensors

A broad definition of a signal is a 'measurable indication or representation of an actual phenomenon', which in the field of biosignals, refers to observable facts or stimuli of biological systems or life forms. In order to extract and document the meaning or the cause of a signal, a physician may utilize simple examination procedures, such as measuring the temperature of a human body or have to resort to highly specialized and sometimes intrusive equipment, such as an endoscope. Following signal acquisition, physicians go on to a second step, that of interpreting its meaning, usually after some kind of signal enhancement or 'pre-processing', that separates the captured information from noise and prepares it for specialized processing, classification and decision support algorithms.

Biosignals require a digitization step in order to be converted into a digital form. This process begins with acquiring the raw signal in its analog form, which is then fed into an analog-to-digital (A/D) converter. Since computers cannot handle or store continuous data, the first step of the conversion procedure is to produce a discrete-time series from the analog form of the raw signal. This step is known as 'sampling' and is meant to create a sequence of values sampled from the original analog signals at predefined intervals, which can faithfully reconstruct the initial signal waveform. The second step of the digitization process is quantization, which works on the temporally sampled values of the initial signal and produces a signal, which is both temporally and quantitatively discrete. This means that the initial values are converted and encoded according to properties such as bit allocation and value range. Essentially, quantization maps the sampled signal into a range of values that is both compact and efficient for algorithms to work with. The most popular biosignals utilized in pervasive health applications are shown in Choudhri (2003), Kifor (2006), Malan (2004) and Gouaux (2004).

In addition to the aforementioned biosignals, patient physiological data (e,g., body movement information based on accelerometer values), and context-aware data (e.g., location, environment and age group information) have also been used by pervasive health applications (Barger, 2005). The utilization of the latter information is discussed in the following sections.

In the context of pervasive healthcare applications, the acquisition of biomedical signals is performed through special devices (i.e. sensors) attached on the patient's body (see Figure 1) or special wearable devices (see Figure 2) (Barger, 2005). The transmission of the collected signals to the monitoring unit is performed through appropriate wireless technologies discussed in the following Section on pervasive networking and communication issues. Regarding the rest multimedia information concerning the patient, most applications are based on data collected from video cameras, microphones, movement and vibration sensors.

Sensor configurations enclosed on wearable clothing have been manufactured in order to enhance usability, comfort and convenience for the users. Many companies have applied this technology to produce high-tech clothing aiming at ameliorating the user's quality of life. Typical examples are the Vivometric's Lifeshirt (see Figure 2c) as well as the Georgia Tech Wearable Motherboard which allow connection to vital signs sensors positioned on different body locations (Vivometrics, 2009). The LifeShirt System is the first non-invasive, continuous ambulatory monitoring system that can collect data on cardiopulmonary function and other physiological patient parameters, and correlate them over time. It contains embedded inductive plethysmographic sensors, accelerometer, and a single-channel ECG.

The Georgia Tech Wearable Motherboard (Georgia Institute of Technology, 2009), is a high tech vest that uses optical fibers to detect bullet wounds and monitor the body vital signs during combat conditions. The Georgia Tech Wearable Motherboard (Smart Shirt) provides an extremely versatile framework for the incorporation of sensing, monitoring and information processing devices. Applications such as the Georgia's Motherboard and the Vivometric's Lifeshirt can incorporate several devices and combine evolutionary technologies for a broader range of health parametric data (breath rate sensor, temperature sensors, ECG electrodes, shoch/fall sensors, global positioning system (GPS) receiver) and more precise outcomes. Smart nanocomposite materials are of particular interest for self-sensing in health monitoring, or self-actuating to improve the performance and efficiency of structures and devices. It has been shown that conductive textiles and piezo-resistive fabric can be integrated into shirts to measure patient movements, peripheral pulse, respiration, and biopotentials (De Rossi et al. 2003). Additional efforts for construction of further high-tech accessories have been made (rings, wrist-watches etc). Reinforced polymers, carbon nanotube solid polymer electrolyte actuator, and piezoresistive sensors have been developed for several potential applications in the sense of miniaturizing the monitoring devices. The patient monitoring finger ring sensor measures PPG signals, skin temperature, blood flow, blood constituent concentration and or pulse rate of the patient. The data are encoded for wireless transmission by mapping a numerical value associated with each datum to a pulse emitted after a delay of a specified duration, following a fiducial time. Multiple ring bands and sensor elements may be

*Figure 1. Accelerometer, gyroscope, and electromyogram (EMG) sensor for stroke patient monitoring*

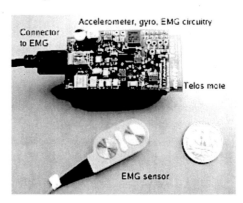

employed for deriving three-dimensional dynamic characteristics of arteries and tissues. A number of research organizations have studied portable and wearable device of physiological signal monitors. Rantanen et al. (2003), developed a smart clothing system that adjusts the clothe temperature in order to facilitate persons living in the arctic environment. The specific smart clothing system measures the heart rate, the humidity and the temperature of body surface. These data may be transmitted wirelessly for further analysis. Significant related work on wearable systems may be found in the literature (Montgomery et al., 2004), (Mangas and Oliver, 2005), (Jafari et al., 2005).

## Pervasive Networking and Communication Issues

In recent years, there has been increased research on commercial mobile health systems based on WiFi (Wireless Fidelity), GPRS (General Packet Radio Service) and 3G UMTS (3rd Generation Universal Mobile Telecommunications System) networking technologies. These technologies have been utilized in the deployment of emerging healthcare systems (Istepanian, 1999; Jones, 2005). The introduction of high speed data rate, wide bandwidth, digital and encrypted commu-

*Figure 2. Wearable medical sensor devices: (a) A 3-axis accelerometer on a wrist device enabling the acquisition of patient movement data, (b) A ring sensor for monitoring of blood oxygen saturation, (c) The Vivometric's Lifeshirt System*

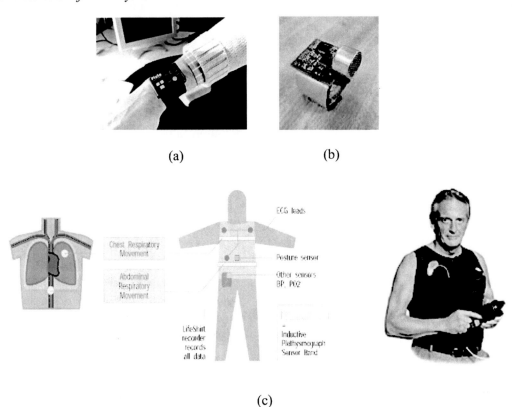

(a)            (b)

(c)

nication technology, makes possible the delivery of audio, video and waveform data to wherever and whenever needed. It is hoped that the current deployment of 3G based systems with global operational morphologies will improve some of the limitations of the existing wireless technologies and will provide a well-organized platform for mobile healthcare services. The shifting of telemedicine from desktop platforms to wireless and mobile configurations has a significant impact on future healthcare. Obstacles for healthcare services are time and space between the providers and the patients. Wireless technology came to encompass the e-health monitoring everywhere from any given location. The benefits of wireless technology have been illustrated in a number of different examples and applications (Pattichis,

2002). Today, patients at rural areas, at accident scenes etc. are often physically remote to suitable healthcare providers.

Broadband connectivity is rapidly evolving around the globe using a diversity of means involving wire-line (e.g. Asynchronous Digital Subscriber Line - ADSL), wireless (e.g. Wi-Fi, WiMax) and satellite interconnections. Multimedia-rich services provided via broadband connections can potentially change the way of communicating ideas, doing business, or acting in the modern digital world. In this framework, European Space Agency (ESA) has initiated the Digital Video Broadcasting with Return Channel via Satellite (DVB-RCS) technology enabling almost all potential locations - even the most geographically dispersed and isolated ones - to gain access to broadband services using low-cost Satellite Interactive Terminals (SITs). Nowadays, the DVB-RCS technology enhanced with the DVB-S2 knowledge is a mature broadband communications technology with comparable implementation and operational costs to the other broadband terrestrial technologies, effectively satisfying the Quality of Service (QoS) requirements of high demanding applications in electronic healthcare.

## E-Health via High-Speed Satellite Networks

In the era of mobile computing the trend in medical informatics is towards achieving two goals: the availability of software applications and medical information anywhere and anytime and the invisibility of computing, while the computing modules are hidden in multimedia information appliances. The DVB-RCS technology seems capable of providing such pervasive e-health services. DVB-RCS is an ETSI (European Telecommunications Standards Institute) standard that specifies the provision of the interaction channel for interactive (two-way) satellite networks using Return Channel Satellite Terminals referred to as RCST or simply SITs. The DVB-RCS Hub is vital for the operation of the DVB-RCS satellite communications network and essentially manages the network operation: it enables SIT access to the satellite network, assigns bandwidth to SITs, relays traffic between SITs inside the satellite network and between the SITs and other networks (e.g. Internet) and also monitors the operation of the SITs.

Tele-medicine provided via satellite communications is an evolving area of healthcare services and provision of medical information, which utilizes the new developments in satellite networks such as DVB-RCS. In fact, satellite communication systems are considered an attractive networking solution for telemedicine platforms, since they have the advantage of worldwide coverage and offer a variety of data transfer rates, even

though satellite links involve high operating costs. However, with the application of the DVB-RCS technology, the operating costs of satellite links tend to be significantly reduced.

The topology of a typical interactive satellite network is star with the central gateway, known simply as DVB-RCS Hub, at its center and the SITs around the DVB-RCS Hub. The DVB-RCS Hub is vital for the operation of the DVB-RCS satellite communications network and essentially manages the network operation: it enables SIT access to the satellite network, assigns bandwidth to SITs, relays traffic between SITs inside the satellite network and between the SITs and other networks (e.g. Internet) and also monitors the operation of the SITs. Note that data communication between two SITs can only take place through the DVB-RCS Hub, thus effectively being a two-hop communication. For the sake of simplicity in this book chapter from this point forward, the transmission from the DVB-RCS Hub towards all SITs will be referred to as Forward Link (FL) and the transmission from each SIT towards the DVB-RCS Hub will be referred to as Return Link (RL). Data rates on the FL can reach 45 Mbps and data rates on the RL can reach 2 Mbps. Bandwidth allocations on both FL and RL can be guaranteed (constant rate) or dynamic, depending on the available bandwidth at certain time periods.

Tele-medicine applications span the areas of emergency healthcare, homecare, patient tele-monitoring, tele-cardiology, tele-radiology, tele-pathology, tele-dermatology, tele-ophthalmology, tele-psychiatry and tele-surgery (Kyriacou, 2003; Maglogiannis, 2004). These applications enable the provision of prompt and expert medical services in underserved locations, like rural health centers, ambulances, ships, trains, airplanes as well as at homes (homecare) (Pattichis, 2002; Shimizu, 1999; Istepanian, 2004; Maglogiannis, 2006). The combination of the medical profession's advanced procedures and equipment with regional healthcare communication networks, may offer complete, integrated healthcare de-

*Figure 3. Satellite tele-medicine network architecture*

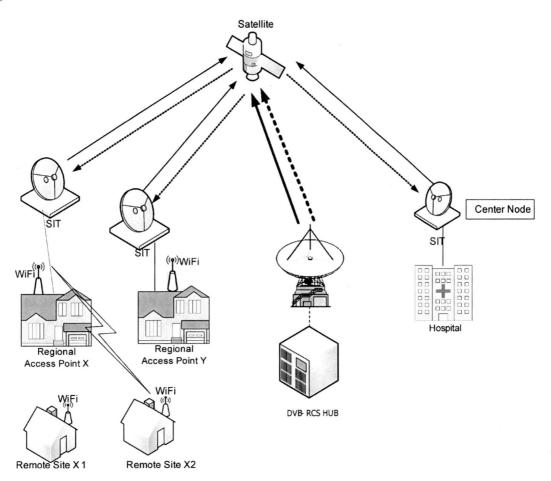

livery systems made up of hospitals, outpatient services, pharmacies and large rural home health operation. From the patient's perspective, that means not only having the necessary technology at hand, but also a centralized environment that is comfortable, convenient and dedicated to the care of their specific condition.

The general topology of a tele-medicine system using satellite network is depicted in Figure 3. The architecture of the systems is hierarchical, involving an access network based on the Wi-Fi technology and a core network based on DVB-RCS. The DVB-RCS satellite core network can gain access by any satellite provider using the expensive but necessary satellite bandwidth (satellite transponder) in order to provide SIT and DVB-RCS Hub

interconnection. The only limitation of the network is the satellite coverage footprint (coverage map) (Brady, 2002; Breynaert, 2005).

The platform may consist of one or more Remote Sites (RSs) placed in several remote areas. Every RS can be equipped with appropriate communication devices (i.e. videoconference units, videophones, patient tele-monitoring unit, IP phones etc). Optionally, the communication device at the RS may have the capability to connect to medical data acquisition units collecting various biosignals and physical data. Each RS has access (Ethernet IP connection) to a wireless access point that utilizes the Wi-Fi technology (IEEE 802.11g), through which the RS is wirelessly connected to a Regional Access Point (RAP). The range of communication between a RS and a RAP is generally less than 1 km. The RAP concentrates video/voice/data from a number of RSs and communicates through the corresponding (located at the site) DVB-RCS SIT, the utilized communication satellite and the available DVB-RCS Hub of the satellite network, with the Center Node (CN), essentially being a hospital or a medical center. Naturally, the equipment of the CN, among others, includes a SIT for communication with the satellite network. The medical personnel (physicians and nurses) at the CN can communicate and provide help to the patients with health incidents as well as potentially realize regular and irregular medical examinations from distance using the platform. The locations of the RSs, RAPs and CN are assumed to be random. Considering the characteristics of the equipment used in the framework of the proposed tele-medicine platform, teleconference/VoIP communication with the patients, tele-monitoring, glucose level and blood pressure measurements, supervision of injuries, monitoring and/or confrontation of hypoglycemia or hyperglycemia symptoms, confrontation of possible heart attack incidents as well as monitoring of the respiratory system of patients can be efficiently performed using the tele-medicine platform described in this book chapter.

Each Remote Site (RS) is equipped with a communication unit that utilizes a VoIP, a special integrated videoconference and/or a medical data acquisition unit. The medical personnel, through the embedded teleconference capability of the device, is able to communicate with the patients using VoIP, real-time video, as with a simple videophone, even permitting the realization of regular and irregular medical examinations from distance.

The required infrastructure at the Center Node (CN) consists of one data Collector Personal Computer (C-PC), one Database Computer (DB-PC), one Multipoint Conference Unit (MCU), two or more Videoconference Units (VCUs), two or more IP phones, two or more TV monitors, one Ethernet Hub or Switch and one SIT to communicate with the RAPs. The C-PC is used for the communication with the special videoconference/medical data collector units located at the RSs. Special software consolidate and process all the medical data coming from the aforementioned units and it will update the medical records of the patients. The DB-PC is used to facilitate the communication to the C-PC and support the database, where the medical history data of the patients will be contained. The VCU gives the opportunity to the doctor at the CN to communicate with his patient (or patients) using real-time video.

There are several situations that this platform can integrate. The first situation concerns a patient, who recently was discharged from hospital after some form of intervention, for instance, after a cardiac episode, cardiac surgery or a diabetic coma. These types of patients are less secure and require enhanced care even at home. However, the home offers a considerably different environment than a hospital or a health unit. The patient or elder will mainly require except video surveillance, also monitoring of his vital signals (i.e., ECG, blood pressure, heart rate, breath rate, oxygen saturation and perspiration).

The second situation concerns a patient, who suffers from saccharoid diabetes and he exhibits hypoglycemia symptoms (e.g. abstractness and ephidrosis). Supposing the patient is located at the RS X2, equipped with a videoconference/medical data collector unit, connected to a glucose meter, allowing a direct connection with a physician at a Center Node (CN), upon his request. The attached glucose meter measures the level of blood glucose and sends the results to the CN. The doctor gains access to these medical data and he also retrieves the patient's medical history from an EHR (Electronic Health Record) relational database system. According to the examination results, the symptoms described by the patient following to the doctor's questions and the patient's medical history, the doctor decides if further medical attention is needed (i.e. if an ambulance has

*Table 1. HSDPA parameters*

| HS-DSCH category | A maximum number of HS- DSCH codes | Peak throughput, Mbit/s | QPSK/16QAM | A number of software bits per channel |
|---|---|---|---|---|
| 1 | 5 | 1.2 | Both | 19200 |
| 2 | 5 | 1.2 | Both | 28800 |
| 3 | 5 | 1.8 | Both | 28800 |
| 4 | 5 | 1.8 | Both | 38400 |
| 5 | 5 | 3.6 | Both | 57600 |
| 6 | 5 | 3.6 | Both | 67200 |
| 7 | 10 | 7.2 | Both | 115200 |
| 8 | 10 | 7.2 | Both | 134400 |
| 9 | 15 | 10.2 | Both | 172800 |
| 10 | 15 | 14.4 | Both | 172800 |
| 11 | 5 | 0.9 | QPSK | 14400 |
| 12 | 5 | 1.8 | QPSK | 28800 |

to be sent to the patent's home or not) and then provides appropriate advise in order to address his uncomfortable condition.

## E-Health via High-Speed Mobile Networks

HSPA (High Speed Packet Access) for uplink and downlink, together with 3G and 4G systems are expected to enforce the m-health applications and overcome the boundaries between time and space. High usability, support for multimedia services with good reliability and low transmission cost, personalization of the services, more capacity and spectrum efficiency are some of the key features of the evolving mobile technologies. Such technologies will make available both mobile patients and end users to interactively get the medical attention and advice they need, when and where is required in spite of any geographical obstructions or mobility constrains.

HSPA is an evolution of WCDMA-UMTS technology, achieving greater bit rates and reduced delays. Responsible for the standardization of HSPA is 3GPP (www.3gpp.org; 3GPP TS 25.308, 2004; 3GPP TR 25.896, 2004). The commercial

utilization of this technology is rather new. New HSDPA (downlink) networks are launched by European providers continuously, while the first Enhanced Uplink (HSUPA - uplink) networks were implemented during the last months. Theoretically, on the downlink the maximum achieved bitrate is about 10.7 Mbps using 16-QAM modulation, while on the uplink the maximum bit rate exceeds 5.5 Mbps per Node-B. Currently 3.6 Mbps and around 1.5 Mbps are the common peak bitrates provided by mobile providers for downlink and uplink correspondingly. HSPA incorporates a significant number of innovative features, such as Adaptive Modulation and Coding, short Transmission Time Interval (2 msec), fast Hybrid Automatic Repeat Request (HARQ), customized schedulers for the proper manipulation and routing of the data, as well as the possibility for a Multiple Input Multiple Output (MIMO) add-on. HS-DSCH (High-Speed Downlink Shared Channel) is also used in HSDPA to send packets on the downlink to the user equipments. The downlink and uplink characteristics of HSPA are depicted in Tables 1 and 2 correspondingly.

Due to the increased capacity that HSPA is able to offer and its packet based nature, the

*Table 2. Enhanced uplink parameters*

| Enhanced Uplink Category | Max Uplink Speed |
|---|---|
| Category 1 | 0.73 Mbps |
| Category 2 | 1.46 Mbps |
| Category 3 | 1.46 Mbps |
| Category 4 | 2.93 Mbps |
| Category 5 | 2.00 Mbps |
| Category 6 | 5.76 Mbps |
| Category 7 (3GPP Release 7) | 11.5 Mbps |

implementation of a variety of applications over cellular networks is now feasible (Holma, 2006). Typical applications may be Voice over IP, browsing, video on demand, mobile TV and video or radio streaming, interactive services, data and music download etc. The ability of HSDPA to serve simultaneously a sufficient number of mobile terminals running multiple demanding applications while keeping the end to end delay low, makes it an ideal candidate for a vast number of new services. Considering the constant geographical expansion and technical development of HSPA networks, they should be soon ready to credibly host e-health services, emphasizing on mobile e-health, emergency and follow-up applications. Figure 4 depicts the HSPA architecture and the interconnection of the fundamentals elements, such as the Radio Network Controller (RNC), the 3G base station (Node-B) and the user equipments (UEs).

The ability of HSPA to serve simultaneously a sufficient number of mobile terminals running multiple demanding applications while keeping the end to end delay low, makes it an ideal candidate for a vast number of new services. Due to the increased capacity that HSPA is able to offer and its packet based nature, the implementation of a variety of applications over cellular networks is now feasible (Holma, 2007; Holma, 2006). Considering the constant geographical expansion and technical development of HSPA networks, they

should be soon ready to credibly host e-health services, emphasizing on mobile e-health, emergency and patient follow-up applications.

Electronic healthcare applications, including those based on wireless technologies span the areas of emergency healthcare, telemedicine in various forms (telecardiology, teleradiology, telepathology, teledermatology, teleophthalmology and telepsychiatry) and electronic access to health records. The range and complexity of telecommunications technology requirements vary with specific medical or health applications. Except for medical images and running through full motion video, the majority of biosignal medical devices require relatively low data transmission rates (Ackerman, 2002; Maglogiannis, 2006).

There are several healthcare applications that can serve via the 3.5G communication technology. For instance, for emergency services in case of accidents and the support of transport healthcare units (i.e. ambulances) or primary care units (i.e. rural centers) in case of accidents. Since, for practical and financial reasons primary care or transport healthcare units cannot be staffed by specialized physicians, general doctors can only rely on directions provided to them by experts. An m-health service in this case allows specialized physicians located at a hospital site, to coordinate remote located primary care or ambulance services paramedical staff via telediagnosis and interactive teleconsultation means.

For teleconsultation collaborative sessions between moving physicians, a teleconsultation session implements a collaborative working environment for physicians in dispersed locations, by enabling; a) electronic exchange of medical data, b) voice/video/chat communication and c) common workspace management (i.e. common image processing toolbox, annotations etc). In case one at least of the commuting doctors is moving or in a random location with no availability of fixed networks a 3.5/4G platform may be used as a communication medium.

*Figure 4. HSPA radio access network architecture*

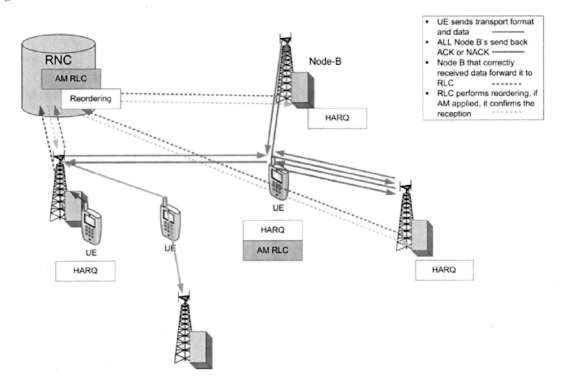

For the transmission of medical information Management service and the mobile access to Electronic Health Records (EHRs), this service is related to applications, enabling the mobile ubiquitous delivery of medical data and implementations of mobile Electronic Health Records (EHR), accessible by PDA's or Tablet PC's. This service is provided to physicians that require immediate access to patient's medical data from random locations. Therefore only broadband cellular systems (i.e 3/4G) may be used due to the corresponding data sizes.

Regarding the transmission of medical images there are essentially no theoretical bandwidth requirements, but lack of bandwidth needs longer transmission time. Yet, high quality medical images such as a single chest radiograph may require from 40 to 50 Megabytes. In practice, it is desirable to transmit medical images during a single patient visit, so as to at-least avoid a follow-up visit. Medical image compression techniques have

primarily focused on lossless methods, where the image has to be reconstructed exactly from its compressed format, due to the diagnostic use. The following section discusses the two basic transmission modes in pervasive healthcare systems; namely real time or synchronous and "Store and Forward" or asynchronous which more or less set the requirements for the underlying network infrastructure.

## SYNCHRONOUS AND ASYNCHRONOUS ELECTRONIC HEALTHCARE SYSTEMS

A basic issue concerning communication is the choice between the transmission of real time multimedia, electronic health record and biosignals data and the "Store and Forward" method with implies asynchronous communication. The "Store and Forward" system is simpler, cheaper and does not require synchronous communication of the two stations. Due to the asynchronous transmission of data the delays of the network are less important and thus lower bandwidth network can be used. Furthermore, the clinical examination procedure is quite easy to program due to the fact that both sides (physician and patient) can interact with the system independently. However "Store and Forward" systems may not be applied for the provision of emergency electronic healthcare services in case of accidents. In addition the physicians seems to prefer in general the synchronous electronic healthcare systems since they offer interactive contact with the patient and simulate better the clinical examination. The most typical scenarios for the provision of pervasive healthcare services are summarized in the following subsections.

## Emergency Services in Case of Accidents

This service refers to the support of transport healthcare units (i.e. ambulances) or primary care units (i.e. rural centers) in case of accidents. Recent studies conclude that early and specialized pre-hospital patient management contributes to emergency case survival. Especially in cases of serious injuries of the head, the spinal cord and internal organs the way of transporting and generally the way of providing care is crucial for the future of the patient. Unfortunately, general practitioners in remote health centres or ambulance personnel, who usually are the first to handle such situations, do not have the required advanced theoretical knowledge and experience. Since, for practical and financial reasons primary care or transport healthcare units cannot be staffed by specialized physicians, general doctors can only rely on directions provided to them by experts. A pervasive health service in this case allows specialized physicians located at a hospital site, to coordinate remote located primary care or ambulance services paramedical staff via telediagnosis and interactive teleconsultation means.

## Follow-Up Service: Patient Telemonitoring

This service is provided to high risk or post surgical patients for monitoring their biosignal data periodically so that if any unusual condition is detected a corresponding alarm rises. Patients recently discharged from hospital after some form of intervention, for instance, after a cardiac incident, cardiac surgery or a diabetic comma are less secure and require enhanced care. The most common forms of special home monitoring are ECG arrhythmia monitoring, post surgical monitoring, respiratory and blood oxygen levels monitoring and sleep apnoea monitoring (Ward, 2006).

## Intrahospital M-Health Services

The use of pervasive health services in hospitals may be divided into two broad categories (Lahtela, 2008). The first one relates to applications, enabling the mobile ubiquitous delivery of medical data and implementations of mobile Electronic Health Records (EHR), accessible by PDA's or Tablet PC's. The second category refers to systems that are used for the monitoring and diagnosis of patients. More details about such systems are presented in Section 3.1.

## Homecare Services

Telehomecare is generally used for rehabilitation of the elder patients to minimize the number of visits for therapists, and thereby, the risk involved in moving the patients (Guang-Zhong, 2004). The elder mainly requires monitoring of his vital signals (i.e., ECG, blood pressure, heart rate, breath rate, oxygen saturation and perspiration). Facilities for medical practice at home are limited by the availability of medical devices suitable for producing biosignals and other medical data (Yang, 2009) (Choudhury, 2008). There is a number of active research and commercial projects developing homecare systems. These systems are surveyed in Section 3.2.

## Medical Information Management Service

This type of services is similar to the first category of the aforementioned intrahospital services related to the mobile access to Electronic Health Records (EHR) (Fei, 2008). This service is provided to physicians that require immediate access to patient's medical data from random locations. Therefore only cellular systems (i.e 2.5/3G) may be used.

## SMALL AND HIGH DATA RATES OF WIRELESS ELECTRONIC HEALTHCARE SYSTEMS

Wireless mobile systems may realize various m-health services. Due the variability of the healthcare scenarios and the extended performance of the mobile and satellite networks in terms of throughput, new m-health services can be implemented. The main restrictions of the potential m-health scenarios can be the functional m-health application, the emergency of the patient's situation, the patient's condition, the territorial state of the patient, etc. Following, there are several prospective scenarios along with their required data rates.

Electronic healthcare applications, including those based on wireless technologies span the areas of emergency healthcare, telemedicine in various forms (telecardiology, teleradiology, telepathology, teledermatology, teleophthalmology and telepsychiatry) and electronic access to health records. In addition, health telematics applications enabling the availability of prompt and expert medical care have been exploited for the provision of healthcare services at understaffed areas like rural health centers, ambulance vehicles, ships, trains, airplanes as well as for home monitoring (Pattichis, 2002; Tachakra, 2003). The range and

complexity of telecommunications technology requirements vary with specific medical or health applications. However, generically defined digital medical devices impose the telecommunications performance requirements. Table 3 illustrates a sampling of several of the more common digital medical devices that may be used in distributed telemedicine. Except for the last few items contained in the table (starting with ultrasounds and running through full motion video).

As long as the transmission of the medical images is concerned, there are no time or bandwidth requirements. In practice, medical image compression techniques have primarily focused on lossless methods, where the image has to be reconstructed exactly from its compressed format, due to the diagnostic use.

About the digital video compression, the Digital Imaging and Communications in Medicine (DICOM) committee has not yet adopted any standard. The adoption of MPEG-2 is possible, but this is limited by the MPEG-2 requirement for constant delay method for frame synchronization. On the other hand, the transmission of offline video is still possible. It is important to distinguish among the requirements for: real-time video transmission, offline video transmission, medical video and audio for diagnostic applications, and non-diagnostic video and audio. Real-time video transmission for diagnostic applications is clearly the most demanding. Offline video transmission is essentially limited by the requirement to provide patient doctor interaction. Real-time diagnostic audio applications include the transmission of stethoscope audio, or the transmission of the audio stream that accompanies the diagnostic video. A typical application will require a diagnostic audio and video bit stream, in addition to a standard teleconferencing bit stream (ITU-D Study Group 2, 2004; LeRouge, 2002).

Future challenges in m-health systems are already mentioned in Istepanian (2004). In general m-health applications may be categorized in two

*Table 3. Data rates of typical devices used in telemedicine*

| Digital device | Signal or Image Resolution | | Data rate required |
|---|---|---|---|
| | Temporal / Spatial (No. of samples per second) | Contrast / Resolution (bits per sample) | |
| Digital Blood Pressure Monitor (sphygmo-manometer) | 1 | x16 | < 10 kbps |
| Digital thermometer | 5 | x16 | < 10 kbps |
| Respiration | 50 | x6 | < 10 kbps |
| Heart rate | 25 | 24 | < 10 kbps |
| Body Temperature | 5 | 16 | 80 kbps |
| Common workspace management controls | - | - | ~ 10 kbps |
| Digital audio stethoscope (Heart Sound) | 10000 | x12 | ~ 120 kbps |
| Galvanic skin response (GSR), or skin conductance response (SCR), | 40-100 | x16 | < 10 kbps |
| Patient movement (accelerometers, gyroscopes and tilt sensors for movement tracking) | 1000 | x11 | ~ 110 kbps |
| On–body microphone Patient sound | 44000 | x8 | ~ 300 kbps |
| Electrocardiogram ECG | 1250 | x12 | ~ 15 Kbps |
| Electroencephalogram EEG | 350 | x12 | < 10 Kbps |
| Electromyogram EMG | 50000 | x12 | ~ 600 Kbps |
| Ultrasound, Cardiology, Radiology | 512x512 | x8 | 256 KB (image size) |
| Magnetic resonance image | 512x512 | x8 | 384 KB (image size) |
| Scanned x-ray | 1024x1250 | x12 | 1.8 MB (image size) |
| Digital radiography | 2048x2048 | x12 | 6 MB (image size) |
| Mammogram | 4096x4096 | x12 | 24 MB (image size) |
| Compressed and full motion video | - | - | 384 kbps to 1.544 Mb/s (speed) |
| Recording of Endoscopic Video | - | - | 256 kbps |
| Demographic Data | - | - | 100 KB (text size) |
| Laboratory and Clinical Data, Medical History | - | - | 1 MB (text size) |

groups depending on the required transmission mode:

- **Real time applications:** These are referred to multimedia connections between centers and moving vehicles including audio and video exchange, biomedical signals and vital parameters transmission, such as electrocardiogram (ECG) signal, blood pressure, oxygen saturation, etc.

- **Near Real Time applications:** These correspond to applications enabling access to administrative files and Electronic Patient Report (EPR) transfer (from medical data exchange between centers and moving vehicles or specialty sections), clinical routine consults during accesses to databases, queries to medical report warehouse, etc.

# PERSONAL AREA NETWORKS: ON-BODY (WEARABLE) AND OFF-BODY NETWORKS

Through the tremendous spread of wireless sensors networks (Mukhopadhyay, 2004) and wireless network systems (WLAN, WMAN, UMTS, Bluetooth, etc.), the wireless user interfaces components increased the abilities and consequently the applications of WPANs (e.g., wearable networks) to medical applications. Infrastructure, topology, coverage, connectivity, heterogeneity, size, lifetime and quality of service are some of the specifications that have to be investigated for selecting the proper wireless user interface component and wireless network.

Wireless sensors are being used to monitor vital signs of patients in home and hospital environment (Baldus, 2004). Compared to conventional approaches, solutions based on wireless sensors are intended to improve monitoring accuracy while also being more convenient for patients. Seven vital signals are presented henceforward. Each provides different and complementary information on the well being of the subject and for each specific examinee the anticipated range of signal parameters is different. For example, heart rate may vary between 25 and 300 beats/min for normal people in different circumstances; likewise, breathing rate could be between 5 and 50 breaths/min. EEG, ECG, and EMG are considerably more complex signals with spectra spanning up to 10 kHz. Voltage levels of the recorded signals vary from less than 1 $\mu$V to tens of millivolts. Not all the signals are required for each examinee.

There are two main networking technologies that the networks can be categorized according to their topology: *on-body* (wearable) and *off-body* networks. The notion of a wearable network of interactive devices aiding users in their day-to-day activities is extremely appealing, but still a lot of open issues need to be addressed by researchers. Recent technological advances have made possible a new generation of small, powerful, mobile computing devices.

A wearable computer must be small and light enough to fit inside clothing. Occasionally it is attached to a belt or other accessory, or is worn directly like a watch or glasses. At the same time, it must be able to accommodate various electronic devices—sensors, cameras, microphones, wireless transceivers, and so on—along with a microprocessor, a battery, memory, and a convenient and intuitive user interface. It must also be able to convey information even when not in use, such as a new e-mail alert. Unlike intelligent wristwatches, wearable radios, and other similar devices, wearware can be reconfigured as required, which greatly widens the scope of applications (Ramachandran, 2008).

An important factor in wearable computing systems is how the various independent devices interconnect and share data. An off-body network connects wearware to other systems that the user does not wear or carry, while an on-body or personal area network connects the devices themselves—the computers, peripherals, sensors, and other subsystems. The advent of portable computers and wireless communication technologies such as IEEE 802.11 has ensured reasonable anytime, anywhere connectivity.

For the area of e-health applications, various low-cost sensor networks have been developed taking into account different technical issues (Ghasemzadeh, 2009). Energy, size, cost, mobility, infrastructure, network topology, connectivity and coverage are some of the requirements that the developer must take into consideration. The most important is size and power consumption. Varying size and cost constraints directly result in corresponding varying limits on the energy available, as well as on computing, storage and communication resources. Low power requirements are necessary both from safety considerations and because in mobile communications the battery lifetime must be commensurate with the application, often several hours. Hence, the energy and other resources available on a sensor node may also vary greatly from system to system. Power may be either stored or scavenged from the environment (e.g., by solar cells).

Mobility is another major issue for pervasive e-health applications because of the nature of users and applications and the easiness of the connectivity to other available wireless networks. Both off-body and personal area networks must not have line-of-sight (LoS) requirements. Consumers generally prefer wireless devices because wires can tangle, restrict movement, be tripped over, and get caught on other objects. Devices such as WPAN wristwatches would not be accepted commercially if wired to other wearables.

The various communication modalities can be used in different ways to construct an actual communication network. Two common forms are infrastructure-based networks and ad hoc networks. The effective range of the sensors attached to a sensor node defines the coverage area of a sensor node. With sparse coverage, only parts of the area of interest are covered by the sensor nodes. With dense coverage, the area of interest is completely (or almost completely) covered by sensors. The degree of coverage also influences information processing algorithms. High coverage is a key to robust systems and may be exploited to extend the network lifetime by switching redundant nodes to power-saving sleep modes.

There are many ad-hoc multi-hop routing algorithms, where network routes are discovered through a self-organizing process. Similarly, many multi-hop routing components are among the most diverse and numerous implementations. These are divided into three classes: *tree-based collection*, where nodes route or aggregate data to an endpoint, *intra-network routing* where data is transferred between in-network end-points, and *dissemination*, where data is propagated to entire regions. Essentially applications use some form of broadcast or dissemination to convey commands, reconfigure, or control in-network processing.

## Off-Body Networks

Off-body communications rely on wireless local area network (LAN) technologies and, increasingly, Manets. There is no single ideal solution, with each varying according to data-rate requirements. Improvements in the area of tiered networks and wireless metropolitan area networks (WMANs) will integrate voice, data, and other multimedia services. Table 4 summarizes the current off-body wireless networking solutions.

High-speed applications such as wireless multimedia delivery and digital imaging require higher and more guaranteed data rates than Bluetooth can offer. On the other hand, WLAN technologies are too costly for many commercial application systems. To fill this gap, IEEE802.15 task group 3 (TG3) has worked since 2000 with the aim of established PHY and MAC level standard for high-rate (20 Mbit/s or greater) wireless personal area networks. Besides the high data rate, the target of the IEEE802.15 TG3 is a low-power and low-cost technology addressing the needs of portable consumer devices (IEEE802.15 TG3), (WiMedia).

To support the work of IEEE802.15 TG3 and promote commercial application systems based on the standard, the WiMedia alliance has been launched in September 2002. The WiMedia alliance is a non-profit open industry association formed to promote personal area range wireless connectivity and interoperability among multimedia devices in a networked environment. The current IEEE802.15.3 standard version supports communication on the same unlicensed frequency band as the Bluetooth (2.4 GHz) with five selectable data rates 11, 22, 33, 44 and 55 Mbit/s. The transmit power is approximately 8 dBm, and the communication range 5 - 55 m. The modulation formats are BPSK, QPSK and QAM. Power management, security, coexistence with Bluetooth and WLAN, and Quality of Service (QoS) capabilities have been incorporated to support high-quality multimedia transport, portable devices and ad hoc

*Table 4. Off-body networking technologies*

| Technology | Operational spectrum | Maximum data rate | Coverage | Power level issues | Price |
|---|---|---|---|---|---|
| *Wireless LANs* | | | | | |
| • IEEE 802.11b | 2.4 GHz | 22 Mbps | 100 m | < 350 mA current drain | **Medium (< $100)** |
| • HomeRF | 2.4 GHz | 10 Mbps | > 50 m | < 300 mA current drain | **Medium (< $100)** |
| • HiperLAN2 | 5 GHz | 32-54 Mbps | 30-150 m | Uses low-power states such as "sleep" | **High (> $100)** |
| *Cellular telephony* | | | | | |
| • CDMA2000 1x Ev-DO | Any existing frequency; band with 2/1 × 3.75 MHz channels | 2 Mbps | Area of a cell | Sophisticated power control with different classes of operation | **Very high (> $1,000)** |
| • UMTS (WCDMA) | 1,920-1,980 MHz and 2,110-2,170 MHz; 2 × 5 MHz channels | 2.048 Mbps | Area of a cell | Sophisticated power control with different classes of operation | **Very high (> $1,000)** |
| *Wireless MANs* | | | | | |
| • IEEE 802.16 | 10-66 GHz; line of sight required; 20/25/28 MHz channels | 120/134.4 Mbps for 25/28 MHz channel | Typically a large city | Complex power control algorithms for different burst profiles | **Not available** |

networking. The products will be more expensive than Bluetooth products but less expensive than WLAN products. Concerning power consumption, the IEEE802.15.3 based products will be between the Bluetooth and WLAN products (Gandolfo, 2002).

## On-Body Networks

Personal Area Networks are generally classified as wire-based, infrared-based, or radio-frequency-based, with wired solutions being the predominant technology for wearware. Many off-body solutions could be used on a smaller scale for on-body communications but would involve a colossal waste of resources. Current on-body networking solutions are summarized in Table 5.

With many small devices such as simple sensors and actuators, continuous communication with high data rate is not usually necessary. Occasional wireless communication through interconnections with the maximum data rate of a few, a few tens or a few hundreds of kilobits per second, and the maximum communication range of a few tens of meters, can facilitate the portability or installation of this kind of devices. Compared to maximizing the data rate, it is usually more important to minimize costs, physical size and power consumption. Many applications belong to the cost critical consumer market. In many places, the electronics should be non-visible.

Power supply through the mains, or recharging or replacing the batteries weekly or even monthly is impossible. Instead, the power supply has to be based on energy scavenging (Rabaey, 2000) or a small battery lasting several months or years. This often calls for average power consumption far below one milliwatt per device. Since the year 2000, IEEE802.15 task group 4 (TG4) has worked to standardize a physical and a MAC-layer applicable in very low-power wireless application systems, which should be able to operate at least

*Table 5. On-body networking technologies*

| Technology | Operational spectrum | Maximum data rate | Coverage | Power level issues | Interference | Price |
|---|---|---|---|---|---|---|
| IrDA | Infrared; 850 nm | 4 Mbps | < 10 m | Distance-based | Present | Low (<$10) |
| BodyLAN | Not available | 32 Kbps | < 10 m | 5.4 mA | Present | Not available |
| IEEE 802.15.1 (Bluetooth) | 2.4 GHz ISM band | Up to 1 Mbps | < 10 m | 1 mA-60 mA | Present | Low (< $10) |
| IEEE 802.15.3 | 2.402-2.480 GHz ISM band | 11-55 Mbps | < 10 m | < 80 mA | Present | Medium (< $50) |
| IEEE 802.15.4 | 2.4 GHz and 868/915 MHz | 868 MHz-20 Kbps, 915 MHz-40 Kbps, and 2.4 GHz-250 Kbps | < 20 m | 20-50 pA | Present | Very low(< $5) |

several months on a battery without replacement (IEEE802.15 TG4). In parallel with IEEE802.15 TG4, the ZigBee alliance has been founded, now incorporating about twenty industrial companies and aimed at establishing open industry specifications for unlicensed, untethered peripheral, control and entertainment devices requiring the lowest cost and lowest power consumption communications between compliant devices anywhere in and around the home. The target for the power consumption is 0.5 to 2 year's operation with two AA-size batteries. According to the alliance, the first commercial products appeared on the market in 2003 (ZigBee).

The IEEE 802.15.4 standard defines two PHYs representing three license-free frequency bands that include sixteen channels at 2.4 GHz, ten channels at 902 to 928 MHz, and one channel at 868 to 870 MHz. The maximum data rates for each band are 250 kbps, 40 kbps and 20 kbps, respectively. The 2.4 GHz band operates worldwide while the sub-1 GHz band operates in North America, Europe, and Australia/New Zealand. The IEEE standard is intended to conform to established regulations in Europe, Japan, Canada and the United States.

Both PHYs use Direct Sequence Spread Spectrum (DSSS). The IC contains a 900 MHz physical layer (PHY) and portion of the media access controller (hardware-MAC). The remaining MAC functions (software-MAC) and the application layer are executed on an external microcontroller. All PHY functions are integrated on the chip with minimal external components required for a complete radio. A low-cost crystal is used as a reference for the PLL and to clock the digital circuitry. To optimize energy consumption in sleep mode while still keeping an accurate time base, a Real Time Clock reference can be used.

Some extra features of the PHY include receiver energy detection, link quality indication and clear channel assessment. Both contention-based and contention-free channel access methods are supported with a maximum packet size of 128 bytes, which includes a variable payload up to 104 bytes. Also employed are 64-bit IEEE and 16-bit short addressing, supporting over 65,000 nodes per network. The MAC provides network association and disassociation, has an optional super frame structure with beacons for time synchronization, and a guaranteed time slot (GTS) mechanism for high priority communications. The channel access method is carrier sense multiple access with collision avoidance (CSMA-CA).

ZigBee defines the network, security, and application framework profile layers for an IEEE 802.15.4-based system. ZigBee's network layer supports three networking topologies; star, mesh,

*Table 6. Wireless standard comparisons*

| | ZigBee™ 802.15.4 | Bluetooth™ 802.15.1 | WiFi™ 802.11b | GPRS/GSM 1XRTT/ CDMA |
|---|---|---|---|---|
| **Application Focus** | Monitoring & Control | Cable Replacement | Web, Video, Email | WAN, Voice/Data |
| **System Resource** | 4KB-32KB | 250KB+ | 1MB+ | 16MB+ |
| **Battery Life(days)** | 100-1000+ | 1-7 | .1-5 | 1-7 |
| **Nodes Per Network** | 255/65K+ | 7 | 30 | 1,000 |
| **Bandwidth(kbps)** | 20-250 | 720 | 11,000+ | 64-128 |
| **Range(meters)** | 1-75+ | 1-10+ | 1-100 | 1,000+ |
| **Key Attributes** | Reliable, Low Power, Cost Effective | Cost, Convenience | Speed, Flexibility | Reach, Quality |

(Source: Helicomm)

and cluster tree as shown in Picture 3. Star networks are common and provide for very long battery life operation. Mesh, or peer-to-peer, networks enable high levels of reliability and scalability by providing more than one path through the network. Cluster-tree networks utilize a hybrid star/mesh topology that combines the benefits of both for high levels of reliability and support for battery-powered nodes. To provide for low cost implementation options, the ZigBee Physical Device type distinguishes the type of hardware based on the IEEE 802.15.4 definition of reduced function device (RFD) and full function device (FFD). An IEEE 802.15.4 network requires at least one FFD to act as a network coordinator.

As an alternative to ZigBee, Nokia has proposed a Bluetooth evolution to IEEE 802.15 TG4. Nokia's proposal takes Bluetooth as the basis but suggests relaxation of some parameters such as data rate, transmitted power, receiver sensitivity and frequency hopping to enable very low-power implementation. One of the main ideas of the proposal is to use standard Bluetooth RF parts as far as possible, which would enable better integrability to the mobile phone environment (IEEE 802.15 TG4b). Table 6 provides a comparison between different wireless standards related to various attributes of the specific networks.

## CASE STUDIES OF EXISTING PERVASIVE HEALTH SYSTEMS

Nowadays, the utilization of modern biomedical data acquisition devices and the deployment of fast wireless networks have enabled the introduction of several pervasive health systems. Hereafter, we review some of the most representative pervasive health applications found in the literature.

In Takizawa (2001), a mobile healthcare unit was implemented utilizing a Ku-band satellite system. The mobile unit consists of a van that houses a spiral computed-tomography (CT) machine and various telecommunications equipment. The unit allows medical examination, CT scanning, and on-line two-way transfer of image data / teleconferencing to a medical center for consultation with various specialists. For trauma cases during the game period of Olympic Games of 1998, images of CT scans were uploaded at an efficient transmission speed of 437.5 kb/s, over a period of 5 min. Video conferencing was achieved at a transmission speed of 384 kb/s. As already mentioned, the major disadvantage of such system is the high cost of the satellite link.

In Salvador (2005)0, a platform built around three information entities (patient, healthcare agent, and central station) was designed to enable patients with chronic heart disease to complete specifically defined protocols for out-of-hospital follow-up and monitoring. The patients were provided with portable recording equipment and a cellular phone that supported data transmission (electrocardiogram - ECG) and wireless application protocol (WAP). The data rate limitations due to the GSM network operation are once again obvious.

The goal of the MobiHealth project (Bults, 2004) was to develop mobile health services using GPRS and UMTS for connection of patient's body area network and hospital servers. Body Area Network (BAN) comprises of various healthcare sensors wirelessly connected to a mobile phone or a PDA. A mobile phone or a PDA acts as a gateway towards wide area networks, thus providing access to remote databases or doctors in charge. For the emergency cases, trials have been conducted showing tele-trauma care both for patients and for health professionals (ambulance paramedics). The trauma patient BAN measured vital signs which were transmitted from the scene to the members of the trauma team located at the hospital.

Finally Chu (2004) have presented a cost-effective portable tele-trauma system was introduced that can assist the healthcare in pre-hospital trauma care. With the commercially available 3G wireless link, the system can simultaneously transmit video, still-ultrasound images, and vital signals. The system enables the trauma physician to continuously monitor the patient's situation during the pre-hospital routine through visual communication (e.g., video) in addition to voice and vital signs information exchange.

## In Controlled Environment (Hospitals, Medical Centers)

As mentioned in Section 2.3.3 the use of pervasive systems in controlled environments, such as hospitals and medical centers may be divided into two broad categories. The first one relates to applications, enabling the mobile ubiquitous delivery

of medical data and implementations of mobile Electronic Health Records (EHR), accessible by PDA's or Tablet PC' s in a hospital equipped with Wireless LAN infrastructure (Finch, 1999). Several research groups (Hall, 2003; Maglogiannis, 2004) have experimented on the use of handheld computers of low cost and high portability, integrated through a wireless local computer network within the IEEE 802.11 or Bluetooth standards. Regarding the medical data exchange, DICOM (www.dicom.org) and HL7 (www.hl7.org) standards are used in the data coding and transmission via mobile client/server applications capable of managing health information.

On the other hand, pervasive systems are used for the monitoring and diagnosis of patients. A wide range of medical monitors and sensors may enable the mobile monitoring of a patient, which is able to walk freely without being tied to the bed. Pervasive systems in a hospital environment are mostly based in Bluetooth communication technology. For example, Khoor (2001) have used the Bluetooth system for short-distance (10m-20m) data transmission of digitized Electrocardiograms (ECGs) together with relevant clinical data. Hall (2003) have demonstrated a Bluetooth based platform for delivering critical health record information in emergency situations, while Andreasson (2002) have developed a remote system for patient monitoring using Bluetooth enabled sensors. The above examples show that the merging of mobile communications and the introduction of handhelds along with their associated technology has potential to make a big impact in emergency medicine. Moreover, many market projections indicate that mobile computer is both an emerging and enabling technology in healthcare (Finch, 1999). Each biosignal provides different and complementary information on a patient status and for each specific person the anticipated range of signal parameters is different. For example, heart rate may vary between 30 and 250 beats/min for normal people in different circumstances; likewise, breathing rate could be between 5 and

50 breaths/min. Electroencephalogram (EEG) and Electrocardiogram ECG are considerably more complex biosignals with spectra up to 10 KHz (Gouaux, 2003).

## In Random Locations - Home Care Systems

Facilities for medical practice in non hospital settings are limited by the availability of medical devices suitable for producing biosignals and other medical data. There is a number of active research and commercial projects developing sensors and devices, which do not require local intervention to enable contact with a clinician remote from the care environment. These new systems provide automated connection with remote access and seamless transmission of biological and other data upon request. Pervasive systems in non hospital systems aim at the better managing of chronic care patients, the controlling of health delivery costs, the increasing quality of life and quality of health services and the provision of distinct possibility of predicting and thus avoiding serious complications.

The patient or elder will mainly require monitoring of his vital signals (i.e., ECG, blood pressure, heart rate, breath rate, oxygen saturation and perspiration). Patients recently discharged from hospital after some form of intervention, for instance, after a cardiac incident, cardiac surgery or a diabetic comma are less secure and require enhanced care. The most common forms of special home monitoring are ECG arrhythmia monitoring, post surgical monitoring, respiratory and blood oxygen levels monitoring and sleep apnoea monitoring. In the case of diabetics, the monitoring of blood sugar levels resigns the patient to repeated blood sampling which is undesirable and invasive. One possible solution is the development of implantable wireless sensor devices that would be able to give this information quickly, and in a continuous fashion. Current conditions where home monitoring might be provided include: hy-

pertension, diabetes (monitoring glucose), obesity (monitoring weight), CHF (monitoring weight), asthma and COPD (monitoring spirometry/peak flow), and, in the near future, conditions utilizing oximetry monitoring. Other home monitoring conditions might include pre-eclampsia, anorexia, low birth-weight infants, growth abnormalities, and arrhythmias. Most chronic health conditions in children and adults could be managed and/or enhanced by home monitoring.

In most applications two monitoring modes are foreseen: the Batch and the emergency mode. Batch Mode refers to the every day monitoring process, where vital signs are acquired and transmitted periodically to a health monitoring centre. The received data are monitored by the doctor on-duty and then stored into the patient's electronic health record maintained by a Healthcare Centre. The Emergency Mode occurs because the patient does not feel well and, thus, decides to initiate an out-of-schedule session, or because the monitoring device detects a problem and automatically initiates the transfer of data to the corresponding centre. Application emergency episode detection and the corresponding alarm processing are important for the protection of the patient. An alarm represents a change in status of a physiological condition or a sensor reading state outside of agreed limits.

Telemonitoring of patients at home: a software agent approach (Rialle, 2003) is an article that describes the general architecture, the various components of the model, and methodology that has been used. It concretely faces the problem of depiction in the object-oriented system of various dimensions of the included systems: the natural world of sensors of domestic biological signals, the numerical world of software experts and everything relative with the internet, and the world of doctors and patients and all-purpose practitioners. In this system, the main part of information passes from the biophysical world of patients in the house, in the social-medical world of experts of care of persons from a chain of appli-

*Figure 5. Computer architecture of the software agent approach*

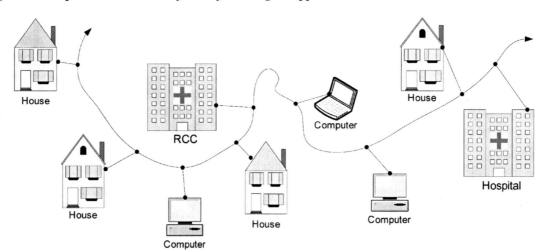

ances including sensors, network of local region, domestic computer, distant central computer, and server computers. Each appliance of software is specialized with different levels of knowledge and complexity. The technologies of Internet and Java provide the structural units of drawn telecontrol of software. The laboratorial experiments have been realized using complete equipped smart home for the telecontrol. This system allows multiple communications of the computers simultaneously and sharing of information among patients, as can be seen in Figure 5 (Rialle, 2003).

A Portable Real Time Homecare System Design with Digital Camera Platform (Kao, 2005) presents a low-cost homecare system based on a platform of digital camera. According to the multimedia functions of recording a digital camera, such as JPEG and MPEG-1/MPEG-4 recording, the proposed system can be further elaborated and depress the mark of a phono cardio graph (PCG).

An ideal portable system homecare as shown in Figure 6 (Kao, 2005), should provide the following characteristic traits:

- diagnostics collection and treatment of data,

- television and acoustic contact between the doctor and the patient for the communication in real time,
- portable appliances with batteries so the doctor can check the patients everywhere and
- the wireless contact of communication.

Due to the limitation of wireless bandwidth communication, the audio and TV data and the vital data should first be compressed before transmitted. The main difficulty in constructing this ideal homecare system is the limited capacity of the battery of the mobile devices.

Figure 7 (Kao, 2005) presents a proposed portable embedded system, based in a platform of digital cameras. The platform incorporates the basic elements of multimedia such as CCD, A/D converter, D/A converter and other processors for the compression of the elements. The microphone and the speaker can also be used for communication between the patients and the doctors, if the wireless appliances are incorporated in the system. Based on this platform, the remainder issues develop a good quality algorithm in order to establish the calculating ability and in order to

*Figure 6. Portable system architecture*

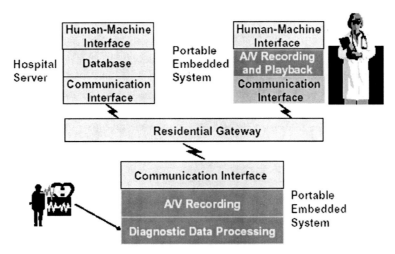

completely use the calculating resources from the software, so as the acoustic/television recordings can be accomplished simultaneously with the treatment diagnoses.

*CodeBlue* (Malan, 2004) is a wireless infrastructure intended for deployment in emergency medical care, integrating low-power, wireless vital sign sensors, PDAs, and PC-class systems. CodeBlue will enhance first responders' ability to assess patients on scene, ensure seamless transfer of data among caregivers, and facilitate efficient allocation of hospital resources. Intended to scale to very dense networks with thousands of devices and extremely volatile network conditions, this infrastructure will support reliable, ad hoc data delivery, a flexible naming and discovery scheme, and a decentralized security model.

CodeBlue is designed to provide routing, naming, discovery, and security for wireless medical sensors, PDAs, PCs, and other devices that may be used to monitor and treat patients in a range of medical settings. CodeBlue is designed to scale across a wide range of network densities, ranging from sparse clinic and hospital deployments to very dense, ad hoc deployments at a mass casualty site. CodeBlue may also operate on a range of wireless devices, from resource-constrained motes to more powerful PDA and PC-class sys-

tems. CodeBlue is depicted in Figure 8 (Malan, 2004) and offers a scalable, robust "information plane" for coordination and communication across wireless medical devices. It provides protocols and services for node naming, discovery, any-to-any ad hoc routing, authentication, and encryption. CodeBlue is based on a publish/subscribe model for data delivery, allowing sensing nodes to publish streams of vital signs, locations, and identities to which PDAs or PCs accessed by physicians and nurses can subscribe. To avoid network congestion and information overload, CodeBlue will support filtration and aggregation of events as they flow through the network. For example, physicians may specify that they should receive a full stream of data from a particular patient, but only critical changes in status for other patient on their watch.

*Wealthy* (Paradiso, 2005) it is a fabric surface filled with sensors, electrodes and connections in fabric moulds that give signals for technical and modern telecommunications systems. The sensors, the electrodes and the connections are realized through conductive and durable threads. The ability of the system to acquire simultaneous various biomedical signals (e.g. electrocardiogram, respiratory activity) has been discovered and compared with a standard system. Moreover, two

*Figure 7. The proposed portable embedded system based in a platform of digital cameras*

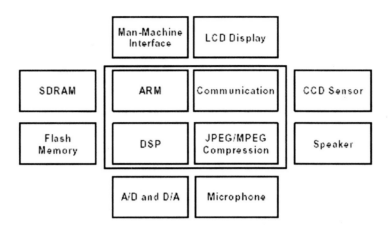

different techniques are presented for the acquisition of respiratory signal with fabric sensors. The proposed system is designed to monitor individual components that are influenced by cardiovascular disease, particularly during the recovery phase. The system can also help workers affected by physical or psychological stress and / or environmental and occupational health risks.

Wealthy will become completely acceptable if it is an appliance easy to use and adaptable to the needs of each customer without he or she feeling depression, specifically in his daily activities. The fabric approaches the application of sensor elements that exists in the clothes allowing firstly at low cost to achieve a long-lasting control ill and an easy adaptation in the configuration of sensor of each customer, according to their needs.

This device helps to prevent an acute crisis or heart problems of workers in conditions of extreme stress. Simultaneous replication of critical signals allows the export of the parameters specifying a new link to all the signals that contribute to risk messages, adding data to the personal health records of patients. In the wealthy appliance, the electrocardiogram signals are sampled at 250Hz. Special treatment is applied to parameters such as heart rate and duration of the QRS with a respectable number of samples. In order to reduce the amount of data transferred via GPRS, the

ECG signals have been cut to prevail samples of 100Hz. The activities of breathing and movement result from the sensors that have been sampled at 16Hz. The portable system of the patient (PPU) is designed by a simple surface with two LEDs, a button aiming at the warning of the user and a button that gives the option to the user of regulating manually the alarm. The communication of this appliance is based on the GPRS protocols. The central system is comprised by:

- Web server
- Database Application module
- Central Control module
- Doctor's desktop/laptop module

## FUTURE RESEARCH DIRECTIONS

The technological advances of the last few years in mobile communications, biomedical data acquisition and mobile computing have facilitated the introduction of pervasive healthcare applications. Healthcare can benefit from pervasive computing benefits in at least four ways:

- Enabling distributed access and processing of medical data;

*Figure 8. The CodeBlue communication substrate*

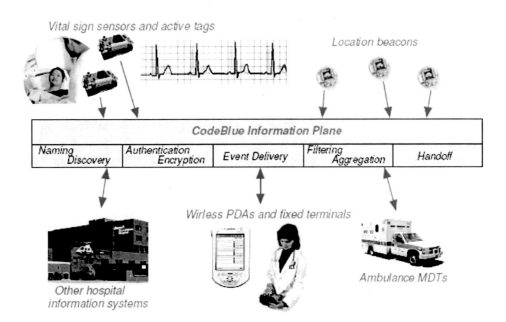

- Lowering costs by getting appropriate care to the people who need it much faster than previously possible;
- Making expert care accessible to more people, thereby increasing the scale at which first-rate healthcare is applied and
- Making healthcare more personalized, prompting individuals to take more responsibility for maintaining their health.

However there are still issues and challenges that have to be addressed. The most significant according to our view is the fact that the vast majority of the existing implementations do not interoperate sufficiently, resulting in segmented solutions. Moving to a fully pervasive system would be a complex transition requiring several steps and incremental budgetary increases to create the necessary infrastructure. This process should not interfere with the basic functioning of the current systems. In addition the introduction of more intelligent approaches and methods, like context-awareness and agent environments is a desired feature of the forthcoming pervasive health systems that might help in overcoming obstacle such as interoperability and collaboration issues. Privacy and security are also potential problems. Healthcare data should be available anytime anywhere, but only to authorized persons. This important aspect of pervasive health systems has not yet been dealt sufficiently in existing systems. The usability of pervasive healthcare solutions is another challenge, at least in the near future. Those who are less technically savvy are generally willing to use pervasive mobile devices if these devices enrich their lives, give them more independence, and offer intuitive interfaces. Training healthcare professionals as well as patients to use such devices will become less problematic as handhelds and other wireless products become commonplace in society.

## CONCLUSION

In this chapter book we analyzed the tremendous impact of wireless technology in the homecare and healthcare environments. We described a number of different case studies of the existing pervasive heath systems, showing great performance and the biosensors that will mark swift growth in the future and will become integral part of our life. There are appliances easy in their use precious and very important for the patient, contributing to the improvement and in the prevention of his or her health.

The use of new technologies for the applications of telemedicine and concretely the homecare system appears today as an obligatory solution: the wireless systems have become a standardized infrastructure for access in the complex applications of telemedicine from substantially any machine and functional system. Such standardized platform of communication guarantees the advantages of possibility of access and possibility of utilization both in the customers and in the suppliers (patients and general practitioners). In other words we can declare that the use of these technologies offer to the patients who typically fill the chambers and the corridors of hospitals, services of high quality and efficiency, outweighing the provisional cost.

Although wired communication technologies, such us ATM (Asynchronous Transfer Mode) and optical communication, are widely used, the key aspect for pervasive healthcare communication is the transfer of high-speed and ubiquitous health data in every place in earth securely and promptly. Wireless technology came to encompass the e-health monitoring everywhere from any given location, providing the so-called m-health services. During the last years, there has been increased research efforts on the production of commercial mobile health systems based on WiFi (Wireless Fidelity), GPRS (General Packet Radio Service) and 3G UMTS (3rd Generation Universal Mobile Telecommunications System) networking technologies. The introduction of high speed data rate, wide bandwidth, digital and encrypted communication technology, makes possible the delivery of audio, video and waveform data to wherever and whenever needed. It is anticipated that the current deployment of wireless-based

systems with global operational morphologies will improve some of the limitations of the existing wireless technologies and will provide a well-organized platform for mobile healthcare services.

Such wireless technologies will make available both mobile patients and end users to interactively get the medical attention and advice they need, when and where is required in spite of any geographical obstructions or mobility constrains. Consequently, it can serve as a new generation technology for mobile health systems providing immediate and ubiquitous health care in a range of different circumstances, as it may handle a variety of telemedicine needs, especially in the fields of emergency health care provision in ambulances, rural hospital centers or any other remote and dispersed located health center and intensive care patients monitoring.

The management of integrated electronic health records and other telemedicine applications and services the system supports, is now internationally well known and has been repeatedly showed interest in the transfer of technology and the know-how to other regions of Europe. Nevertheless, various questions exist that should be discussed in-depth, regarding to the applications relative with the benefit of attention in the distance, called today telecare applications. In the telecare applications the role of patient becomes vital, through the actively inclusion in the stage of management of treatments and care, and through the responsibility for the collection of certain measurements and relative information.

The technologies of today are tools for a high-quality coordination procedure. Their capabilities are improving rapidly from time to time and their cost decreases exponentially with their use. What is needed is coordination of relevant concepts, attitudes and best practices, so that we can seize the great opportunities that they provide.

# REFERENCES

3GPP TR 25.896. (2004). *Feasibility Study for Enhanced Uplink for UTRA FDD, Release 6, v6.0.0.*

3GPP TS 25.308. (2004). *High Speed Downlink Packet Access; Overall Description; Stage 2, v6.3.0.*

*3rdGeneration Partnership Project.* (n.d.). Retrieved from www.3gpp.org

Ackerman, M., Craft, R., Ferrante, F., Kratz, M., Mandil, S., & Sapci, H. (2002). Telemedicine Technology. *Telemedicine Journal and e-Health, 8*(1), 71–78.

Andreasson, J., Ekstrom, M., Fard, A., Castano, J. G., & Johnson, T. (2002). Remote system for patient monitoring using Bluetooth/spl trade. *IEEE Sensors, 1,* 304–307.

Baldus, H., Klabunde, K., & Muesch, G. (2004). Reliable Set-Up of Medical Body-Sensor Networks. In *Proc. EWSN 2004,* Berlin, Germany.

Barger, T. S., Brown, D. E., & Alwan, M. (2005). Health-Status Monitoring Through Analysis of Behavioral Patterns. *IEEE Transactions on Systems, Man, and Cybernetics, 35*(1), 22–27.

Brady, M., & Rogers, M. (2002). DVB-RCS Background Book. Technical Report, Nera Broadband Satellite AS (NBS), Publication no. 102386.

Breynaert, D. (2005). *2Way-Sat: A DVB-RCS Satellite Access Network. Technical Report, Newtec Cy N.V.* Belgium: NTC.

Bults, R. (2004). Body Area Networks for Ambulant Patient Monitoring Over Next Generation Public Wireless Networks. In *Proceedings of the 13th IST Mobile and Wireless Communications Summit,* Lyon, France, (pp. 181-185).

Choudhri. A., Kagal, L., Joshi, A., Finin, T. & Yesha, Y. (2003). PatientService: Electronic Patient Record Redaction and Delivery in Pervasive Environments. In *Fifth International Workshop on Enterprise Networking and Computing in Healthcare Industry.*

Choudhury, T. (2008). The Mobile Sensing Platform: An Embedded Activity Recognition System. *IEEE Pervasive Computing / IEEE Computer Society [and] IEEE Communications Society, 7*(2), 32–41.

Chu, Y., & Ganz, A. (2004). A Mobile Teletrauma System Using 3G Networks. *IEEE Transactions on Information Technology in Biomedicine, 8*(4), 456–462.

De Rossi, D., Carpi, F., Lorussi, F., Mazzoldi, A., Paradiso, R., Scilingo, E. P., & Tognetti, A. (2003). Electroactive fabrics and wearable biomonitoring devices. *AUTEX Research Journal, 3*(4), 180–185.

Fei, H., Meng, J., Wagner, M., & De-Cun, D. (2007). Privacy-Preserving Telecardiology Sensor Networks: Toward a Low-Cost Portable Wireless Hardware/Software Codesign. *IEEE Transactions on Information Technology in Biomedicine, 11*(6), 619–627.

Finch, C. (1999). Mobile computing in healthcare. *Health Management Technology, 20*(3), 63–64.

Flores-Mangas, F., & Oliver, N. (2005). *Healthgear: A realtime wearable system for monitoring and analyzing physiological signals.* Technical Report MSR-TR-2005-182, Microsoft Research.

Gandolfo, P. & Allen, J. (2002). *802.15.3 Overview/Update.*

Georgia Institute of Technology. (n.d.). *The Aware Home.* Retrieved from http://www.cc.gatech.edu/fce/ahri/projects/index.html

Ghasemzadeh, H., Guenterberg, E., & Jafari, R. (2009). Energy-Efficient Information-Driven Coverage for Physical Movement Monitoring in Body Sensor Networks. *IEEE Journal on Selected Areas in Communications, 27*(1), 58–69.

Gouaux, F., Simon-Chautemps, L., Adami, S., Arzi, M., Assanelli, D., Fayn, J., et al. (2003). Smart devices for the early detection and interpretation of cardiological syndromes. In *Proceedings 4th International IEEE EMBS Special Topic Conference on Information Technology Applications in Biomedicine*, (pp. 291-294).

Guang-Zhong, Y., Lo, B., Wang, L., Rans, M., Thiemjarus, S., Ng, J., et al. (2004). From Sensor Networks to Behavior Profiling: A Homecare Perspective of Intelligent Building. In *Proceedings of the IEE Seminar for Intelligent Buildings*.

Hall, E. S., Vawdrey, D. K., Knutson, C. D., & Archibald, J. K. (2003). Enabling remote access to personal electronic medical records. *IEEE Engineering in Medicine and Biology Magazine*, 133–139.

Holma, H., & Toskala, A. (Eds.). (2006). *HSDPA/HSUPA for UMTS*. New York: Wiley.

Holma, H., Toskala, A., Ranta-aho, K., & Pirskanen, J. (2007). High-Speed Packet Access Evolution in 3GPP Release 7. *IEEE Communications Magazine, 45*(2), 29–35.

*IEEE802.15 TG4b*. (2001). IEEE802.15 TG4 Contributions, WPAN-LR Call For Proposals for Session #13/Portland, Plenary, Bob Heile.

IEEE802. *15 TG3, IEEE 802.15 WPAN Task Group 3* (TG3). (n.d.). Retrieved from http://www.ieee802.org/15/pub/TG3.html

International Telecommunication Union. (2004). *Telecommunication Development Bureau, ITU-D Study Group 2. "Question 14-1/2: Application of telecommunications in health care, technical information - A mobile medical image transmission system in Japan", PocketMIMAS*. Rapporteurs Meeting Q14-1/2 Japan.

International Telecommunication Union. (2004). *Telecommunication Development Bureau, ITU-D Study Group 2. Question 14-1/2: Application of telecommunications in health care, technical information - A mobile medical image transmission system in Japan, PocketMIMAS*. Rapporteurs Meeting Q14-1/2 Japan.

Istepanian, R. S. H., & Chandran, S. (1999). Enhanced telemedicine applications with next generation of wireless systems. In *Proc. First Joint BMES/EMBS IEEE International Conference of Engineering in Medicine and Biology*, Atlanta.

Istepanian, R. S. H., Jovanov, E., & Zhang, Y. T. (2004). Guest Editorial Introduction to the Special Section on M-Health: Beyond Seamless Mobility and Global Wireless Health-Care Connectivity. *IEEE Transactions on Information Technology in Biomedicine, 8*(4), 405–414.

Jafari, R., Encarnacao, A., Zahoory, A., Brisk, P., Noshadi, H., & Sarrafzadeh, M. (2005) Wireless Sensor Networks For Health Monitoring. In *Second ACM/IEEE International Conference on Mobile and Ubiquitous Systems*.

Jones, V., Van Halteren, A., Widya, I., Dokovsky, N., Koprinkov, G., Bults, R., et al. (2005). Mobihealth: Mobile Services for Health Professionals, In R.S.H. Istepanian, C.S. Pattichis & S. Laxminarayan (Ed.), M-Health Emerging Mobile Health Systems, (pp. 237-246, Topics in Biomedical Engineering International Book Series). Berlin: Springer.

Kao, W. C., Chen, W. H., Yu, C. K., Hong, C. M., & Lin, S. Y. (2005). Portable Real-Time Homecare System Design with Digital Camera Platform. *IEEE Transactions on Consumer Electronics, 51*(4), 1035–1041.

Khoor, S., Nieberl, K., Fugedi, K., & Kail, E. (2001). Telemedicine ECG-telemetry with Bluetooth technology. In *2ⁿᵈ Annual Conference of Computers in Cardiology,* Rotterdam, Holland, (pp. 585–588).

Kifor, T., Varga, L., Vazquez-Salceda, J., Alvarez, S., Miles, S., & Moreau, L. (2006). Provenance in Agent-Mediated Healthcare Systems. *IEEE Intelligent Systems, 21*(6), 38–46.

Kyriacou, E., Pavlopoulos, S., Berler, A., Neophytou, M., Bourka, A., & Georgoulas, A. (2003). Multi-purpose HealthCare Telemedicine Systems with mobile communication link support. *Biomedical Engineering Online, 2*(7).

Lahtela, A., Hassinen, M., & Jylha, V. (2008). RFID and NFC in healthcare: Safety of hospitals medication care. In *Second International Conference on Pervasive Computing Technologies for Healthcare,* (pp. 241–244).

LeRouge, C., Garfield, M. J., & Hevner, A. R. (2002). Quality Attributes in Telemedicine Video Conferencing. In *Proceedings of the 35th Hawaii International Conference on System Sciences,* Hawaii.

Maglogiannis, I. (2004). Design and Implementation of a Calibrated Store and Forward Imaging System for Teledermatology. *Journal of Medical Systems, 28*(5), 455–467.

Maglogiannis, I., Apostolopoulos, N., & Tsoukias, P. (2004). Designing and Implementing an Electronic Health Record for Personal Digital Assistants (PDAs). *International Journal for Quality of Life Research, 2*(1), 63–67.

Maglogiannis, I., Delakouridis, K., & Kazatzopoulos, L. (2006). Enabling collaborative medical diagnosis over the Internet via peer to peer distribution of electronic health records. *J Medical Systems, Springer, 30*(2), 107–116.

Maglogiannis, I., Karpouzis, K., & Wallace, M. (2007). Image, Signal and Distributed Data Processing for Networked eHealth Applications. *IEEE Engineering in Medicine and Biology Magazine, 26*(5), 14–17.

Malan, D., Jones, T. F., Welsh, M., & Moulton, S. (2004). CodeBlue: An Ad Hoc Sensor Network Infrastructure for Emergency Medical Care. *MobiSys, Workshop on Applications of Mobile Embedded Systems.*

Montgomery, K., Mundt, C., Thonier, G., Tellier, A., Udoh, U., Barker, V., et al. (2004) Lifeguard - A Personal Physiological Monitor For Extreme Environments. In Proceeding of 26th annual International of IEEE EMBS, (pp. 2192-2195).

Mukhopadhyay, S., Paniyrahi, D., & Dey, S. (2004). Data aware, Low cost Error correction for Wireless Sensor Networks. In *IEEE Wireless Communications and Networking Conference,* Atlanta, (pp. 2492-2497).

Paradiso, R., Loriga, G., & Taccini, N. (2005). A Wearable Health Care System Based on Knitted Integrated Sensors. *IEEE Transactions on Information Technology in Biomedicine, 9*(3), 337–344.

Pattichis, C. S., Kyriacou, E., Voskarides, S., Pattichis, M. S., Istepanian, R., & Schizas, C. N. (2002). Wireless Telemedicine Systems: An Overview. *IEEE Antennas and Propagation Magazine, 44*(2), 143–153.

Rabaey, J. M., Ammer, M. J., da Silva, J. Jr, Patel, D., & Roundy, S. (2000). PicoRadio Supports Ad Hoc Ultra-Low Power Wireless Networking. *Computer, 33*(7), 42–48.

Ramachandran, R., Ramanna, L., Ghasemzadeh, H., Pradhan, G., Jafari, R., & Prabhakaran, B. (2008). Body Sensor Networks to Evaluate Standing Balance: Interpreting Muscular Activities Based on Inertial Sensors. In *The 2nd International Workshop on Systems and Networking Support for Healthcare and Assisted Living Environments (HealthNet)*, Breckenridge.

Rantanen, J., Impio, J., Karinsalo, T., Malmivaara, M., Reho, A., Tasanen, M., & Vanhala, J. (2002). *Smart clothing prototype for the arctic environment. Personal and Ubiquitous Computing.* Berlin: Springer.

Rialle, V., Lamy, J. B., Noury, N., & Bajolle, L. (2003). Telemonitoring of patients at home: a software agent approach. *Computer Methods and Programs in Biomedicine, 72*(3), 257–268.

Salvador, C. H. (2005). Airmed-Cardio: A GSM and Internet Services-Based System for Out-of-Hospital Follow-Up of Cardiac Patients. *IEEE Transactions on Information Technology in Biomedicine, 9*(1), 73–85.

Shimizu, K. (1999). Telemedicine by Mobile Communication. *IEEE Engineering in Medicine and Biology Magazine, 18*(4), 32–44.

Tachakra, S., Wang, X. H., Istepanian, R. S. H., & Song, Y. H. (2003). Mobile e-Health: The Unwired Evolution of Telemedicine. *Telemedicine Journal and e-Health, 9*(3), 247–257.

Takizawa, M. S. (2001). Telemedicine System Using Computed Tomography Van of High-Speed Telecommunication Vehicle. *IEEE Transactions on Information Technology in Biomedicine, 5*(1), 2–9.

VivoMetrics. (2009). *VivoMetrics LifeShirt System Technology.* Retrieved from http://www.vivometrics.com

Ward, J. A., Lukowicz, P., Troster, G., & Starner, T. E. (2006). Activity Recognition of Assembly Tasks Using Body-Worn Microphones and Accelerometers. *IEEE Transactions on Pattern Analysis and Machine Intelligence, 28*(10), 1553–1567.

*WiMedia Alliance.* (n.d.). Retrieved from http://www.wimedia.org.

Yang, A.Y., Jafari, R., Sastry, S.S., & Bajcsy, R. (2009). Distributed Recognition of Human Actions Using Wearable Motion Sensor Networks. *Journal of Ambient Intelligence and Smart Environments.*

ZigBee. (n.d.). Retrieved from www.zigbee.org

## ADDITIONAL READING

Axisa, F., Gehin, C., Delhomme, G., Collet, C., Robin, O., & Dittmar, A. (2004). Wrist Ambulatory Monitoring System and Smart Glove for Real Time Emotional, Sensorial and Physiological Analysis, Proceedings of the 26th Annual International Conference of the IEEE on Engineering in Medicine and Biology Society, San Francisco, CA, USA, 2161-2164.

Bellazzi, R., Montani, S., Riva, A., & Stefanelli, M. (2001). Web-based telemedicine systems for home-care: technical issues and experiences, International Conference on Advances in Delivery of Care, London, *64*(3), 175-187.

Bolaños, M., Nazeran, H., Gonzalez, I., Parra, R., & Martinez, C. (2004). A PDA-based Electrocardiogram/Blood Pressure Telemonitor for Telemedicine, Proceedings of the 26th Annual International Conference of the IEEE EMBS, San Francisco, CA, USA, 2169-2172.

Bricon-Souf, N., Beuscart-Zephir, M. C., & Beauscart, R. (2001) A helpful framework for the organisation of the homecare, 23rd Annual International Conference of the IEEE on Engineering in Medicine and Biology Society, 4, 3567-3570.

Poon, C.C.Y., Wong Y.M., & Zhang, Y.T. (2006). M-Health: The Development of Cuff-less and Wearable Blood Pressure Meters for Use in Body Sensor Networks, Life Science Systems and Applications Workshop, 1-2.

Rhee, S., Yang, B. H., Chang, K., & Asada, H. H. (2006). The Ring Sensor: a New Ambulatory Wearable Sensor for Twenty-Four Hour Patient Monitoring, 20th Annual Conference of the IEEE on Engineering in Medicine and Biology Society, 4, 1906-1909. The association of telehealth service providers; http://www.atsp.org

Wealthy Project: Wearable Health Care System, IST 2001 – 3778, Commission of the European Communities; http://www.wealthyist.com

Wilson, C. B. (1999). Sensors in Hospitals. *BMJ (Clinical Research Ed.), 319*(7220), 1288.

www.tech-faq.com

# Chapter 11
# Lessons from Evaluating Ubiquitous Applications in Support of Hospital Work

**Monica Tentori**
*UABC, México*

**Victor M. González**
*University of Manchester, UK*

**Jesus Favela**
*CICESE, México*

## ABSTRACT

*The evaluation of ubiquitous computing (Ubicomp) applications presents a number of challenges ranging from the optimal recreation of the contextual conditions where technologies will be implemented, to the definition of tasks which often go well beyond the model of human-computer interaction that people are used to interact with. Many contexts, such as hospitals and healthcare which are frequently explored for the deployment of Ubicomp raise additional challenges as a result of the nature of the work where human life can be in risk, privacy of personal records is paramount, and labor is highly distributed across space and time. For the last six years the authors have been creating and pilot-testing numerous Ubicomp applications in support of hospital work and healthcare (Ubihealth). In this chapter, they discuss the lessons learned from evaluating these applications and organize them as a frame of techniques that assists researchers in selecting the proper method and type of evaluation to be conducted. Based on that frame the authors discuss a set of principles that designers must consider during evaluation. These principles include maintaining consistency of the activities and techniques used during the evaluation, give proper credit of individual benefits, promote replication of the environment, balance constraints and consider the level of pervasiveness and complexity.*

DOI: 10.4018/978-1-61520-765-7.ch011

## INTRODUCTION

The ubiquitous computing vision aims at surrounding users with a comfortable and convenient information environment that merges physical and computational infrastructures into an integrated habitat (Weiser, 1991). As Weiser stated *"the most powerful things are those that are effectively invisible in use [...] They weave themselves into the fabric of our everyday life until they are indistinguishable from it"* (Weiser, 1998). Indeed, Ubicomp technologies may be embedded in the environment, embedded in objects, worn, or carried by the user throughout everyday life. Interactions may be implicit or even sensed, unlike the explicit and intentional interactions typical of user interfaces in desktop environments. Ubicomp technologies may be used in unpredictable situations, changing contexts, and highly mobile applications. These issues and the invisibility posed by Weiser's vision alter the relationship between humans and technology posing multiple challenges for the evaluation of ubicomp.

While there are currently available an ample set of techniques and examples of ubicomp evaluation following traditional HCI approaches (Consolvo et al., 2007), using traditional techniques for evaluating ubicomp systems is quite challenging as we need to consider other issues. Among these issues include the ambiguity, scalability, and context of use of an ubiquitous application (Carter & Mankof, 2004). For example, a context-aware system can assume that every object of interest will be tagged with an RFID to automatically adapt the information shown to a user. Researchers have only recently begun to address the development of evaluation techniques that meet ubicomp's demands (Carter & Mankof, 2004; Consolvo et al., 2007; Mankoff et al., 2003). One reason for this is the relatively slow development and gradual evolution of methods and techniques that allow researchers to evaluate ubiquitous applications at different stages of their implementation. Among those efforts we can found the Wizard of Oz as one of the most popular techniques adopted (Consolvo et al., 2007). This distance from the real work practice and context means that much has to be done to understand how to apply qualitative or quantitative evaluation methods for Ubicomp.

The challenges to evaluate Ubicomp are emphasized in a healthcare domain. Hospitals represent a fruitful area to study the evaluation of Ubicomp and many researchers have focused on providing solutions for this particular context. Indeed, some elements of ubicomp are gradually being introduced in hospitals. These range from wireless networks, PDAs (Chin, 2005), RFID tags for patient tracking (O'Connor, 2006), voice-activated communication devices (Stanford, 2003), and sensors for patient monitoring (Pentland, 2004). However, given the critical nature of hospital work, the creation of such an Ubihealth environment needs to be gradual. This will allow confidence on the technology to build and lessons-learned to be incorporated into such environment. These issues in Ubihealth raise new challenges that go beyond those posed by ubicomp. Those challenges involve the level of integration of an Ubihealth application with existing systems deployed in the hospital, the context of use of such system that must be replicated when evaluating the system, as well as, the level of risk involved in case of system failure. As others researcher have pointed before, we regret the lack of techniques that allow us to cope with the evaluation issues faced when evaluating Ubihealth systems.

In this chapter we discuss our lessons learned from evaluating three Ubihealth applications. We organize our lessons a set of design principles that assist researchers in selecting the proper method and type of evaluation to be conducted. The rest of the chapter is organized as follows: In section II we describe the related work in the area highlighting the challenges for Ubicomp evaluation and why those are more difficult in the healthcare domain. Section III, describes six case studies of the evaluation of three systems. In section IV, we discuss how our lessons learned were organized as a set of principles that allow designers to manage those challenges in the evaluation of Ubihealth applications. Finally, in section V we present our conclusions and directions for future work.

## CASES AND LESSONS LEARNED

For the last six years, we have conducted a number of studies and evaluations at IMSS General Hospital in the city of Ensenada, Mexico a public institution providing health services to a high proportion of the 360 thousand city's habitants. As any other hospital of its size, the IMSS at Ensenada is a working environment, where information is distributed, workers are mobile and many artifacts support the coordination of people. Our relationship with the hospital has been oriented towards designing and pilot-testing different kinds of Ubihealth applications and technologies aimed at supporting the everyday practices of the staff working there, including nurses, medical interns and physicians. In this section, we present and discuss the evaluation of three systems conducted within a period of five years.

## Using Theatrical Representations and Scenario-Based Techniques to Evaluate a Context-Aware Mobile Communication System

The context-aware mobile communication system (CHIS) is an application that evolved and was gradually defined through three versions (Favela, Rodríguez, Preciado, & Gonzalez, 2004; Munoz, Rodriguez, Favela, Martinez-Garcia, & Gonzalez, 2003; Tentori, Favela, & Rodriguez, 2006).

The first version of CHIS (Figure 1b and 1c) aimed at supporting the exchange of messages among co-workers, in a way that the context of the recipient is considered for the delivery. This allows the opportunistic access to relevant information and increases awareness of the whereabouts of hospital workers and resources (Munoz et al.,

2003). For example, a physician can send a message to the doctor responsible for a patient in the next shift when the laboratory results become available (Figure 1b). Similarly, CHIS provides access to information and services according to user context. For instance, when a physician carrying a Personal Digital Assistant (PDA) is near to one of his patients, the system can automatically display that patient's clinical record.

A second version of CHIS integrates public displays that personalize the information shown to the user and offer opportunistic access to clinical information (Favela et al., 2004). For instance, if a physician approaches a public display it detects her presence and provides her with a personalized view of the CHIS system highlighting in the floor map recent additions to clinical records of patients she is in charge of, messages addressed to her, and the services most relevant to her current work activities (Figure 1a). The public display also allows the seamless transfer among heterogeneous devices. For instance, a physician can drag the information shown by the display to her picture to transfer it to his PDA.

A third and final version of CHIS, incorporates mechanisms that let users manage their privacy based on contextual information (Tentori, Favela, & Rodriguez, 2006). For instance, a physician can configure the floor map to only show the room he is in and his role instead of his exact location and name.

CHIS was fully developed but in order to be deployed within the hospital, it still would require integration with the Hospital Information System (HIS) and with the location estimation component (Castro & Favela, 2008). This integration was not possible in part because the current information management in the hospital is mainly paper-based as they do not have a Hospital Information System (HIS) and an Electronic Medical Record (EMR). For this reason, we needed to consider an approach that allows either simulating these components (e.g., the hospital information system) by allowing CHIS to interoperate with them or capturing the

*Figure 1. CHIS presents relevant information and facilitates collaboration (a) The user interacts with the handheld to know the availability and location of users and services (b) and to send context-aware messages (c)*

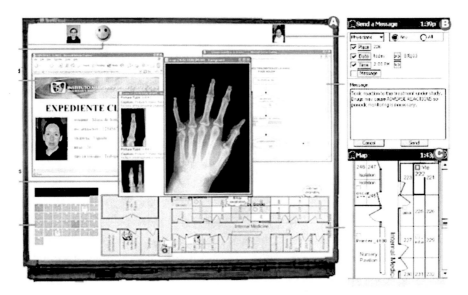

system's context of use, while reducing the cost and the complexities during its evaluation.

## The Evaluation

Within a period of 36 months we designed and evaluated CHIS. We conducted multiple evaluations that were used to inform the re-design of CHIS –including its last two versions. Figure 2a shows the methodology followed.

During these evaluations we evaluated CHIS' core characteristics, the hospital workers' intention to use it, their perception of its utility, ease of use and the privacy threats raised by it. The y-axis of the figure 2 depicts the activities executed during the development of CHIS including: a workplace study to understand hospital workers practices and identify design insights and scenarios of use; the design and the construction of the prototype and; its evaluation along with the analysis of the data. In contrast, the x-axis shows the time in months we spent in each activity. In the following lines

we describe in detail the technique used during the evaluation of each version of CHIS.

## Conducting a Scenario-Driven Evaluation

As Figure 2a shows we evaluated the first version of CHIS for a period of two months at the end of 2003 –once the implementation of the prototype was completed. We conducted a scenario-driven evaluation as proposed by Carroll (1995). Scenario-driven evaluations are typically conducted when the system has not been deployed allowing to vividly show its context of use to potential users.

We created animated slides of how CHIS could be used once deployed and presented them to 28 hospital staff members—13 physicians, 8 nurses, and 7 support staff. We then gave participants a questionnaire to evaluate how realistic they perceived the scenarios, if they would change anything, and if they could envision new scenarios to support their work with context-aware mobile

*Figure 2. (a) Methodology followed during the design and evaluation of the CHIS system (b) Two physicians working with a researcher during the theatrical representation*

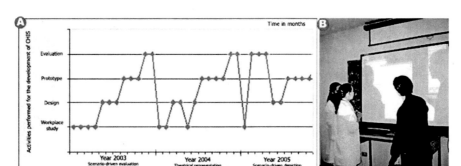

technology. We posed additional questions to validate the findings of our previous workplace study, such as *"Is it useful to have access to the patient's medical records through a handheld computer?"* The results validated most of our findings including assumptions and claims we made during the design process. For instance, all participants agreed that having awareness of the location of colleagues, use context as the basis for sending or receiving messages, and use handheld computers for accessing medical data would improve how they currently performed these activities –locate colleagues, communicate and consult clinical information.

After this exercise, we gave a 15-minute demonstration of the prototype and asked participants to answer a second questionnaire aimed at predicting user acceptance (F. D. Davis & Venkatesh, 1995). The results show that 91 percent of the participants would use the system. Additionally, 84 percent believe that using the system would enhance their job performance—a high degree of perceived usefulness—and 78 percent perceived the system would be easy to use. Nurses gave the lowest ratings for ease-of-use, which could in part be because they are less familiar with Instant Messaging and PDAs in general. We expect that user training before system deployment can help alleviate this aspect.

For the last 20 minutes of the session participants expressed opinions about the envisioned use of the system. Most of their opinions were related to how the system may improve their everyday practices. For instance, a participant made the following comment: *"The system may be used for several reasons [...] For instance, I can use it to register medical notes in a predefined order, share such information and even ask for pending tasks"*. In addition, participants highlighted that having opportunistic access to information and services will have a positive impact in care delivery. For instance, a participant expressed: *"... most of the time the laboratory results are available 1 or 2 days later and the most important thing for care delivery is to have opportunistic access to the information of a patient"*. On the other hand, other participants discussed problems they might face in using the system in practice and in a real setting. For instance, a participant expressed that the system does not guarantee the delivery of a message, he explained: *"I can leave my indications and the nurses may ignore them or not read them"*. However, other participants expressed that this problem might be solved if the recipient, once he had read the message, sends an acknowledge message back. This type of feedback helped us to improve the design of CHIS and such improvements were incorporated in its next version. In general, most of the participants agreed that the system will improve the practical issues raised by the use of a paper-based medical record enhancing the communication within the hospital and the access to opportunistic information.

## Performing a Theatrical Representation

The evaluation of the second version of CHIS was conducted for two months at the end of 2004 –once the implementation of the public display was completed (Figure 1a). It is important to note that the way this version of CHIS was designed differs from the way the first version was. As Figure 2a shows, the time invested in each activity during the development of the first version of CHIS was increasing exponentially; while, for the second version was executed through iterations between the study and the design –reducing at the same time the amount of time invested during the design process. This happened because the results of our first evaluation guided the design of the new version of CHIS. In this case, when we started the design of the public display we already had some scenarios of use that were generated from the insights gathered during our first evaluation. Despite the importance of the results of our first evaluation, we found out that showing only a pre-defined set of scenarios did not gave us enough information about what participants want, need or never even considered before by acting in and upon the new environment proposed. Hence, we could not capture issues regarding the potential adoption of the system, only feedback for its improvement. For this reason, we decided to complement our scenario-driven evaluation with a theatrical representation. A theatrical representation allows the participant to interact with the system following a specific scenario, which could be either pre-defined by the researcher or improvised by the participant. We found this technique an ideal mechanism to go beyond current practices while at the same time letting users to get involved in the design process. Consequently,

users may envision novel schemes of application while remaining the evaluation study relatively simple and inexpensive. To this aim, we showed video sequences to the participants and conducted a theatrical representation showing them a live demo of the system –we asked participants to also situate themselves in a role (Santana et al., 2005). Figure 2b shows two physicians and a researcher during a theatrical representation. After this exercise, we gave a 15-minute demonstration of the prototype and asked participants to answer a second questionnaire aimed at predicting user acceptance (F. D. Davis & Venkatesh, 1995). The entire session was videotaped and comments while using the devices were also collected.

We found out that hospital workers felt that the Ubihealth technology shown to them would be significantly better that their current solution. To this aim, we asked participants to assess the usefulness of the environment to address threes significant problems they face everyday in their working environment: asking for a second opinion; locating co-workers; and sending and receiving alerts the availability of the results of clinical tests. They all agreed that these are actual problems they face everyday and are not adequately addressed by current technologies. Eighty percent of them believe that using the system would enhance their job performance and 75 percent perceived the system would be easy to use, which indicates that they might indeed use the technology. Most of the opinions of the participants highlighted that the system will help them to improve performance. For instance a physician made the following comment: *"[the system] will help us to save time, effort and allow us to be more productive [...] will even increase collaboration among colleagues"*. We also discover the main obstacles foreseen by participants in the use of the proposed technology. These obstacles include the lack of training of many hospital workers, uncertainties in terms of the hospital being able to acquire the technology, the availability of appropriate technical support and privacy issues related to the use of the system by hospital workers. For instance a physician made the following comment: *"you will be fighting against people who do not want to learn how to use it"*.

## Conducting a Scenario-Driven Depiction

The evaluation of the third prototype was conducted for three months at the beginning of 2005 –before the implementation of the system was completed (Figure 2a). This version of CHIS differed from the way we designed the first two versions. This change of approach came as a result of an initial study conducted to evaluate the potential privacy risks raised by the use of CHIS (where six hospital workers were observed and interviewed), where we surprisingly found that they were not concerned about their privacy or those risks that a Ubihealth environment might raise (Tentori, Favela, & Gonzalez, 2006). We thought that we required a more direct approach to study these issues as people often do not care about privacy risks until an invasion to their privacy occurs (Palen & Dourish, 2003). For instance, a nurse might do not have problem to share her exact location with a colleague; however the reaction can be different, if she realizes that the system can be used to notify her supervisor that she has been most of their time in the dinning room. Therefore, we decided to conduct an evaluation of CHIS highlighting possible privacy issues that participants might face when using such system and we confronted them with situations that seemed to invade their privacy. To this aim we conducted a scenario-driven evaluation of CHIS and presented a pre-defined set of scenarios depicting a limiting functionality of the system. We showed to twenty-seven medical interns two scenarios as reported in (Tentori, Favela, & Rodriguez, 2006). The subjects were asked to situate themselves in a specific role within the scenario. After each scenario, they were asked to complete a survey to evaluate the threats raised by the technology to their privacy.

As a result of our evaluation, we encountered a mismatch between what they *perceived* as privacy violation and what they actually *did*, apparently ignoring privacy issues. They explained that some situations are not allowed under any circumstances, because they compromise the privacy of patients and hospital workers. However, they admit that there are times when they ignore privacy issues and justify their decisions based on circumstances. In this case the interns manage their privacy balancing the risks and benefits associated to their decisions. Thus, privacy was not major concern when raised *a priori*. An intern explains: *"At the beginning, I was more careful, for example, I wouldn't leave the hospital during my shift. But with time I learned how to move around. I learned with which hospital staff I could bend the rules and with whom I couldn't"*. Additionally, we identified the main privacy risks experienced by our participants during their everyday practices. These risks are related to CHIS ability to invisibly track the locations of hospital workers, the lack of feedback about how and with whom this information is being shared and for how long it is stored. For instance a medical intern made the following comment: *"This sensor just estimates my position, right? Can anybody hear what I am saying? If so I would like to be informed about what type of information I am sharing with the system"*. These results were later used to re-design CHIS to incorporate privacy-aware mechanisms (Tentori, Favela, & Rodriguez, 2006). This solution takes into account contextual information to enforce a privacy policy previously specified by a user. We re-designed the CHIS client to display the roles, rather than the names, of those they are not acquaintance with. The design made a compromise between letting the user know that someone is around without revealing her identity. Thus, in need for help, the user might know that a nurse is nearby and ask her for help, but under normal circumstances her identity will remain undisclosed to the user.

## Lessons Learned

A key advantage of scenario-driven or theatrical representation evaluations is that important design and system requirements can be discovered before much development effort has been put into building the underlying system. We consider that this process is fundamental for Ubicomp when applied to large spaces of interaction such as hospitals. As Figure 2 shows each evaluation of the CHIS system helped to improve the design of the system. Therefore, this technique allows researchers to easily perform iterative design sessions with end-users increasing thus user experience.

Also, scenario-driven evaluations helped us see that only when people have a representation of their work can then provide details beyond what we can be described from their memories. For instance, during the evaluation of CHIS participants validated the scenarios presented and provided us with additional insights and opportunities for applying our technology—for example, to schedule a surgery by tracking the availability of the operating room and the specialists involved. However, showing a set of pre-defined scenarios constraint the ability of participants to envision other opportunities and discover new breakdowns to apply the technology being presented to them. In contrast, theatrical representation evaluations contribute to get a realistic feel for what it would be like to actually use the technology as part of their everyday lives. This type of evaluation also helps researchers and participants to consider other challenges beyond those purely technical. They can also be used to help potential users to discover other potential benefits or threats never even considered before by envisaging others acting in and upon the environment. We found that despite that during an initial study of the use of CHIS users did not identify privacy threats, when we made those threats more evident through scenarios they did find a wide range of risks in using such system.

In addition, the type of activities conducted during the evaluation and the way they were conducted did not change all the way through the period of this case. For the tree evaluations, participants were shown a set of scenarios, they were asked to situate themselves in a specific role and then we asked them to fill a questionnaire based on the same model. This allows having a level of consistency that can be easily extended across evaluations. Therefore, a researcher might only need to learn an evaluation technique that can be applied to different systems under different conditions, increasing learnability and memorability for researchers and participants.

The CHIS system is highly complex as it supports an ample range of activities and requires a high degree of integration with the hospital infrastructure. When fully deployed, the CHIS system integrates an electronic health record system, lab results, a location-estimation service and smart phones wore by the hospital staff, supporting several hospital activities. The evaluation of such technology in the hospital is a considerable challenge. The technology itself needs to be robust; there is no room for errors in an environment where people treat with the health and life of human beings. Despite of this, a scenario-driven or theatrical representation allows to consolidate a well-informed evaluation without requiring the researchers to cope with the complexities associated in fully deploying such system.

## Replicating the Nature of Work to Evaluate the Use of Electronic Patient Records and Nurse Charts

We developed two applications with the goal of facilitating the capture of patients' information while physicians and nurses are on the move (Silva, Zamarripa, Strayer, Favela, & González, 2006; Zamarripa, Gonzalez, & Favela, 2007).

MedNote is a mobile application designed to provide physicians quick and easy access to their annotations about a patient's condition,

*Figure 3. (a) A screenshot of MedNote (b) A nurse using the augmented patient chart*

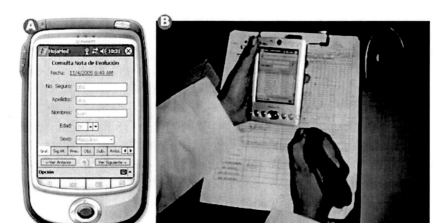

reducing the time and effort involved in generating the official medical notes to be integrated to a patient's medical record (Silva et al., 2006). MedNote keeps annotations in a database on the mobile device from which the user may access them for its review or modification. These notes are associated with patients in such a way that a physician may select a specific patient from a list and then be able to retrieve all notes related to that patient from the database –such notes are displayed in a chronological order (Figure 3). The system provides a dropdown list menu so the user may quickly select an option. On fields where a menu is not available, the user enters text directly on a textbox, in which case the user may use a predictive option where the application suggests words that match what he has entered so far. For this predictive functionality, three glossaries are used: common medical terms, drug names, and a general language dictionary. Notes are kept in the mobile device from where they can be transferred to a desktop computer to be completed, filled and integrated to a patient's medical record.

In a similar direction, the augmented patient chart system allows nurses to easily update a nurse chart by preserving the use of paper while digitalizing its content through a digital pen based on the Anoto™ technology (Zamarripa et al., 2007). Anoto™ technology uses a digital pen with an embedded camera that takes pictures as the device moves across the surface while making annotations on the paper. The paper contains a special printed dotted pattern that works with the camera to identify the exact position of the paper where the annotation is made. Our system chart design replaced manually generated graphs with a set of widgets to annotate accurate values used to plot graphs every time a new patient chart is created. The nurse annotates information on the chart and then she digitalizes it by placing the pen in its base. Then, all the information stored in the memory of the pen is transferred to the Hospital Information System. Nurses may review such information and confirm it in order to minimize errors in the information captured resulting from the lack of fidelity of the written notes.

Both systems were evaluated through a modified version of controlled experiments. When conducting laboratory experiments we need to consider that such experiments must recreate conditions similar to those faced by users during their everyday practices. The aim of this is to put in context the use of the technology to users, and moved from controlled experiments to a type of evaluation that replicates the conditions of the environment –we call this technique *in replica.* In

*Figure 4. (a) Interns creating medical notes with MedNote following a scene of a ward round (b) Nursing students walking throughout workstations to evaluate the patient augmented chart*

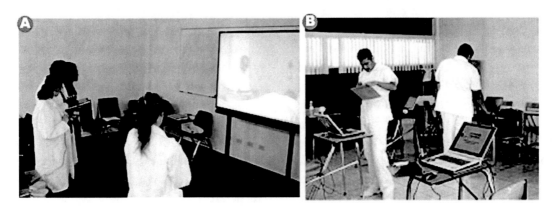

the following lines we illustrate two evaluations following this approach.

## The Evaluation

We conducted an *in replica* experiment to assess the degree to which MedNote helps medical interns in creating medical notes when compared with other forms of interaction (Silva et al., 2006). Seven interns created notes using MedNote in a PDA, with a tablet PC and on plain paper. We assembled an experimental setting where work conditions were recreated: interns were standing and wearing robes and a video projection of three clinical cases was shown (Figure 4a). Prior to the experiment, our research team consulted an attending physician working in the hospital to select three real clinical cases which were suiTable 1n clinical content for the medical interns to take notes. The same physician portrayed in the videotape is the attending physician who assesses patients' condition by providing a clinical summary of the clinical case being observed –as it is executed in real life. The video was recorded within hospital facilities to include all the routine artifacts used by the staff during a typical ward round. We had a member of our team posing as a bedridden patient, while the physician reviewed the case using artifacts such as stethoscope, x-rays,

ECGs, and medical records. While the clinical cases were based upon actual admitted patients to the hospital, all identifiers such as names and other personal information were omitted to protect patients' privacy. After viewing all three cases, participants were required to elaborate an official medical note with the help of their personal notes as they normally do in their everyday practice, using a desktop computer. We then measured the following variables: time to complete the tasks, number of tasks completed, and perception of difficulty and comfort when using each device. At the end of the experiment a questionnaire was applied and a focus group was conducted.

We found out that using MedNote on a PDA reduced the time physicians spent elaborating medical notes but decreased their quality when compared with the use of paper. First, using the application proved to be faster in elaborating the official note when compared against the use of paper: PDA users were 22.65% faster and Tablet PC users 19.15% faster. An analysis of the session shows that the improved performance was due to the fact that when using paper, the interns had to type the whole medical note, while PDA and Tablet PC users began with the digital version of the notes they took while watching the videos. Additionally, we found out that participants find it more comfortable to use a PDA than a Tablet PC.

According to the questionnaire applied at the end of the experiment, using a seven-point Likert scale with anchors ranging from strongly disagree(1) to strongly agree(7), we observe a wide difference between users' perception of comfort between these two devices. For the PDA the average of users' opinions was 5.0, showing that they slightly agree with the idea of the PDA being comfortable for taking notes during ward rounds. On the other hand, the average user opinion about the Tablet PC being comfortable was 2.6 (between disagree and slightly disagree). We also noticed that paper received a rating of 6.4 which means they think that using paper is the most comfortable way for taking notes.

Participants were very motivated during the experiment, they felt that it would not be difficult to learn how to use the application, they thought that it would help them improve their general performance at work and that they showed disposition to adopt the technology in their workplace. Participants also made some suggestions for improving the application, such as adding more medical vocabulary to the word prediction functionality, allow for the use of letter recognition data entry, reduce the number of open fields replacing them with option menus, and even incorporating voice notes and digital pictures of the patients' cases.

Using also the *in replica* technique we evaluated the augmented patient chart (Zamarripa et al., 2007). To evaluate the system, we arranged three workstations[1] where nurses were confronted with a clinical case and were asked to consult and fill the corresponding patient chart. The main working tasks that our evaluation aimed at exploring were: (1) reading of information on the format that was captured by another colleague during the previous work shift, and (2) annotation of information on the format as it would be done during the interaction with the patient. Both tasks were performed by each participant using the traditional and the new augmented patient chart formats. In order to minimize learning effects, we divided the participants and assigned them randomly to one of two groups. The first group (12 participants) started the evaluation using the digital format, and then used the traditional one. Participants' movement among workstations simulated the movement nurses have between patient rooms or beds and the tasks they perform during their everyday practices. The task was performed with two patients, one using a traditional chart and another one with the augmented one.

The results of our evaluation indicate that participants experienced a significant reduction in the number of errors while reading information related to vital signs when using the augmented patient chart. On average, those participants using the traditional patient chart obtained significantly less correct answers (6.05 s.d. 1.35) compared to those using the new patient chart format (7.5, s.d. 1.79) ($t=3.864$, $p<0.001$). We also found a significant increment of the accuracy while responding to the three tasks involving the annotating of data related to vital signs. On average, the participants using the new patient chart format had more correct answers (5.18, s.d. 1.68) than those using the previous version of the format (3.68, s.d. 2.70) ($t = 2.28$, $p<0.05$). A trend towards less time spent while annotating data on the digital paper was observed. On average, those participants using the previous version of the format spend slightly more time (9.74 min. s.d. 3.01 min.) completing the tasks than those using the new digital format (9.10 min s.d. 2.52 min). Clearly, the difference is small, but still provides some evidence of the advantages of the new design.

Furthermore, based on the results from the TAM questionnaire, we found that the perceptions of participants with regards to the augmented patient chart's usefulness are very encouraging: they recognize the advantages of the solution, but more important, the new interface does not appear to be either challenging or fundamentally modifying the essence of the task performed with the artifact. Overall, our results indicated a significant reduction in the number of errors while reading information and a significant increment on the accuracy while annotating data.

## Lessons Learned

As we discussed, *in situ* evaluations are quite complex and expensive. However, conducting them allow researchers to consider other aspects that go beyond those pure technical including for instance physical arrangement of devices and artifacts, sequential order of work practices, and other socio-technical and or economic issues. As shown in both evaluations of MedNote and the augmented patient chart, *in replica* evaluations allow researchers to consider to some extent these issues. Designing and setting up an *in replica* evaluations demands researchers to consider similar aspects in order to built-on in the experiment the context of work participants face during their everyday practices. For instance, during the evaluation of the augmented patient chart we need to even consider the distance between workstations to simulate the movement nurses experienced during their everyday practices. This allows taking the advantages offered by controlled lab experiments combined with *in situ* evaluations.

This approach however has the downside that researchers must make significant efforts to design and implement the evaluation. In some cases researchers' effort even surpasses the one they might invest in conducting an *in situ* evaluation. For instance, when we evaluated the MedNote application we made a video to simulate a ward round. In order to allow interns feel like they were taking notes as if they were following an attending physician on a typical ward round in the hospital. This took a lot of time ranging from the selection of the clinical case to be taped, setting up the environment and editing the video. Therefore, the important issue of the overall amount of time invested and the rigid schedule required of the researchers to effectively simulate the conditions of the hospital became clear from this evaluation.

## Conducting an Evaluation *In Situ* of a Persuasive Virtual Community Network that Promotes a Healthy Lifestyle

The pHealthNet is a persuasive virtual community that was designed to support the PREVENIMSS program[2] (Gasca, Favela, & Tentori, 2008). pHealthNet uses a pedometer and a mobile phone that work together with a virtual persuasive site (Figure 5). The site allows users to maintain community cohesion, challenge friends about nutritional habits and physical activities while providing activity awareness and gives adequate feedback of the benefits obtained in using the system (e.g., the amount of weight lost). Users might use a smart phone to maintain a connection with relevant events in the site, as well as, easily and quickly upload the amount of steps walked during the day. pHealthNet is self-contained which means that it does not need to interoperate with other systems; reducing thus, the cost and the complexities associated in evaluating it. However, we needed to consider other variables such as the experience of the participants with computers, their social background and how committed are the owners of the program with the use of the system.

## The Evaluation

We evaluated pHealthNet core characteristics, participant's intention to use the system, their motivation, their lifestyle habits, as well as the impact of the system in the program. We deployed the system for a period of three months, were twelve participants of two SODHi groups used the system –eight sessions in total. In the first group (Group A) a total of six participants used pHealthNet from June to August 2008, attending to SODHi the entire month of June and them maintaining contact with the community through pHeatlhNet for the following months. In contrast, the second group (Group B) used pHealthNet from July to

*Figure 5. The control SODHi (a) A participant receives a challenge notification in her mobile phone (b) She reviews her goals through a timeline*

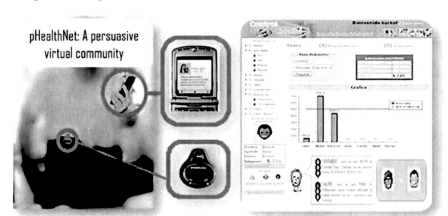

August 2008, attending SODHi during July and maintaining contact through pHealthNet for the following months.

The structure of each SODHi session was changed to incorporate pHealthNet. In each session an amount of time was set aside to allow patients to use the system and learn new features. Figure 6 shows how participants were introduced to pHealthNet during SODHi. The y-axis of the figure depicts the tools of pHealthNet that were introduced for each session of SODHi (x-axis). These activities include the use of tools aim at promoting:

- *Individual commitment,* allowing a participant to interact with the site in an individual manner, by uploading recipes, steps, diet plans, comments and testimonies.
- *Community attachment,* allowing a participant to interact with his community by inviting friends, asking questions to specialists and sending or receiving messages to and from them –including SMS ones.
- *Lifestyle changes through persuasion,* persuading a participant to change their lifestyle habits by challenging each other, creating goals and using persuasive games.

For both groups in the first session, pHealthNet was introduced to each patient and they were given internet access and their userID to log into the system. All the participants of the SODHi group were included in their social network. Though, it is interesting to note that the rest of the activities were introduced differently from one group to another (Figure 5). For Group A, individual tools were introduced at the first session, following from community ones (second session) and finally, those that promote persuasion (third session). In contrast for Group B, community tools were introduced at the first session, following from those tools that promote persuasion (second session) and finally, individual ones (third session). The session when the pedometer was given to participants also differs from one group to another. While the pedometer for Group A was given in the second session for Group B it was given in the first one. We made these changes since we noticed with Group A that the pedometer had an important motivating factor while giving participants a reason to log into the system everyday to register the number of steps they have walked. For both groups, in the fourth and final session, we conducted a focus group and a brainstorming session to gather feedback and capture their experiences with pHealthNet. We logged some of the user events specifying which

*Figure 6. Methodology followed during the evaluation of pHealthNet*

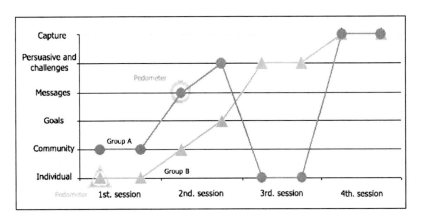

features were used and at what time, throughout both evaluations.

The use of the system has been rather heterogeneous due to patients' computing skills and computer access. All patients had a mobile phone; however, some of them didn't have internet access or even knew how to use a computer. For instance, in four weeks Participant A (PA) published nine diets, twenty three recipes, two comments and one testimony. She registered nineteen times her footsteps and updated her weight seven times. On the other hand, Participant B (PB) only published three recipes, one goal and registered fourteen times her footsteps during the same period. In contrast with participant PA, PB didn't have access to a computer at home. However, she kept a paper-based journal of their activities and brought it along with recipes to the session to be assisted in recording the data. In total, patients recorded their footsteps seventy four times, added four comments, nine diets, twenty-seven recipes, ten goals, one question to the specialist, one testimony and updated their weight twelve times.

Comparing the information during and after SODHI, it is interesting to note that the amount of activities that involve collaboration (such as steps goals, messages, Q&A to specialists) decreased after SODHi while the individual activities (such as steps, weight, diets) increased –the amount of activities that involve collaboration decreased from 39.3 to 33 and the individual ones increased from 63.5 to 231. From this, one can infer that despite the fact that participants engaged with the site, a long lasting relationship among the team members of the SODHi group wasn't created. However, half of the individual activities that increase in their total amount after SODHi aimed at promoting collaboration –including recipes, comments and testimonies (this activities increased from 51 to 319). Related to this, patients repeatedly expressed that the system kept them motivated by connecting their goals and problems with those of others. For instance, a patient made the following comment: *"you are used to skip exercise at home, but with the [site] you know that you aren't alone and that motivates you"*. Another patient stated that: *"A [rivalry] in a good way exists because you could see the amount of exercise others have been doing but that cheers you up because you don't want to be left behind"*. As a result of the use of our system, three of the participants decided to continue with the program to become part of a larger community with the group that started the following month.

A second analysis was conducted to evaluate the patients' perceived usefulness of the system and ease of use based on the TAM model (Fred D. Davis, 1989). We found that 85% of the patients completely agreed that the use of the system increases the level of physical activities and 71%

completely agreed that the system helps them maintain their dietary plan. All patients agreed that the system promotes a healthier lifestyle by allowing them to better control their dietary and exercise habits. In addition, 71% of the patient completely agreed that the system was flexible and understandable and 57% completely agreed that system was easy to use. Overall, the results of our evaluation show an increased engagement of the patients with the program due to the use of the system while helping them to abide to their plans. In addition, patients' viewed the application as useful, efficient, and generally appealing. pHealthNet was qualified by patients as the main motivator to follow the program.

## Lessons Learned

It is important to give proper credit of the individual benefit participants might earn as a consequence of the constant use of the system, which then can act as a source of motivation for them to engage with it and discover new ways to interact with the system. For instance, lack of internet access was the main obstacle in using pHealthNet. Despite of this, some participants asked family members to upload their information for them. These "assistants" ended up registering themselves to the system and participating in it as well.

Conducting *in situ* evaluations it is hard work. For instance, during the evaluation of pHealthNet, a researcher had to call participants up to five times per day from the early morning until late evening every day for four deployments, each of which lasted for 2 months. This schedule included weekends, nights, and holidays. In addition, when conducting *in situ* evaluations the conditions of the environment and participants often change. For instance, one participant of the SODHi group left the program during our evaluation. Hence, we need to cope with rapidly changing physical environments –finding another participant and start from scratch. For instance, when we evaluated pHealthNet the activities we followed during

the evaluation of Group A were changed with the ones followed by Group B to mitigate how the environment conditions might change for the second evaluation.

## DISCUSSION

In addition to the lessons learned that are specific to each evaluation we conducted – and their related techniques–, we have also learned lessons that apply more generally to collecting data for designing purposes. In the following lines we discuss a framework that depicts some evaluation principles that researchers might need to take into account when evaluating Ubihealth applications.

## Maintain Consistency

This principle promotes the design evaluations that have similar activities and use similar techniques for assessing a system. In particular, a consistent evaluation is one that follows the same activity and uses the same techniques for data gathering and analysis. For instance, we maintained consistency in the activities and the techniques used when we evaluated the CHIS system, while for the pHealthNet we changed some of these elements. One of the benefits of consistent evaluations is that they are easier to learn and use. Researchers have to learn only a single mode of operation that is applicable to the system under different conditions and for different users. This principle works well in evaluating systems for which their implementation has been completed and which behavior is somewhat predictable. However, it can be more problematic to apply the concept of consistency aimed at understanding problem spaces, or evaluating systems at early stages or their implementation. Maintaining consistency will help to gather results without a high variance when replicating the evaluation on different occasions under the same circumstances increasing the reliability of the results.

## Balance Constraints

The concept of constraining refers to determining ways of restricting the types of user interaction that can take place at a given moment with a given application. We argue that researchers must include constraints in their evaluation balancing such constraints based on the feedback they expect to capture. For instance, when we evaluated the first version of the CHIS we restricted participants' perception of the system use by showing a set of pre-defined scenarios restricting them to show just a few features provided by the system. As a result of this we could not gather feedback related to how participants foresee user experience with the system as a whole. However, for the evaluation of the second version of CHIS system we unrestricted the type of scenarios presented and we were able to capture issues that go beyond those merely technical. The main advantage of this form of constraining is that it allows researchers to depict the type of user experience they might need to portray and evaluate. For instance, we constrained the scenarios of the CHIS system to identify its privacy risks. Techniques that allow increasing or decreasing constraints in the evaluation are those based on scenarios and theatrical representation, respectively.

## Aim at Providing Benefits for Individuals

Researchers must provide feedback about the individual or personal benefits participants may obtain in return of the effort they might need to invest in evaluating a system. Feedback is about sending information about what are the benefits they obtained and what has been accomplished, allowing participants to continue through the evaluation. For instance, pHealthNet congratulates and gives credit for sending SMS messages (we call this credit *healthypesos*). The scheme rewards the amount of time participants interact with the site, by uploading recipes, goals, chal-

lenging friends, etc. We found out that this type of rewarding scheme and related information was one of the main motivations that kept participants engaged with the system. We argue that any Ubi-health system to be evaluated must incorporate an amount of feedback in this direction providing the necessary visibility of human experience. If we provide the appropriate credit of individual benefits it does not matter if the effort or the barriers in using the technology being evaluated is significant. Participants, just by being aware of such benefits, would find ways to cope with these challenges.

## Consider the Level of Pervasiveness and Complexity

Evaluation is integral to the design process. It collects information about potential users' experiences when interacting with a prototype—it focuses on both the usability and on the users' experience. However, when choosing the techniques for the evaluation it is necessary to consider if the system needs to be fully integrated with other technology within the environment (including devices or systems) or if it is self-contained, as well as, the stage of the design process when it would be evaluated. It is important to evaluate throughout the design process as we exemplified with the design of CHIS. However, if the system is not self-contained conducting an evaluation *in situ* could be very difficult and time-consuming delaying the design process. In those cases using other techniques (such as scenarios and theatrical representation) allows to evaluate prototypes at early stages of the design. It is important to note that when using other techniques the evaluation must replicate the conditions of the environment. Thus we must promote the replication of the environment for each system to be evaluated. This will allow researchers to discover unseen opportunities to improve the design and issues in deploying such a system.

## BACKGROUND: CHALLENGES FOR UBICOMP EVALUATION IN HOSPITALS

In this section we discuss several cases showing the evaluation of Ubicomp environments and applications using a varied number of techniques. These cases range from those evaluations where researchers have used techniques that allow evaluating prototypes at early stages of design (i.e. before implementation is completed) to those that conduct *in situ* evaluations with a robust and the final version of the application. Some of these cases include multiple evaluations conducted to evaluate one system or several versions of it.

The main goal of previous efforts has been to implement techniques that reduce the cost and the complexities in conducting an evaluation of Ubicomp environments, while at the same time supporting the evaluation of prototypes which implementation has not been completed, yet. Consolvo and colleagues discuss further insights from their evaluation of Ubicomp applications at early stages of design, in particular Wizard of Oz and Experience Sampling methods (Consolvo et al., 2007). Consolvo and Walker (2003) introduce the experience sampling method (ESM) as a way to evaluate Ubicomp applications, *in situ*, by multiple users, over time and collecting both quantitative and qualitative data (Consolvo & Walker, 2003). In Consolvo and Walker's version of ESM, a self-reporting technique, was implemented in a PDA to be used by participants who received 10 randomly scheduled alerts per day asking about their locations, resources available around them, and asking them to take pictures of their surroundings. Consolvo and colleagues (2007) found that conducting *in situ* evaluations, letting people experience the applications in a day-to-day basis, modifies initial reactions of users towards the technology, making them more aware of its implications, and what it would be like to use it. However, they also found that using mobile devices to support *in situ* evaluations presents

some challenges from the cost of the equipment and other resources, to the most practical one such as the duration of batteries, and response times of devices. They argue for the use of *in situ* studies to cope with the unpredictable, mobile and rich nature of activities supported by Ubicomp applications.

In a similar direction, Carter and Mankoff (2005) present their experiences while balancing the quality of evaluation with the easy or prototyping Ubicomp applications, and highlight interactivity as the most important factor (Carter & Mankoff, 2005). Their experiences with paper-prototyping found value in terms of getting early feedback from users, but limitations to test interactivity, peripherally, synchronous activities, and testing errors and ambiguity. Similarly, several evaluations studies in Ubicomp have borrowed traditional usability testing techniques and tailored them for the evaluation of ubiquitous applications. For instance, Mankoff et al, (2003), discuss the use of a heuristic evaluation technique for ambient displays. The formal heuristic evaluation method involves having usability specialists judging whether each dialogue element follows established usability principles –that is "heuristics" (Nielsen, 1994). They successfully adapted techniques typically used on desktop application to the content of Ubicomp, identifying 40-60% of issues with displays (Mankoff et al., 2003). Likewise, others have modified traditional approaches based on meetings, inspections or cognitive walkthroughs to apply them for the evaluation of Ubicomp. For instance, Intille et al.'s automated method for asking users about what is going on during a moment in time captured by a video camera (Intille, Kukla, & Ma, 2002). This technique has the advantage of requiring little ongoing effort from end users or researchers. However, it depends upon extensive infrastructure to capture images and send them to the user. This highlights the point that one may need a tool complex enough to be considered an Ubicomp environment in its own right to easily evaluate this type environments. This technique could be seen as an intersection between *pluralistic walkthroughs* where users, developers, and humans step through a scenario, discussing each dialogue element (Bias, 1991) and *feature, consistency or standard inspection* were a list of features is used to accomplish typical tasks, checks for long sequences, cumbersome steps, and steps that require extensive knowledge/ experience in order to assess a proposed feature set (Wixon, Jones, Tse, & Casaday, 1994).

Others have tailored or developed models that allow researchers to test specific metrics of ubiquitous applications. The most popular model used for the test of ubiquitous applications is the Technology Acceptance Model (TAM) (Fred D. Davis, 1989; F. D. Davis & Venkatesh, 1995). Such model suggests that when users are presented with a new technology, their perceived usefulness and ease-of-use of the system influence adoption (i.e., their decision about how and when they will use it). Based on such model a specific one was created for the evaluation of ubiquitous system –Ubiquitous Computing Acceptance Model (Spiekermann, 2008). Zaad and Allouch used it to investigate how the level of control influences elders' intention of use of an intelligent system that helps them to live independently (Zaad & Allouch, 2008). They found that the acceptance of ubiquitous technology in a care setting is not completely comparable with the acceptance process of intelligent devices that are not meant directly for care settings. As these case studies highlight, and as pointed out by (Carter & Mankof, 2004), Ubicomp systems are difficult to evaluate as a result of their ambiguity, scalability, and context of application. In addition, while a variety of methods are available for the evaluation of desktop applications (Carter & Mankof, 2004) there is currently a lack of evaluation measures and techniques for use at early stages of the design of Ubicomp applications. Therefore, it is important to highlight the importance of selecting adequate usability metrics (e.g., privacy, comfort, predictability, control), the application of participatory design, and the need of constantly adapt the solutions given that it is not possible to obtain complete feedback before deployment.

The evaluation of Ubicomp environments and applications is quite challenging in general, but particularly more in the healthcare domain. Bardram and colleagues describe their experiences from an ongoing deployment of a suite of context-aware technologies and applications in a hospital environment, including a context-awareness infrastructure, a location tracking system, and two context-aware applications running on interactive wall displays and mobile phones (Bardram, Hansen, Mogensen, & Soegaard, 2006). During an *in situ* evaluation they spent days conducting field studies with the purpose of analyzing work, identifying problems, and registering changes in work practices. They also applied questionnaires and conducted interviews before and after the deployment of such systems. In spite of their efforts, they found out that the type of context-aware computing that they designed and deployed in the hospital ended up mainly providing context-awareness instead of performing automated action. This result is explained by them pointing to a number of factors. One of the main challenges faced during this evaluation was the integration of such systems with those systems already used in the hospital (e.g., a patient medical record and a schedule calendar). To reduce complexities Bardram and colleagues decided to replace the schedule calendar with the one provided by the context-aware suite being deployed. To this aim a head nurse closely followed the daily schedule making adjustments to the operation schedules and ensuring a smooth flow of work by coordinating all the involved clinicians. Therefore, with Ubicomp for healthcare (Ubihealth), designers face the general challenge that most of the systems proposed need to be semi or completely integrated into existing Hospital Information Systems (HIS).

Similarly as in the Ubicomp literature, Ubihealth systems have been evaluated at different stages of system development. For instance, the

*Table 1. A comparison of the evaluation methods*

| Type of evaluation | Cost: effort & time (lightweight or heavyweight) | Where (Real, Anywhere, Controlled or simulated) | When (Early or prototype) | What type of data (Qualitative, Quantitative or Both) | Feedback (Measures, user experience or problems) | Who (potential users or experts) |
|---|---|---|---|---|---|---|
| In situ* | heavyweight | real | prototype | Both | user experience | potential users |
| Experience sample | heavyweight | real | prototype | Both | user experience | potential users |
| Easy prototyping | heavyweight | real | early | Both | user experience | potential users |
| Usability experiments | heavyweight | controlled | prototype | quantitative | measures | potential users |
| Wizard of oz | heavyweight | controlled | prototype | quantitative | measures | potential users |
| In replica* | lightweight | simulated | prototype | both | user experience | potential users |
| Analytic evaluation | lightweight | anywhere | prototype | qualitative | problems | experts |
| Heuristic Evaluation | lightweight | anywhere | early | qualitative | problems | experts |
| Scenario-driven* | lightweight | controlled | early | both | problems | potential users |
| Theatrical representation* | lightweight | controlled | early | both | problems | potential users |

Houston is a software application that promotes healthy lifestyles in social groups, allowing users to register physical activities and send instant messages (Sunny, Katherine, Ian, & James, 2006). Houston uses a pedometer to measure the physical activity and mobile phones for members of the social group to communicate. It offers services to record physical activity, set goals, exchange messages with friends and visualize activity for a period of time. Participants of the evaluation of Houston were divided in two groups. For the first group computer and internet access was provided while for the other no technology support was given. After six months of evaluation, participants perceived the application useful and having a meaningful impact on the quality of people's lives under circumstances of stress and social isolation. They highlight that the conditions of the environment influence how the application is perceived –comparing one group with technology support and the other without it.

In our own experience, we have seen that to be effective, evaluation of Ubihealth applications demand the recreation of task context with some detail, as this influences the way such applications will be used once they are deployed (Zamarripa et al., 2007). For instance, while a physician is writing a note he is normally standing. Hence, his position will affect the way he is carrying a computing device and how long he will be able to carry it out. The evaluation of Ubihealth face the challenge of recreating relevant work conditions in an experimental setting (mobility, interruptions, patient care, collaboration) (Zamarripa et al., 2007). This often requires the integration of the services being evaluated with other applications and artifacts currently used by practitioners (i.e. electronic health record, patient monitoring systems, etc.), since many healthcare settings, notably hospitals, already make extensive use of technology without which the Ubiheath solution being proposed might seem unrealistic, thus hampering the evaluation itself.

Table 1 shows a comparison of the evaluation methods discussed throughout the paper. It is interesting to note that lightweight techniques are mostly used in an early stage of the prototype to identify design problems that could be effectively and opportunistically incorporated in the deployment of the system. In contrast, heavyweight techniques are used when the prototype is available with the aim at gathering user attitudes towards the system. It is interesting to note that the *in replica* evaluation is the only lightweight technique that can provide feedback regarding user experience; however, it couldn't be used at an early stage of the implementation of a product. By comparing the lightweight techniques we proposed with the others available in the literature it is clear that the available ones are by no means focused on potential users. Therefore, the goal of problems identified with each will vary. While the problems identified by potential users will be most likely related to the barriers for the system's adoption the problems identified by experts will be mostly related to the design of the system. As the table shows, we are not implying that one technique is better that another one but that one technique will be definitely more suitable for our specific goal and stage of design.

## CONCLUSION

As Rogers *et. al.* stated *"Ubicomp applications are inherently difficult to evaluate due to their context of use"* (Rogers et al., 2004). Healthcare, hospitals in particular, impose significant demands to the deployment and evaluation of Ubicomp technologies. This is due not only to the critical nature of the work, but also, to the conditions in which this work is conducted (high mobility of the staff, frequent task switching, need to coordinate tasks and collaborate, and so forth). For the last six years, we have conducted a series of studies in a hospital to better understand hospital workers' practices and envision ubiquitous technologies to support their work. We have evaluated those applications with diverse approaches such as pre- and post-study interviews, questionnaires,

controlled *in replica* experiments and *in situ* evaluations. In this chapter, we present six cases showing the evaluation of three systems that we conducted within a period of five years. Based on our lessons learned during the evaluation of those applications we discuss a set of principles that must be taking into account during the design and execution of Ubihealth evaluations. Given the challenges raised by the evaluation of Ubihealth systems, we believe that existing evaluation techniques would benefit from modifications before being applied to Ubicomp applications.

## REFERENCES

Bardram, J., Hansen, T. R., Mogensen, M., & Soegaard, M. (2006). *Experiences from Real-World Deployment of Context-Aware Technologies in a Hospital Environment.* Paper presented at the Ubicomp, Orange County, CA, USA.

Bias, R. (1991). Walkthroughs: Efficient collaborative testing. *IEEE Software, 8*(5), 94–95. doi:10.1109/52.84220

Caroll, J. (1995). Scenario-Based Design: Envisioning work and technology in system development. New York.

Carter, S., & Mankof, J. (2004). *Challenges for Ubicomp Evaluation.* EECS Department UC Berkeley.

Carter, S., & Mankoff, J. (2005). Momento: Early-Stage Prototyping and Evaluation for Mobile Applications. In n. o. C. a. Berkeley (Ed.).

Castro, L. A., & Favela, J. (2008). Reducing the Uncertainty on Location Estimation of Mobile Users to Support Hospital Work. *IEEE Transactions on systems, man and cybernetics--Part C: Applications and Reviews.*

Chin, T. (2005, January, 17 2006). Untapped power: a physician's handheld. *AMNews.*

Consolvo, S., Harrison, B., Smith, I., Chen, M. Y., Everitt, K., & Froehlich, J. (2007). Conducting In Situ Evaluations for and With Ubiquitous Computing Technologies. *International Journal of Human-Computer Interaction, 22*(1-2), 103–118. doi:10.1207/s15327590ijhc2201-02_6

Consolvo, S., & Walker, M. (2003). Using the Experience Sampling Method to Evaluate Ubicomp Applications. *IEEE Pervasive Computing Magazine: The Human Experience, 2*(2), 24–31. doi:10.1109/MPRV.2003.1203750

Davis, F. D. (1989). Perceived Usefulness, Perceived Ease Of Use, And User Acceptance Of Information Technology. *Management Information Systems Quarterly, 13*(3), 318–323. doi:10.2307/249008

Davis, F. D., & Venkatesh, V. (1995). *Measuring User Acceptance of Emerging Information Technologies: An Assessment of Possible Method Biases.* Paper presented at the 28th Hawaii Int'l Conf. System Sciences.

Favela, J., Rodríguez, M. D., Preciado, A., & Gonzalez, V. M. (2004). Integrating Context-aware Public Displays into a Mobile Hospital Information System. *IEEE Trans. IT in BioMedicine, 8*(3), 279–286.

Gasca, E., Favela, J., & Tentori, M. (2008). *Persuasive Virtual Communities to Promote a Healthy Lifestyle among Patients with Chronic Diseases.* Paper presented at the In Proc. of CRIWG, Omaha, Nebraska, September, 14-18.

Intille, S., Kukla, C., & Ma, X. (2002). *Eliciting user preferences using image-based experience sampling and reection.* Paper presented at the Extended Abstracts of the Conference on Human Factors in Computer Systems.

Mankoff, J., Dey, A. K., Hsieh, G., Kientz, J., Lederer, S., & Ames, M. (2003). *Heuristic Evaluation of Ambient Displays.*

Munoz, M., Rodriguez, M. D., Favela, J., Martinez-Garcia, A. I., & Gonzalez, V. M. (2003). Context-Aware Mobile Communication in Hospitals. *IEEE Computer, 36*(9), 38–46.

Nielsen, J. (1994). Heuristic evaluation. In *Usability Inspection Methods.* New York: John Wiley & Sons.

O'Connor, M. C. (2006). Testing Ultrasound to Track, Monitor Patients. *RFID Journal, 1*(31), 2.

Palen, L., & Dourish, P. (2003). *Unpacking 'privacy' for a networked world.* Paper presented at the Conference on Human factors in computing systems.

Pentland, A. (2004). Healthwear: Medical Technology Becomes Wearable. *IEE Computer, 37*(5), 42–49.

Rogers, Y., Connelly, K., Tedesco, T., Hazlewood, W., Kurtz, A., Hall, R. E., et al. (2004). *Why It's Worth the Hassle: The Value of In-Situ Studies When Designing Ubicomp.* Paper presented at the Mobile Human-Computer Interaction – MobileHCI 2004.

Santana, P. C., Castro, L. A., Preciado, A., Gonzalez, V. M., Rodriguez, M. D., & Favela, J. (2005). *Preliminary Evaluation of Ubicomp in Real Working Scenarios.* Paper presented at the 2nd Workshop on Multi-User and Ubiquitous User Interfaces MU3I, January 9, 2005, San Diego, USA.

Silva, J., Zamarripa, S., Strayer, P., Favela, J., & González, V. (2006). *Empirical Evaluation of a Mobile Application for Assisting Physicians in Creating Medical Notes.* Paper presented at the Proceedings of the 12th Americas Conference on Information Systems (AMCIS 2006), Acapulco, Mexico, August 4-6, 2006.

Spiekermann, S. (2008). *User Control in Ubiquitous Computing: Design Alternatives and User Acceptance*. Aachen, Germany: Shaker Verlag.

Stanford, V. (2003). Beam Me Up, Doctor McCoy. *IEEE Pervasive Computing / IEEE Computer Society [and] IEEE Communications Society, 2*(3), 13–18. doi:10.1109/MPRV.2003.1228522

Sunny, C., Katherine, E., Ian, S., & James, A. L. (2006). Design requirements for technologies that encourage physical activity, *Proceedings of the SIGCHI conference on Human Factors in computing systems*. Montreal, Quebec, Canada: ACM.

Tentori, M., Favela, J., & Gonzalez, V. (2006). Quality of Privacy (QoP) for the Design of Ubiquitous Healthcare Applications. *Journal of Universal Computer Science, 12*(3), 252–269.

Tentori, M., Favela, J., & Rodriguez, M. (2006). Privacy-aware Autonomous Agents for Pervasive Healthcare. *IEEE Intelligent Systems, 21*(6), 55–62. doi:10.1109/MIS.2006.118

Weiser, M. (1991). The Computer for the 21st Century. *Scientific American, 265*(3), 94–104.

Weiser, M. (1998). The future of ubiquitous computing on campus. *Communications of the ACM, 41*(1), 41–42. doi:10.1145/268092.268108

Wixon, D., Jones, S., Tse, L., & Casaday, G. (1994). Inspections and design reviews: Framework, history, and reflection. In *Usability Inspection Methods*. New York: John Wiley & Sons.

Zaad, L., & Allouch, S. B. (2008). *The Influence of Control on the Acceptance of Ambient Intelligence by Elderly People: An Explorative Study*. Paper presented at the Proceedings of the European Conference on Ambient Intelligence, Nuremberg, Germany.

Zamarripa, M. S., Gonzalez, V. M., & Favela, J. (2007). *The Augmented Patient Chart: Seamless Integration of Physical and Digital Artifacts for Hospital Work*. Paper presented at the HCI.

## KEY TERMS AND DEFINITIONS

**Ubihealth:** The term stands for Ubiquitous Healthcare and refers to a computing infrastructure of applications, systems and devices distributed over a physical space and orchestrated to provide services healthcare providers and users.

**Scenario-Driven Evaluation:** Evaluation using scenarios to represent the situated use of interactive systems.

**In Situ Evaluation:** Evaluation of interactive systems conducted at the place where the system is used when it is deployed.

**Context-Aware Mobile Communication system (CHIS):** A system that provides communication functionality based on the constant monitoring of the location of people and artifacts.

**Hospital Information System (HIS):** A system used to support hospital services.

**In Replica Evaluation:** Evaluation of interactive systems using methods to replicate the actual conditions experienced by people where the system is used when it is deployed.

**Theatrical Representation Evaluation:** Evaluation of interactive system where simulated performance of real activities is used as a method to replicate the actual conditions experienced using the system.

## ENDNOTES

[1] A workstation is a desk equipped with a laptop where a clinical case of a patient is projected simulating a patient bed in the hospital

[2] The PREVENIMSS support program is a federal program in Mexico aiming at preventing diseases. The SODHi group is a part of PREVENIMSS aimed at promoting a healthy life style by organizing informational sessions where a group of health specialists (nutritionist, exercise trainer, physician and psychologist) assesses a patient's health condition to design a personalized diet and exercise plan.

# Section 3
# Methodologies and Frameworks

# Chapter 12
# Model–Driven Prototyping Support for Pervasive Healthcare Applications

**Werner Kurschl**
*Upper Austria University of Applied Sciences, Austria*

**Stefan Mitsch**
*Johannes Kepler University, Austria*

**Johannes Schoenboeck**
*Vienna University of Technology, Austria*

## ABSTRACT

*Pervasive healthcare applications aim at improving habitability by assisting individuals in living autonomously. To achieve this goal, data on an individual's behavior and his or her environment (often collected with wireless sensors) is interpreted by machine learning algorithms; their decision finally leads to the initiation of appropriate actions, e.g., turning on the light. Developers of pervasive healthcare applications therefore face complexity stemming, amongst others, from different types of environmental and vital parameters, heterogeneous sensor platforms, unreliable network connections, as well as from different programming languages. Moreover, developing such applications often includes extensive prototyping work to collect large amounts of training data to optimize the machine learning algorithms. In this chapter the authors present a model-driven prototyping approach for the development of pervasive healthcare applications to leverage the complexity incurred in developing prototypes and applications. They support the approach with a development environment that simplifies application development with graphical editors, code generators, and pre-defined components.*

## INTRODUCTION

Pervasive computing is a fast-growing area: technical advancements in the fields of sensor and actuator hardware miniaturization, low-power wireless communication and processors, and machine learning algorithms have the capacity to make the vision of smart environments come true. Pervasive healthcare utilizes pervasive computing to improve quality of life by assisting individuals in living

DOI: 10.4018/978-1-61520-765-7.ch012

autonomously. To exemplify the complexity of pervasive healthcare applications and to point out the specific challenges we intend to tackle in this chapter we reflect on the application of pervasive healthcare in the domain of eldercare. As a system that is fully integrated into the lives of people in order to support them in daily tasks and help them in critical situations, customization (i.e., the system needs to be exactly tailored to the individual's needs), non-obtrusiveness, ease of interaction, and integrating end users into the development lifecycle are key to the success of such applications (Demiris et al., 2008). Yet pervasive healthcare applications are still far from being commercially available: to date numerous research projects work on enabling technologies like wireless sensor network platforms, body sensor networks, routing protocols, time synchronization algorithms, signal processing, data fusion, and machine learning algorithms. Other projects utilize these base technologies to develop isolated solutions for single use cases like item tracking and searching, warning of household dangers (e.g., slippery floor, unattended stove, or running water taps), recognizing alarming situations (e.g., collapse, or sleep disorders), or remote health monitoring. All of them are important enablers of pervasive healthcare systems; the challenge now is to integrate the findings from these projects into a compound system. The coherent information thereby provided potentially increases the scope of detectable situations and realizable use cases, improves the system's fault tolerance, and could lead to a much richer user experience. But the distributed nature of such highly interconnected pervasive healthcare systems leads to an increased system complexity. New development concepts and tools are required to reduce complexity during design, development, deployment, and maintenance.

Many of the domain's envisioned use cases demand context-awareness (Dey, Salber, & Abowd, 2001): their goal is to collect information on the system's surroundings with sensors, interpret the sensor data to ultimately understand the observed situation, and then take appropriate actions. A popular approach is pattern recognition, defined by (Duda, Hart, & Stork, 2001) as "the act of taking in raw data and making an action based on the 'category' of the pattern" (p. 1). If such systems additionally combine data from several sources describing different entities, they are termed to be situation-aware (Baumgartner, Retschitzegger, Schwinger, Kotsis, & Schwietering, 2007). Although many solutions differ in terms of sensing hardware, programming language, signal processing, feature extraction, or classification algorithms, their architectures show noticeable commonness. They can be structured into six layers: (i) data acquisition, (ii) preprocessing, (iii) interpretation, (iv) aggregation, (v) situation inference, and (vi) application. The data acquisition layer collects information on a system's surroundings (context data) with wired or wireless sensors. This information not only comprises environmental data, like temperature, sound, or acceleration, but also measurements on a person's behavioral patterns and health status, e.g., heart rate, blood pressure, or gait posture. The massive amount of raw data needs to be restricted in the preprocessing layer before it can be interpreted: distracting background noise or undesired phenomena can be ignored, and distinctive features must be selected to enable robust and efficient classification. The interpretation layer categorizes incoming data with machine learning algorithms and thereby derives semantics (e.g., 25°C means "hot" in the context of room temperature). Semantics from different data sources combined in the aggregation layer enable the situation inference layer to detect relations and to derive comprehensive situations. This knowledge can be utilized in different applications to, e.g., interact with the environment with actuators that execute appropriate actions, to visualize context information, or to report to connected software systems (application layer).

Every layer can be realized with different hardware platforms, programming languages, frameworks, and algorithms. Because the field of pervasive computing is still evolving we lack a mature and commonly agreed development paradigm; each project follows its own, mostly hardware-driven low-level programming approach. Pervasive healthcare systems are therefore hard to develop, integrate, often tightly coupled to the implemented use case, and not reusable in different settings. Moreover, domain experts and other non-programmers with knowledge on the application domain are thereby excluded from the development process. This technical approach may lead to systems not being accepted by the user, because the system's applications may perform well in isolation but integrate improperly with others, or because the system does not exactly meet the user's individual needs. Especially in pervasive healthcare we face the challenge of systems exactly tailored to a single user and, therefore, the effort of integrating off-the-shelf components to a working system is extremely high. If we could abstract from the low-level implementation details and specify system functionality independent from the hard- and software platform, we would increase reusability, simplify integration, and promote cooperation between domain experts and programmers. Stankovic, Lee, Mok, & Rajkumar (2005) claim that "Raising the level of abstraction for programmers will be key to the growth of wireless sensor networks. Currently programmers deal with too many low-level details regarding sensing and node-to-node communication." (p. 29). We therefore propose formal models as a possible abstraction from hardware and implementation details. These models should not only serve documentation purposes, but rather be integrated into the development process as first-class artifacts (Bézivin, 2005), which is the main idea of Model-Driven Software Development (MDSD).

Based on a pervasive healthcare application survey the chapter discusses problems developers currently face to achieve the goals of customization, non-obtrusiveness, and ease of interaction mentioned above. We merge common architectural styles into a reference architecture for such applications, and show how MDSD can base on the architecture to hide the complexity of pervasive healthcare application development, and how domain experts and software engineers with knowledge from different fields in computer science can work together in a compound development process. The chapter introduces formal meta-models that reflect the reference architecture, discusses development support in the form of automatic transformations between models and code, and shows in an exemplary use case how such a development environment simplifies the creation of pervasive healthcare applications.

## BACKGROUND

The following sections introduce related work in context awareness, wireless sensor networks, and MDSD, followed by a survey on pervasive healthcare projects. By applying an evaluation framework commonalities as well as shortcomings between the reviewed projects are identified. The results of the survey are the foundation for our approach.

## Context-Awareness, Machine Learning and Pattern Recognition Basics

Knowledge on the application's surroundings (context-awareness) is the basis for pervasive healthcare applications that should support or act on behalf of the user. We use the definition of Dey, Salber, & Abowd (2001): "context is any information that can be used to characterize the situation of entities (i.e., whether a person, place or object) that are considered relevant to the interaction between a user and an application, including the user and the application themselves" (p. 107). Context must be collected automatically with sensors to unburden the user from entering it manually. Sensors, however, do not deliver symbolic context information; instead, they provide a digital representation of the observed phenomenon's measured side-effect (e.g., a capacitive accelerometer outputs a voltage between 0-5V proportional to the ratio "current acceleration to maximum measureable acceleration", which is then converted with an Analog-Digital-Converter into a digital representation – often an integer value). We call this digital representation raw sensor data, which is characterized by high data volumes and may contain portions of undesired other phenomena or noise (e.g., an accelerometer not only measures an object's acceleration, but at the same time the earth's gravity). Often, a sensor can only measure a particular side-effect (i.e., it only detects a portion of the phenomenon). Its data can therefore not unambiguously distinguish between the desired phenomenon and other phenomena that show a similar side-effect (but which may, nevertheless, differ in other side effects not measured by the particular sensor). Thus, we are interested in fusing raw data from different sensors and automatically deriving symbolic context information (i.e., semantics) with machine learning and pattern recognition algorithms.

In Duda, Hart, & Stork (2001) pattern recognition systems are structured into five steps: sensing, segmentation, feature extraction, classification, and post-processing. Sensing collects raw sensor data, segmentation filters raw data to remove noise and undesired measuring, and feature extraction then reduces the data volume and prepares data as feature vectors for the classifier (it makes classification easier and more efficient; an ideal feature extraction algorithm would make classification trivial). Classifiers decide to which category (symbolic context) a given feature vector most probably belongs to, as perfect classification can, due to ambiguous raw data, often not be achieved. During post-processing we can use domain knowledge to enhance the classifier's output and evaluate the costs that are incurred if we follow its decision. For detailed information

on different context-awareness frameworks and context-aware systems please refer to (Baldauf, Dustdar, & Rosenberg, 2004).

The Context Recognition Network (CRN) Toolbox (Bannach, Amft, & Lukowicz, 2008) describes a C++ framework integrating hardware abstraction, filter algorithms, feature extraction components and classifiers in a configurable runtime to support rapid development of context recognition applications. It is designed for deployment to embedded devices that support the POSIX runtime environment.

## Wireless Sensor Networks Basics

Wireless Sensor Networks (WSNs) play a key role in pervasive healthcare systems as every smart environment relies on sensory data from the real world (Lewis, 2005). WSNs consist, typically, of a multitude of cooperating sensor nodes to cover a particular area. Often sensor nodes are deployed rather spontaneously and therefore form an ad-hoc-network and must make use of self-organizing algorithms and protocols (Karl & Willig, 2005). WSNs can be used for the sensing step in pattern recognition systems. There are many hardware and software platforms available using different programming languages. TinyOS (Hill, Szewczyk, Woo, Hollar, Culler, & Pister, 2000) is a component-based operating system for wireless sensor networks, which can be programmed using nesC (Levis, et al., 2005). It is widely used in developing applications for the popular Crossbow hardware. Just recently the Sentilla platform (formerly Moteiv) emerged, which hosts a virtual machine on its motes (called JCreate) allowing programmers to run Java programs (Sentilla Corporation, 2009). The .NET Micro Edition allows programmers to write applications for embedded devices, which must run a restricted version of the Common Language Runtime, using managed C# code (Kühner, 2008). The .NET Micro Edition additionally provides a hardware emulator for rapid prototyping and debugging.

Originally motes were designed to be deployed randomly (possibly by air plane) in areas that cannot be reached easily by individuals and to be able to work independently for a long period of time (e.g., for watching wildfires (Chaczko & Ahmad, 2005). As there is no permanent power supply available in such scenarios motes rely on battery power and preserving energy is therefore a critical issue. In pervasive healthcare we face similar problems because sensors can be wearable or attached to moveable apartment interior, e.g., chairs. As communication requires a lot of energy research focuses on energy efficient routing and communication protocols. A broad range of routing algorithms for the commonly used communication stack IEEE 802.15.4, called ZigBee (Zhao & Guibas, 2004) exist: AMRIS (Wu & Tay, 1999), SPIN (Kulik, Heinzelman, & Balakrishnan, 2002), Directed Diffusion (Intanagonwiwat, Govindan, & Estrin, 2000), Energy Aware Routing, Geographic Hash Tables (Ratnasamy, et al., 2002), Greedy Perimeter Stateless Routing (Karp & Kung, 2000). They, however, cause additional effort, when one of these routing algorithms, instead of multihop broadcasting, should be configured into an application.

The CodeBlue project described in (Shnayder, Chen, Lorincz, Fulford-Jones, & Welsh, 2005) aims at developing a robust, scalable software framework for deploying sensor networks in medical settings; it provides support for device discovery, location tracking, data querying, and a publish/subscribe multihop routing protocol implemented in nesC.

## Model-Driven Software Development Basics

Model-Driven Engineering (MDE) is a development approach using abstract models to describe systems; these models are systematically transformed to concrete implementations (France & Rumpe, 2007). Besides MDE the terms Model-Driven Software Development (MDSD), Model-Driven Development (MDD) and Model-Driven Architecture (MDA) are often used. MDE and MDD are the most general terms describing the underlying principles independent from the engineering domain. In contrast, MDSD focuses on providing building blocks for software development processes. In (Stahl, Völter, Efftinge, & Haase, 2007) MDSD is defined as a general term for techniques that generate executable software from formal models. MDA, a specification of the OMG, is an MDSD approach based on the Meta Object Facility (MOF) to ensure interoperability between models. Furthermore it emphasizes the separation between Platform Independent Models (PIMs) and Platform Specific Models (PSMs) as stated in (Miller & Mukerji, 2006). Although we introduce PIM and PSM in the following section we do not explicitly focus on standards and interoperability, but instead on the simplification of the software development process using models. Therefore, we prefer the term MDSD through the rest of the chapter.

Gaps between different models are bridged with transformations. Czarnecki & Helsen (2006) differentiate between transformations generating lower-level models from higher-level models (e.g., a PIM to PSM transformation) and mapping models at the same level of abstraction (e.g., PIM to PIM transformation). Current research in model transformation focuses on graph transformations or specific transformation languages. Graph-based approaches make use of the fact that object-oriented software models are often expressed as graphs which allows the application of graph theory. Examples for graph-based transformation tools are Triple Graph Grammars (Köngis, 2005) or Attributed Graph Grammar (Taentzer, 2004). Transformation Languages can roughly be categorized into imperative, declarative, or hybrid languages. Imperative approaches are similar in use to traditional programming languages and allow the programmer to explicitly manipulate transformation execution state and control flow. Declarative approaches are typically based on rules that are interpreted by an execution engine to produce the desired result. Hybrid approaches mix up declarative and imperative features and thus increase flexibility. The Query-View-Transformation specification (QVT, 2008) of the OMG includes a declarative part (QVT Relational) and an imperative part (QVT Operational). The Eclipse Modeling project (2009) includes an implementation of QVT Operational, whereas mediniQVT (2009) provides an implementation of QVT Relational. A prominent hybrid approach is the Atlas Transformation Language (ATL), which we use for model transformation (Jouault & Kurtev, 2005). Another interesting approach makes use of Colored Petri Nets for model transformation (Reiter, 2008). The work's main focus is to provide reusable transformation components (in terms of Petri Nets) to simplify specification of transformations and to cover recurring structural heterogeneities in model transformation.

## Survey on Pervasive Healthcare Projects

This section gives a short overview about significant research projects in the domain of pervasive healthcare. The survey bases on an evaluation framework and details the requirements for the proposed MDSD approach. SOPRANO Consortium (2007) discusses in a related survey the state-of-the-art in ambient assisted living, smart homes, semantic meta-models, context models, and sensor technology. Muras, Cahill, & Stokes (2006) introduce a taxonomy for pervasive healthcare systems to exemplarily evaluate five projects. Both surveys compare current projects on the basis of their implemented features and used technologies with respect to the user's needs and preferences; they do not concentrate on the development process itself. We therefore focus in our survey on criteria in the context of MDSD.

## Evaluation Framework

We structure our evaluation criteria into three categories: (i) context processing, (ii) MDSD, and (iii) utilized technology; each criterion comprises a name, an acronym, a definition, and characteristics.

## Context Processing

Context processing (e.g., vital and environmental data like blood pressure, temperature, or acceleration) is a major part of pervasive healthcare applications. The listed criteria evaluate the context processing capabilities implemented or envisioned in projects and thereby show the heterogeneity of platforms; the criteria are based on the definitions of Schwinger, Grün, Pröll, & Retschitzegger (2008).

*Data Acquisition Scope (C.DAS):* Distinguishes projects by the scope of acquired data: (i) environmental parameters, (ii) vital parameters, or (iii) Activities of Daily Living (ADL), e.g., daily routines like eating, sleeping, and bathing habits. For each of these characteristics the recorded time dimension, in terms of (i) historical, (ii) current, and (iii) anticipated future context data, is of interest. We further evaluate whether the data acquisition scope can be extended to integrate future context parameters.

*Analysis and Decision Making Mechanism (C.ADM):* The analysis mechanism may either be (i) initiated on demand or (ii) it may continuously monitor context data (eager). We are additionally interested in the projects' decision making approaches (e.g., pattern recognition, static thresholds, or manual inspection).

*Action Execution (C.AE):* Systems may need to execute an action in accordance with a decision made. The criterion evaluates the degree of automatism in this process. Criteria characteristics are: (i) not implemented, (ii) manual (i.e., an expert needs to initiate the action), (iii) semi-automatic (i.e., the system suggests an action, the expert needs to authorize or overrule the action), or (iv) automatic.

## Model-Driven Software Development

The diversity and heterogeneity of hardware and software platforms utilized in the development of pervasive healthcare applications suggests, according to Stankovic, Lee, Mok, & Rajkumar (2005), an MDSD approach. Project artifacts modeled platform-independently could then be applied to specific platforms via transformations. The evaluation criteria presented in this section were first introduced in (Schauerhuber, Schwinger, Retschitzegger, Wimmer, & Kappl, 2007) to evaluate Web modeling approaches for ubiquitous Web applications.

*Language Definition (M.L):* Distinguishes projects according to their level of adoption of application definition languages: (i) no language definition, (ii) grammar, (iii) explicit meta-model, or (iv) ontology.

*Model Transformation Types (M.T):* In MDSD models may be transformed to other, typically more specific models: (i) between platform independent models (PIM2PIM), (ii) platform independent to platform specific model (PIM2PSM), (iii) platform independent model to multiple platform specific models (PIM2MultiPSM, i.e., the application is composed of multiple platform specific application parts), (iv) models to text (M2T), e.g., platform specific model to code.

*Platform and Deployment Description Model (M.PDD):* Evaluates whether the project uses an explicit platform description model to represent a platform's attributes, or if these attributes are implicitly recorded in the transformation rules. Additionally, we evaluate to which extent projects formally model the system's deployment: (i) not defined, (ii) informally defined, or (iii) formal model.

## Utilized Technologies

The projects' technical details give insight into current development practices, design decisions, and technical preferences. We use these criteria to later highlight potential problems in developing pervasive healthcare applications.

*Architectural Style (T.AS):* Describes the system's architectural style with respect to well-established design patterns. Becker (2008) lists important styles: (i) Service-Oriented Architecture (SOA), (ii) Peer-to-Peer (P2P), (iii) Event-Driven Architecture (EDA), (iv) Component and Connector (C2), (v) Multi Agent System (MAS), and (vi) Blackboard.

*Platform (T.P):* Describes the platforms a project's system is built of: (i) proprietary or standards-based, and (ii) single- or multiple-platform.

## Project Evaluation

We have chosen four distinct projects for the evaluation in the domain of pervasive healthcare: SOPRANO aims at establishing a component market for ambient assisted living applications, whereas AlarmNet combines body sensor networks together with environmental sensing. The main focus of TigerPlace is to deploy the system in a retirement community. BelAmi, finally, focuses not entirely on the pervasive healthcare domain, but develops technologies and methods for Ambient Intelligence in general.

### SOPRANO

SOPRANO is an EU-funded project that aims to assist elderly in leading a more independent life in their familiar environment. The project's main contribution is the SOPRANO Ambient Middleware (SAM) described in (Klein, Schmidt, & Lauer, 2007), which is designed to efficiently process sensor input and user commands. Ontologies embedded in the middleware describe sensor information semantically and thereby enable applications to trigger appropriate actions. SOPRANO additionally provides a modeling environment to efficiently build pervasive healthcare systems based on SAM (Varginadis, Gouvas, Bouras, & Mentzas, 2008).

- C.DAS: SOPRANO does not define or restrict the type of context data pervasive healthcare systems process; instead, SAM is explicitly designed, as described in (Wolf, Schmidt, & Klein, 2008) for extensibility with third-party-components (it specifically encourages to provide components which derive high-level context data from other component's data). The context data is, nevertheless, tracked in terms of historical and current context state (Balfanz, Klein, Schmidt, & Santi, 2008). SAM does not by itself anticipate future context data, but it could be extended with such components.
- C.ADM: Due to SAM's extensibility, SOPRANO systems analyze incoming data in an eager fashion (third-party components are notified from data changes, analyze the data, and feed their results back into the system). Besides that, SAM does not prescribe any context reasoning formalism, as stated in (Wolf, Schmidt, & Klein, 2008). Similar to data acquisition components, analysis components can be plugged into SAM as third-party services.
- C.AE: SAM includes, as described in (Balfanz, Klein, Schmidt, & Santi, 2008), an action execution system – the Procedural Manager – based on the Event-Condition-Action cycle: events trigger an action, if specific conditions are satisfied. Again, SAM does not contain actions itself, but third-party components can contribute such actions.
- M.L: SOPRANO provides an explicit meta-model for conceptual models of pervasive healthcare systems based on SAM; a

model authoring environment supports in creating such conceptual models.
- M.T: SOPRANO does not address platform independent modeling; thus it only provides transformations from its platform specific models to machine-readable models (code in the form of XML configurations).
- M.PDD: SOPRANO does not address issues related to modeling the properties of different platforms (it only supports the single platform SAM); it also ignores system deployment issues.
- T.AS: SAM's core architectural style, as described in (Wolf, Schmidt, & Klein, 2008), is a combination of semantic-enabled technologies and service-orientation based on a blackboard. Extensibility is achieved with a service-oriented approach: third-party components – such as sensors or reasoning components – are plugged into SAM as services specified in terms of their semantic service contract. The architectural style, according to the criteria characteristics, is a combination of SOA, EDA, and Blackboard.
- T.P: SOPRANO uses its own proprietary platform named SAM. Third-party vendors can extend the platform with their own components that must strictly adhere to the platform specification.

## Alarm Net

Alarm Net, described in (Virone, et al., 2006), is a medical information system designed for smart healthcare with the focus of continuous, long-term and remote monitoring of an assisted individual's health parameters and life habits. It is based on wireless and body sensor networks for data acquisition. Alarm Net tackles sensor heterogeneity at the hardware level: the project extends or adapts existing hardware to interface with the MICAz platform (Crossbow Technology, Inc., 2008).

- C.DAS: Alarm Net comprises body sensor networks and emplaced environmental sensors, which together collect activity, location, and physiological data, and also motion, temperature, humidity, smoke, dust, gas, and acoustic information (Virone, et al., 2006).
- C.ADM: The system derives a measure on the assisted individual's daily life rhythm from raw sensor data – the so-called Circadian Activity Rhythm described in (Wood, et al., 2006). Besides this, data analysis is left to domain experts, like doctors or nurses, who can manually query the system for data on demand.
- C.AE: Action Execution in Alarm Net is manual (Wood, et al., 2006), i.e., the system alerts experts who then can inspect recorded data in detail and set appropriate actions.
- M.L, M.T, M.PDD: The medical information system is exactly tailored to the chosen hardware platform and the deployment area Smart Living Space (Virone, et al., 2006). Therefore, modeling is not an issue.
- T.AS: Alarm Net follows a multi-tiered approach: body and environmental sensors provide data, which is aggregated in the backbone network in one or more central storage and processing nodes (Blackboard).
- T.P: Alarm Net is built using two standard platforms: TinyOS-enabled Crossbow MICAz motes host the body and environmental sensing system, whereas Crossbow Stargate single-board computers hosting Linux form the processing backbone.

## TigerPlace

The Center for Eldercare and Rehabilitation Technology at the University of Missouri runs the TigerPlace retirement community, which is designed to promote aging-in-place (Rantz, et al., 2005). TigerPlace also acts as a research venue for pervasive healthcare projects. These projects closely cooperate with the Medical Automation Research Center at the University of Virginia; in fact, the projects base on the smart in-home monitoring system developed there. The cooperation with real residents and a test longevity spanning years are the project's unique features.

- C.DAS: The smart in-home monitoring system comprises motion sensors in every room, stove temperature sensors, a bed activity, and a floor-vibration based gait and fall detector (Tyrer, et al., 2006). Many of these sensors produce Boolean output, which simplifies data analysis at the expense of informative value.
- C.ADM: Rather simple rules, as described in (Dalal, Alwan, Seifrafi, Kell, & Brown, 2005), evaluate the Boolean sensor outputs to infer high-level context in an eager fashion (e.g., IF motion in kitchen AND motion in meal ingredients cabinet THEN a meal is being prepared). Users may further analyze data manually by querying the central database server on demand. The server aggregates raw sensor data, as well as an additional feature called restlessness, which describes the amount of a resident's activity (Tyrer, Aud, Alexander, Skubic, & Rantz, 2007).
- C.AE: Actions are implemented in the form of caregiver alerts, who need to execute appropriate actions manually (Dalal, Alwan, Seifrafi, Kell, & Brown, 2005), (Tyrer, et al., 2006). This restriction is due to the fact that TigerPlace is actually not being used in a test lab, but hosted in a real retirement community.
- M.L, M.T, M.PDD: The smart in-home monitoring system solves problems mostly on hardware level and relies on rather simple rules attached to a static software framework. They do not consider supporting the

development of their applications with MDSD.

- **T.AS:** A wireless sensor network transmits collected data to a local data logger in the apartment, which forwards it to a central server for storing, processing, and analysis (Blackboard), see (Rantz, Skubic, Miller, & Krampe, 2008).
- **T.P:** The projects do not describe technological details on the sensor and server platforms being used. We assume, however, that these platforms are exactly tailored to each other, and that the server demands a common data format.

## BelAmi

The BelAmi project focuses, in contrast to the other three projects, not entirely on the pervasive healthcare domain, but aims at developing technologies and methods for Ambient Intelligence in general. Especially the modeling tools have not been designed with pervasive healthcare in mind.

- **C.DAS:** BelAmi envisions body and home sensor networks to collect environmental and vital data, and aggregate it into situations. Nehmer, Becker, Karshmer, & Lamm (2006) additionally desire situation prediction (anticipating situations), but no implementations were described yet.
- **C.ADM:** Nick & Becker (2007) describe the project's decision making process. Situation assessment classifies situations into being "ok" or "not ok"; the latter ones require proactive treatment. The work, however, does not describe implementation details concerning classification.
- **C.AE:** Treatments (actions) are planned and executed automatically. If expected and actual outcome of treatments differ, a human expert is informed.

- **M.L:** BelAmi describes a formal modeling language based on SDL, which supports platform independent and platform specific models (Kuhn, Gotzhein, & Webel, 2006).
- **M.T:** Their process SDL-MDD supports transformations between PIM and PSM (both directions), and transformations from PSM to code. The project does, however, not include transformations of a single PIM to multiple cooperating PSMs (Kuhn, Gotzhein, & Webel, 2006).
- **M.PDD:** Platform descriptions seem to be incorporated in a platform-specific repository to automate transformations from PIM to PSM, but the modeling approach lacks deployment descriptions, i.e., applications are assumed to run on a single device (Kuhn, Gotzhein, & Webel, 2006).
- **T.AS:** BelAmi investigates a combination of SOA and EDA (Becker, 2008).
- **T.P:** To the best of our knowledge, the project has not yet published or developed a working prototype of its ideas; we can therefore not evaluate this criterion.

## Evaluation Result

We summarize the evaluation results in Figure 1 and discuss the evaluation's implications for this work.

The projects are all developed bottom-up: a hardware platform to develop applications is chosen, which then dictates the development process. In terms of data acquisition scope we see that heterogeneous sensor platforms are very common in this domain. Alarm Net and TigerPlace are directly based on a fixed hardware platform, whereas SOPRANO's SAM is designed as a generic and extensible platform; nevertheless, it relies on a similar architectural style as the other projects, simply to achieve flexibility. BelAmi discusses a model-driven development approach to generate applications exactly tailored to a platform, but did not apply the approach to pervasive healthcare

*Figure 1. Project evaluation results*

| | Alarm Net | BelAmi | SOPRANO | TigerPlace |
|---|---|---|---|---|
| Data Acquisition Scope (C.DAS) | Current Env. + Vital | Current (+ Future) Env. + Vital | Open | Current Env. + Vital |
| Analysis and Decision Making (C.ADM) | Manually | Automatic | Open | Rules + Manually |
| Action Execution (C.AE) | Manually | Automatic + Manually | Automatic | Manually |
| Language (M.L) | n.a. | Meta-model | Meta-model | n.a. |
| Transformations (M.T) | n.a. | PIM2PSM, M2T | M2T | n.a. |
| Platform and Deployment Description (M.PDD) | n.a. | Platform only | n.a. | n.a. |
| Architectural Style (T.AS) | Blackboard | SOA + EDA | SOA + EDA + Blackboard | Blackboard |
| Platform (T.P) | Multiple + standard | n.a. | Single + proprietary | n.a. |

systems. We argue that tailor-made applications outmatch generic applications in terms of energy consumption, bandwidth requirements, and performance, but they lack platform abstraction and extensibility (see section Issues, Controversies, Problems). Automated data analysis, decision making, and action execution is mentioned to be an issue in all projects, but they tackle it with varying sophistication. TigerPlace and Alarm Net rely on rather simple analysis mechanisms and manual execution to ensure reliability (especially TigerPlace must be robust, because it is used in a real setting). SOPRANO delegates these issues completely to third-party component vendors. BelAmi envisions a sophisticated approach with situation and action assessment, but does not describe reasoning algorithms in detail; in fact, it is unclear whether the described approach has yet been realized. None of the projects uses deployment descriptions, because they assume a fixed platform setting per use case and develop tailor-made applications for it (in the case of Alarm Net and TigerPlace), or they define a platform themselves (SOPRANO). At least SOPRANO

supports developers with a modeling environment to efficiently configure their middleware. BelAmi uses platform descriptions to support transformations from PIM to PSM models.

## MODEL-DRIVEN DEVELOPMENT OF PERVASIVE HEALTHCARE APPLICATIONS

In the following section we introduce a model-driven development approach for pervasive healthcare applications. Based on existing work in the field of context awareness and on the investigation of existing projects we define an architecture for pervasive healthcare applications. We compare possible implementation strategies for the presented architecture, especially concerning data acquisition and deriving semantics from raw data. The main part of the section focuses on the detailed description how to adapt the concepts of MDSD in the domain of pervasive healthcare. The sections conclude with an exemplary use case modeled with the implemented tools.

*Figure 2. Pervasive healthcare application reference architecture*

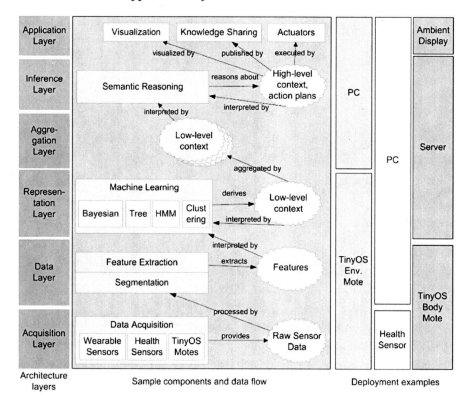

## A Pervasive Healthcare Application Reference Architecture

The main challenge of pervasive healthcare applications is to provide meaningful context out of a huge amount of raw data. Therefore research in pervasive healthcare is tightly knit with context awareness as well as machine learning and pattern recognition. We applied the architectures of Ailisto, Alahuhta, Haataja, Kyllönen, & Lindholm (2002) and Zhang, Gu, & Wang (2005) in the domain of pervasive healthcare. The resulting architecture with typical components/configurations for every layer as well as deployment examples are shown in Figure 2.

The layers defined by Zhang and Ailisto are quite similar, therefore layers from one architecture can be exchanged with the corresponding layer of the other one. We include Ailisto's Data Layer for segmentation and feature extraction (ig-

nored by Zhang). The separation of the Semantic Layer into Representation and Aggregation Layer increases deployment flexibility. The remaining layers of both architectures are only named differently but define the same scope. Therefore our combined architecture comprises six layers: Acquisition Layer, Data Layer, Representation Layer, Aggregation Layer, Inference Layer and Application Layer.

The Acquisition Layer collects different types of measurements (raw sensor data) and delegates them to the next layer. Here the problem arises that different manufacturers provide different sensor and processing boards using different programming languages which need to be integrated. The Data Layer separates raw data from noise and extracts features. Depending on the analysis requirements on raw data different data models can be applied. Strang & Linnhoff-Popien (2004) discuss advantages and restrictions of data models in context applications. Refer to (Kurschl, Mitsch, Schönböck, & Beer, 2008) for a possible solution. The Representation Layer then derives low-level context from features using machine learning and pattern recognition algorithms (e.g., noise level is high or low). The Aggregation Layer combines low-level context information from multiple context sources. The Inference Layer reasons on the aggregated low-level context to deduce high-level context (situations). These situations, if described in terms of an ontology, are the foundation for situation awareness as defined by Endsley (2000). Reasoning on situations permits to assess situations and predict future developments (situation evolution) which could be included in the Inference Layer as well. The Application Layer contains components that utilize situations to adjust their behavior, to issue actions (actuators) or to simply visualize it. Ferscha (2007) proposes to use ambient displays that operate at the periphery of a user's attention (e.g., some artwork). Knowledge sharing with other systems (e.g., medical information systems) may also be implemented here.

Baldauf, Dustdar, & Rosenberg (2004) compare various architectures of context-aware systems: (i) direct sensor access applications tightly integrate sensor access and application, which is useful for small, stand-alone applications, (ii) middleware-based applications use layers to separate sensor details from application details, and (iii) context-server applications additionally permit multiple clients to access shared context data on a server. As context acquisition is an important part of pervasive healthcare systems all three types should be supported within the proposed architecture. Therefore we would like to point out that layers do not depict deployment boundaries. Thus it is possible that powerful sensor platforms host the Acquisition Layer, the Data Layer and the Representation Layer whereas less powerful platforms might only host the Acquisition Layer (see deployment examples in Figure 2). We assume that at deployment boundaries communication between two different platforms

is possible, e.g., using (generated) sender/receiver adapters based on a common data model and communication protocol.

## Issues, Controversies, Problems

The reference architecture introduced in the previous section already highlights the challenges in developing pervasive healthcare applications. Knowledge from different fields of computer science is needed to successfully implement the different layers (Wolf, Schmidt, & Klein, 2008): (i) pervasive computing to gain raw data with sensors, (ii) machine learning and pattern recognition to interpret these data, and (iii) human-computer interaction knowledge to enable implicit interaction with the system. Of course there exist many different approaches to the problems in every layer, and programmers therefore apply different strategies to integrate these approaches. The survey in section Background showed different integration strategies, which are discussed in the following paragraphs.

We face the challenge of integrating many different data sources: examples for such sensors are the TinyOS sensor platform for environmental monitoring, or Bluetooth-enabled blood pressure sensors or heart rate monitors. The question, however, arises how to minimize the integration effort. A possible solution would be to configure or alter the hardware itself to acquire data on additional phenomena. Alarm Net for example modifies existing X10 motion sensors to interface with the Crossbow MICAz platform. These extensions lead to proprietary solutions and have to be adapted if new platforms emerge. Furthermore, these modifications are often tailored to one specific use case and thus can hardly be reused, not even in just a slightly different scenario.

We suggest that the integration of different sensor platforms should therefore be done on a higher level of abstraction, but integration on a software level still raises some problems. A trivial solution, applied by TigerPlace, would be to use the sensor platform only for data acquisition and process data on a powerful server, which hosts abstraction components for every platform and defines a common data format. This approach leads to a high communication effort as every single sensor reading has to be reported to the server. If wireless communication protocols are used for data transfer a lot of energy is consumed (Mini, Loureiro, & Nath, 2005), which is a critical issue on battery powered platforms. Furthermore a permanent connection to the server has to be maintained for data transmission which limits the possible application scenarios. A body network for example could then not be used outdoors without making use of cost-intensive public networks like UMTS or GPRS. As the server is the central processing unit it represents a single point of failure. To eliminate these problems sensors should host local processing components. Preprocessing or even classification could be done locally on a sensor platform and thereby problems concerning permanent data transmission can easily be omitted. Thus specific software for different hardware platforms is needed.

With such an approach the problem, however, arises that the implemented software is now tailored to a specific use case on a specific hardware platform. Moreover, this also determines possible deployment scenarios (e.g., exactly two body sensors that communicate data to a Linux server) and thereby limits software reusability. Concerning sensor networks this is due to the tight integration of the communication protocol with the sensing tasks. For example using a single-hop communication protocol is an efficient solution in a network consisting of two sensor nodes. But if a higher number of nodes should be supported a multi-hop protocol should be used instead. In software engineering strategies like dependency injection and frameworks have been developed to transparently tackle this problem. The SAM platform of SOPRANO uses this approach to integrate different hardware and software components into their server. Unfortunately resource

constrained devices are typically not able to host such frameworks, not least because programming languages for embedded systems do not offer features like object-oriented programming (OOP) these principles heavily make use of. A possible solution is to raise the level of abstraction towards models and to generate source code based on these models to detach deployment specifics from the application code.

What is then still limiting reuse is the specific tailoring of a use case to a certain platform. On the one hand there are several suitable platforms available but make for example use of different programming languages. On the other hand a single platform might not be able to execute the whole code of a use case locally. For example a sensor platform may not be able to execute complex machine learning algorithms. Therefore different hardware and software platforms have to be combined to a common solution. A concept is desired that is able to cope with different platforms, which handles their differences adequately and simplifies application development. Moreover, the wide conceptual gap between functionality specification and implementation details should be minimized. MDSD reduces this gap with systematic transformations of problem-level abstractions to software implementations as stated in (France & Rumpe, 2007). This viewpoint is also supported by Stankovic, Lee, Mok, & Rajkumar (2005) who state that "embedded software components must be designed and reused at an abstraction level independent of the underlying hardware platform, operating system, middleware, and even programming languages"(p. 28). But to date only very few tools supporting an MDSD approach in the domain of context-awareness in general and pervasive healthcare in particular are available (in contrast to, e.g., hardware manufacturers, which successfully use modeling to reduce development costs). Losilla et al. (2007) describe a modeling tool for wireless sensor network applications that supports the software development process with different levels of abstraction: domain experts model WSN applications in a domain model. Implementation is then detailed in a PIM; components are further refined in a PSM, before code for a specific platform is generated. The modeling tool is, however, too focused on wireless sensor networks to be directly applicable to pervasive healthcare applications; it does, e.g., not support cross-platform processing between sensor nodes and coordinators. In fact, their domain model corresponds to the PSM in our approach.

## Solution Overview

Based on the evaluated projects and the issues shown in the previous section we believe that MDSD provides solutions for these issues. To successfully apply the concepts of MDSD to develop pervasive healthcare applications tool support is indispensable (France & Rumpe, 2007). First of all meta-models for describing the context-recognition process are needed; the meta-models define a so-called Domain Specific Language (Stahl, Völter, Efftinge, & Haase, 2007). Tools that automatically transform functionality descriptions into implementation specifications as well as graphical editors speed up development. Finally methods to generate executable code for specific platforms have to be applied.

Developing pervasive healthcare applications includes at least three different stakeholders: hardware vendors, software engineers and domain experts. The hardware components provided by different vendors are characterized with distinct advantages and restrictions (e.g., price level, accuracy or measured phenomenon). A non-trivial pervasive healthcare application therefore includes hardware from different vendors. The software engineer's main focus is to develop efficient software for a use case on a specific hardware platform, e.g., detecting whether the light is on or off using TinyOS motes. The task of the domain experts is to decide which type of application (and thereby which specific components) is suitable in an application setting. Often informal requirements docu-

ments or simple notes for software engineers are used. If domain experts would instead use formal models, errors could be omitted and development time could be reduced. Before going into detail we briefly present a solution overview by exemplarily modeling and transforming a pattern recognition application, as shown in Figure 3.

A platform independent model (PIM) allows domain experts to describe the requirements of an application independent from the implementation platforms (in Figure 3 we see a PIM consisting of two parallel pattern recognition pipes). The PIM is then handed to software engineers who transform it to one or more suitable platform specific models (PSMs). Not all platforms offer enough processing power or memory to process data locally, as the example's body sensors. Therefore low-level context has to be generated on a more powerful platform. In contrast, the TinyOS platform is able to process data locally and therefore submits low-level context instead of raw data. The Eclipse platform processes the body network's raw data and aggregates it with the TinyOS platform's low-level context in a data store. The resulting three PSMs are then used to automatically generate platform specific source code.

We provide a formal meta-model for the PIM as well as for PSMs of common hardware platforms summarized into an IDE based on Eclipse. Additionally automatic model transformation mechanisms are included in the IDE to transform a PIM to PSMs as well as code generator templates from PSMs to source code. The development environment includes a graphical editor to simplify model creation. The following sections describe these concepts in detail.

## Platform Independent and Platform Specific Meta-Model

Meta-models describe how to build models and thereby specify the abstract syntax of the modeling language in terms of, e.g., aggregations and relations between model elements and their at-

*Figure 3. Solution overview by example*

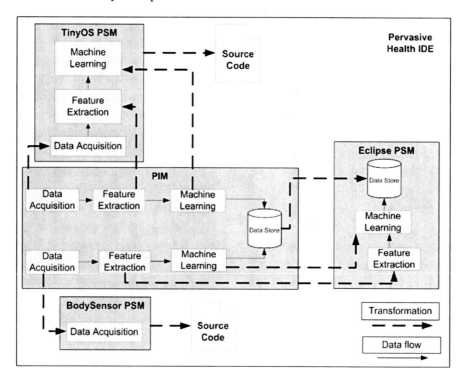

*Figure 4. Platform independent meta-model*

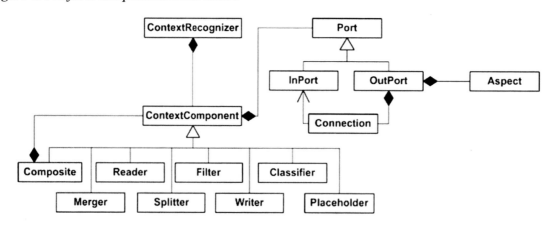

tributes. The platform independent meta-model shown in Figure 4 provides elements to model context-aware applications without depending on and restricting to a certain platform.

In the meta-model we defined components to match the steps listed in section Background: *Readers* are used for sensing, *Filters* for segmentation and feature extractions, *Classifiers* for classification. Post-processing can be realized with filters (e.g., smoothing the sequence of a classifier's predictions) or classifiers (e.g., multiple classification or voting). Their common abstraction *ContextComponent* allows domain experts to arrange them in a pipes-and-filters architectural style (Buschmann, Henney, & Schmidt, 2007). The *ContextRecognizer* component aggregates a pipeline's components in a single model and thus represents a context recognition application. Every context component defines its interface with *In-* and *OutPorts* which can be connected to each other.

Readers interact with their environment and deliver selected data on a phenomenon which we call *Aspects*. Depending on the desired application type a reader could, e.g., read from a file or a database, or could make use of environmental sensors. Aspects describe data items with a specific name and a description on how to interpret the data. In the case of environmental monitoring an aspect could be the temperature or the vertical acceleration of an object. The binding how to acquire a specific aspect (like generating an SQL statement for reading from a database) is not done within the PIM – this has to be later refined in a PSM. Filters extract features from aspects and thereby limit the amount of data subsequent classifiers need to process. Depending on the type of application and low-level context to be generated from raw data various different filters can be used. Domain experts need for example different algorithms to extract audio features (e.g., MFCC Filter) or to convert values from time to frequency domain (e.g., Fourier transformations), depending on the use case specifics. Therefore, it is impossible to represent every specific filter within the platform independent meta-model. To gain flexibility we provide two different variants: typed and generic filters. Typed filters represent commonly used filter functions, are predefined in the platform independent meta-model, and can be used out of the box during creation of the PIM (e.g., Minimum Filter or Maximum Filter). For typed filters a specific transformation to a platform (refer to the following section) must be defined. Rarely used filters are defined as so-called generic filters in the PIM. They include a clear description of the filter's purpose (e.g., in terms of a mathematical filter function) specifying how to implement the filter. Classifiers interpret aspects and reason for new ones based on either raw data delivered by readers or features extracted by filters. Within the PIM the domain expert can specify which input aspects a classifier needs to reason about certain output aspects. A property on classifiers is set to use either supervised, unsupervised or reinforcement learning algorithms (Duda, Hart, & Stork, 2001). Furthermore it can be specified if the classification problem consist of a process that unfolds in time suggesting, e.g., a Hidden Markov Model.

Besides the three basic types utility components are needed for efficient modeling. If it is necessary to process only parts of a data packet or to process parts differently, a *Splitter* splits an incoming data packet to create new distinct or partly overlapping output data packets. As the Splitter's inverse function the *Merger* component merges several different data packets to a single one. *Writers* are used to either present aspects to the user, to save them to a persistent storage, or to send them via a network. A *Composite* is a reusable component to hierarchically group other components used to hide complexity. To enable reuse of components composites define interface contracts with required and provided ports in terms of aspects they need and aspects they produce. In contrast, *Placeholders* are black-box components that do not specify a concrete assembling at the point of modeling. Imagine that for example a fall detection component is needed in a PIM. There might be several possibilities to implement the needed functionality: for example it is possible to use a fall detector based on acceleration aspects or a different one based on video surveillance. As the PIM does not refer to any specific implementation the placeholder represents an exchangeable composite. Before transforming a PIM to specific platforms contained placeholders have to be resolved by referencing composites.

The PIM allows domain experts to model a context- aware application without respect to a specific platform. As mentioned above many platforms must be supported to efficiently acquire and process data from the environment. Therefore, every platform is described in a PSM meta-model with the specific elements it provides. A PSM combines the specification in the PIM with the details of a particular type of platform (Miller & Mukerji, 2006). We identified that, although platforms differ in implementation details, they still share a lot of commonalities which we aggregate in a meta-model called *PSMBase*. Within this base model the three types (Reader, Filter and Classifier) as well as the utility components are represented again. The platform specific components (e.g., a minimum filter on the TinyOS platform) are defined in their own specific meta-model, which references the PSMBase meta-model; thereby the PSM meta-model represents a formal platform description. Not all platforms have to support every type of component.

The current implementations of the provided meta-models are based on the Eclipse Modeling Framework (Budinsky, Steinberg, Merks, Ellersick, & Grose, 2004) and represented in Ecore. EMF provides rich model validation capabilities which we use to verify our model instances before transformation. In the next section we focus on the automatic transformations from PIMs to PSMs.

## Model Transformation

The separation of the system functionality represented in a PIM and the adaption to specific platforms represented in PSMs requires automatic model transformations. Pervasive healthcare applications often comprise functionality that must be realized with heterogeneous cooperating platforms. For example, if we want to monitor the environment to detect patterns and present them to users, we would certainly use two platforms: a WSN to monitor the environment and a PC to detect patterns and to host the user interface. Therefore, it is necessary to split a single PIM up into several PSMs during model transformation. The problem, however, arises which components of the PIM can be transformed to which specific platform. Additional problems are that multiple

platforms could host a component and that one platform could offer multiple instances of a specific type (e.g. the Eclipse Platform offers the writer types console writer, file writer, and chart plotter). The first issue can be solved with formal platform descriptions, whereas the latter two need to be specified by the user during transformation because in MDSD a 1:1 association between the elements in the PIM and the PSM is assumed (e.g., class A of meta-model M1 is always transformed to class B in meta-model M2). This user-defined transformation specification is captured in a transformation model, which again conforms to a transformation meta-model. Figure 5 shows the model transformation process in detail.

A PIM model that conforms to the PIM meta-model captures the functionality (in this case, an aspect is read, filtered and then presented to the user). At the beginning of the transformation process a transformation model instance is automatically created: it includes the available platform descriptions extracted from the PSM meta-models (the example shows an instance of the transformation model including the Eclipse and the TinyOS platforms as possible transformation target platforms). Platforms are detected automatically using the Eclipse extension point concept allowing simple integration of new platforms. For every platform the concrete implementations of context components are extracted from the PSMs. Annotations in the meta-model components define the type of the PIM concept they implement. In case the PSM meta-model extends the PSMBase meta-model these annotations are already included in base classes. Thereby we can ensure that one type of component in the PIM (e.g. reader) can only be transformed to the corresponding type in a PSM. The extracted transformation model is presented in a graphical wizard to guide the software engineer through the process of selecting possible platform specific realizations. The specified mapping is stored in the transformation model by adding source references. After mappings for every PIM component are specified

*Figure 5. Model transformation*

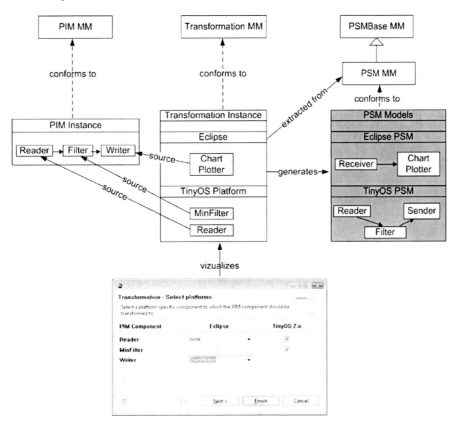

the transformation is executed to generate PSM model instances. In case a PIM is transformed to more than one platform connections that bridge platform boundaries cannot be realized with in-process method calls (in contrast to connections within the same platform). Therefore we generate a *Sender* component on the connection's source platform and a *Receiver* component on the connection's target platform respectively (see generated PSMs in Figure 5). Sender and Receiver handle data marshalling and stream information between the two platforms.

We use the Atlas Transformation Language (ATL), see (Jouault & Kurtev, 2005), for specifying the transformations from PIM to PSM. ATL is a hybrid model transformation language that allows declarative and imperative constructs to be used in transformation definitions. For every supported platform an ATL transformation template from the platform independent meta-model to the platform specific meta-model has to be developed. Models can not only be transformed to other, more specific, models but also to source code. We use the template-based code generation method XPand (for an overview about code generation methods please refer to (Stahl, Völter, Efftinge, & Haase, 2007)) to transform PSMs into source code. The XPand template language would be capable of generating both component code (e.g., the implementation of a minimum filter component) and application code (references between the components implementation, so called wiring). We suggest, however, to rely on prefabricated component code and to generate only application code due to the following reasons: (i) In a pipes-and-filters architectural style the component code does not change in different applications, only the wiring does. (ii) The wiring of compo-

*Figure 6. Graphical editor*

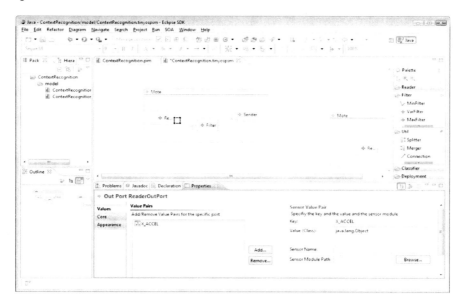

nents is simple to understand and expresses best the model on code level. (iii) Component code can be tested, compiled and used independently from the modeling environment. (iv) It reduces template complexity. This component-based approach allows us to generate applications that can be deployed to hardware without additional programming or configuration effort. But in case of generic filters being used, which lack a formal description, the code generator can only generate the component's interface but leave its implementation to the programmer.

The meta-models as well as the transformations are integrated in a modeling tool. The next section describes how a graphical editor applies these concepts to realize the MDSD approach.

## Graphical Editor

Domain experts do usually not have expert knowledge in programming, but should nevertheless be able to express their domain knowledge in platform independent models. Thus an expressive mapping from the abstract syntax defined by the meta-model to specific machine representations and encodings must be defined: the so called concrete syntax. As we based our meta-model on Ecore using EMF there are several possibilities to specify a concrete syntax. The PIM meta-model and the PSM meta-model are instances of Ecore (meta-meta-model) and are represented as Java classes. A possible concrete syntax would be therefore Java itself: a model can then be created by instantiating the meta-model classes. Doing so would be tedious and error-prone. Moreover, the resulting models are hard to read and programming skills are needed for modeling. Therefore a more expressive and intuitively applicable syntax for non-programmers is needed, for example in the form of a graphical domain-specific language (DSL). The EMF framework includes templates to automatically generate a tree-based editor from Ecore models. Even though this is a simple and efficient graphical editor, it is still quite hard to understand the meaning of a model represented as a tree, especially if relations between objects are modeled. To overcome these limitations the Graphical Modeling Framework (GMF) can be used to define feature-rich graphical editors (Völter, Haase, Efftinge, & Kolb, 2006). In Fig-

*Figure 7. Use case functionality captured in the PIM*

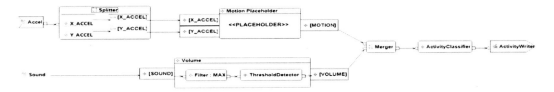

ure 6, which shows a screenshot of our current implementation of the graphical editor, different components (concrete classes in the meta-model) have different graphical representations. With the help of the graphical DSL domain experts are able to quickly define models.

## Application of the MDSD Approach

To conclude this section we apply the concepts presented above to implement a use case for the Eclipse and TinyOS platforms.

## Use Case and Hardware Setup

A major goal of pervasive healthcare systems is to increase or maintain a person's safety or state of health by detecting deviations from normal behavior. Therefore we first need to learn a person's normal behavior (his or her daily routines, also called *activities of daily living* (Bourke & Lyons, 2008)) with machine learning algorithms (situation-awareness according to the reference architecture). The amount of raw data produced by sensors, however, is too large for situation-awareness; we first need to interpret raw data and thereby derive semantics.

The exemplary use case shows how to interpret raw data to distinguish between two common household activities, which are still simple enough to be presented within the chapter: watching TV and vacuum-cleaning. To distinguish between these situations we decided to use two Crossbow MICAz motes equipped with MTS310 sensor boards and TinyOS-2.x. A test person wears one mote at the ankle and the other one at the belt.

We were interested in the acceleration values obtained from the sensor board's orthogonal accelerometers (we call these values x-acceleration and y-acceleration) and the raw sound data that could be used to detect the specific sound of a vacuum cleaner. We assume that it is most likely that a person is sitting when watching TV and walking around when vacuum cleaning a room. During vacuum cleaning the volume level is significantly higher than during watching TV as the worn microphone is closer to the vacuum cleaner than to the TV. We therefore need a component that is capable to decide if a person is walking or standing and another one that interprets the volume. These two activities are quite different but for recognizing them we make use of common low-level components, which points out the advantages of the MDSD process.

## Platform Independent Use Case Modeling

A domain expert captures the user's requirements, preferences and constraints (e.g., a user may dislike image sensors due to privacy reasons but can imagine wearing a sound and accelerometer sensors possibly integrated into clothing). Additionally, the domain expert can observe characteristic behavioral patterns and environmental settings that indicate if a certain implementation is feasible or not. The domain expert's task is now to roughly describe the necessary steps to analyze the input aspects to produce the desired output aspects, as depicted in Figure 7.

The first step in the modeling process is to define the available aspects to the application.

In our case the motes which are worn by the test person deliver the aspects X_ACCEL, Y_ACCEL (horizontal and vertical acceleration values) and SOUND which are modeled in the out ports of the Reader components. Note that we use Readers to group similar aspects, because it is often likely to collect them on a single platform (we could also use a single or three readers; in the PIM readers only specify which data is available to the system). It is quite obvious that sound and acceleration values need to be treated differently and therefore are handled in different components. The *Volume* composite introduced by the domain expert comprises a *Maximum* filter and a *Threshold Detector*. The maximum filter computes a simple closure of the signal which is then used in the threshold detector to decide whether the value is low, medium or high (the threshold detector uses pre-defined static thresholds for its decision). If this kind of composite is already available (e.g., because volume is often needed within the domain) the domain expert can reuse the composite. The detection of motion is a rather complicated task. As our test person is willing to wear one sensor at the belt and another one at the ankle there might be several possibilities to detect whether a person is walking, sitting or standing; the domain expert therefore decides to use a Placeholder that can be specified later. The consumed input aspects (X_ACCEL and Y_ACCEL) and the produced output aspect (MOTION) define the Placeholder's interface. Additional information can be provided in the form of informal descriptions, e.g., "Person is willing to wear up to two sensors, and placement of the sensors is preferably belt and ankle". Usually software engineers and domain experts will cooperate in a refinement cycle to define the placeholder's structure in a composite. Thereby the domain expert gets detailed knowledge about possible implementation strategies and will be able to apply the newly defined composite in future similar use cases and the software engineer is less likely to misinterpret the placeholder's purpose. The newly generated aspects MOTION and

VOLUME (already low-level context) are then merged and fed into the activity classifier. The classifier's decision is finally presented with the ActivityWriter.

## Platform Specific Adaption

The functionality defined in the PIM needs to be transformed to suitable platforms that adapt the use case to the platform. Before an automatic transformation can be executed all placeholders have to be refined with a platform independent composite. The software engineer and the domain expert decide to calculate the variance of the x- and y-acceleration at the person's ankle and use a threshold detector to detect motion. However, this simple classification is not able to distinguish between a person sitting and just moving his/her feet or a person actually walking. Therefore, they introduce a second filter to calculate the angle on basis of the acceleration's gravity portion. Combining the variance features and the angle feature enables a more sophisticated tree-based classifier.

In the next step the transformation target platform and the target component of each component in the PIM has to be selected. The ActivityWriter should present the results on a PC whereas the Readers should acquire raw sensor data with the TinyOS platform; all other components could either run on the motes directly or on a PC. The decision to which platform certain components are transformed and where feature extraction as well as classification is done has enormous influence on the application's performance and life time. Concerning the use case it would for example be possible to send raw acceleration data to a PC and do the feature extraction and classification remotely. Thereby complicated feature extraction and machine learning algorithms could be applied but on the expense of battery life time. At the other end of the spectrum all components are hosted on motes and notifications are only sent when the situation changes from vacuum

*Figure 8. TinyOS model to classify between watching TV and vacuum cleaning*

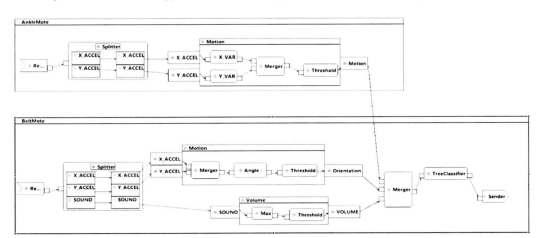

cleaning to watching TV or vice versa. This so called in-network data processing can improve the application's scalability and reduce its energy and other resource consumption, since it may significantly reduce the data volume that has to be routed through the network (Römer, 2005).

The software engineer, in our example, prefers increased battery lifetime and therefore hosts as many components as possible on motes. By selecting the appropriate platforms the PIM is automatically transformed to two PSMs, one for the Eclipse platform hosting the writer on the PC and one for the TinyOS platform hosting the remaining components. The transformation to the TinyOS platform can further be detailed with a deployment description. Typically in WSNs multiple TinyOS (sub) applications hosted on different motes cooperate to implement the functionality, e.g., one sub application collects sensor data whereas the other one acts as a gateway. In the example the software engineer introduces two different applications: one application for motes placed at the ankle which detects the movement of a person, and the other application at the belt, which detects whether a person is standing or sitting. The belt application additionally hosts the components for sound classification and acts as a gateway. It therefore aggregates the data

from the ankle application with its local data and additionally hosts classifiers that finally decide between vacuum cleaning and watching TV (or none of both), depicted in Figure 8. This semantic information is then sent to the Eclipse platform, which can present the result to the user. Note that the PIM's motion composite (which specifies the Motion Placeholder) is partitioned to both motes (i.e., the motes cooperate to implement the composite's functionality).

Platform specific information, which cannot be specified during transformation, needs to be added to complement the PSMs before source code can be generated. The aspects of the PIMs readers are symbolic names and therefore the software engineer must now add the name of the nesC component that is able to read horizontal and vertical acceleration values as well as raw sound data from the sensor board to generate accurate wirings during source code generation. Connections between components hosted on one mote represent local calls, whereas connections between different motes require a wireless communication link. The type of routing protocol (see section Background) can be specified as a property of wireless communication links. The flexibility in terms of changes of one routing protocol allows us to easily adapt the application to certain needs, without changing any part of the processing components and the overall control flow. Finally nesC source code is generated and deployed to the hardware.

## Benefits and Drawbacks

The proposed approach entails the following strengths and benefits: With the help of an MDSD approach in general and with the presented tool in particular a prototyping-oriented development process is supported (Pomberger & Weinreich, 1994). Powerful and universal platforms (like the Eclipse platform) can be used in the very early stages of the development process. Within the Eclipse platform it is possible to execute and debug the model by using chart plotters that visualize data. This is especially useful for finding or testing different kinds of features for classifiers. After analyzing the data programmers can start implementing the application model and transform it to the desired target platform. The proposed approach and the implemented tool help to integrate domain experts into the software development process. By capturing the user's requirements in a formal model (the PIM) a detailed description of the program is established at an early stage in the development cycle. Composites as application building blocks can be easily reused and thus enable rapid development of complex pervasive healthcare applications.

Current pervasive healthcare applications often make use of only one type of sensor or platform. In our opinion this is due to the fact that there are various different programming languages and platforms available but tool support that hides this complexity is missing. Thus programming for specific (hardware) platforms requires expert knowledge which often hinders the use of specific sensors or devices and thus limits the application domain. Additionally, there is intensive research in the field of WSNs leading to new sensor platforms frequently. By applying a MDSD approach the application can be modeled independently form the

underlying hardware or programming language. Abstract models of specific use cases (e.g., the above mentioned ADL detection scenario) within pervasive healthcare applications provide a means to better reuse existing knowledge and therefore increase sustainability. PIMs can subsequently be transformed to specific platforms and finally to source code, thereby integrating multiple platforms that host parts of the application. Besides the separation of platforms MDSD enforces a common architecture. As applications are generated (at least in large part) the architectural style defined in the code generation templates is inherited to every single application. Thereby complex pervasive healthcare applications are documented during development, and therefore easier to understand, extend, and maintain. Security concepts can also be enforced within the templates. Additionally, barriers of manufacturers, which often make switching to platforms of competitors nearly impossible (platform lock-in), are abridged, and comparing or evaluating the performance of an application on different platforms is thereby easily possible. A facilitator for the proposed approach would be a component market place for components adhering to the reference architecture: a steadily increasing component catalog would decrease modeling effort and, hence, time-to-market. Graphical models additionally lower the entry barrier into the domain, which would greatly increase the developer community size and make it possible to examine pervasive healthcare technology also in non-technical teaching classes (e.g., in health care studies).

However, the proposed approach is exposed to the following risks and barriers: Although there are already frameworks available to develop tools that allow the application of MDSD concepts in practice, programming such tools is still very time-consuming and therefore only justified if lots of similar applications are created for a particular platform. If this is the case programmers can fully benefit from the MDSD approach. Although we provide a platform specific base model (PSMBase)

*Figure 9. SWOT analysis of the proposed approach*

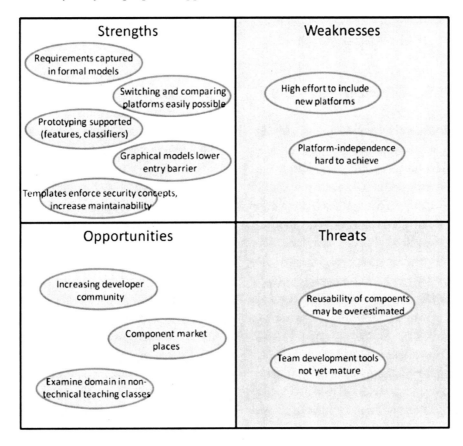

that can be extended by programmers who want to include a new platform programming effort is still high. A formal meta-model of the new platform is needed, which is often hard to define. Furthermore the transformation from the PIM to the new platform has to be specified. Last but not least a concrete (graphical) syntax has to be created to allow efficient modeling. Therefore expert knowledge in the domain of MDSD is needed to successfully extend our tool with new platforms. Additionally, development tools needed for shared development (e.g., version control systems) which treat models on a semantic level are not yet mature (but may evolve in the future, as MDSD gets more widespread). The PIM offers on the one hand the advantage of modeling without respect to a certain platform. On the other hand this leads to the fact that rather abstract concepts need to be applied.

This is especially true when defining placeholders, or readers and their aspects as they represent concrete hardware. Therefore, during modeling the PIM the domain expert has to keep in mind that high-level aspects might only be available on very special platforms, require complex algorithms or shift development efforts into the platform specific modeling phase. The proposed approach suggests simplicity in this issue, but platform-independence is hard to acquire: for example, a placeholder that takes sound as input and produces English text hides a lot of complexity, which usually cannot be realized from scratch easily, or readers with extremely high sampling rates might require a powerful processor board and therefore be very expensive. Additionally, reusability of complex components may be overestimated, leading to unnecessary effort put into making components platform-independent. Figure 9 recapitulates the discussed benefits and drawbacks in a SWOT-style analysis.

## FUTURE RESEARCH DIRECTIONS

To date the development environment only includes three concrete platforms (Java, Eclipse, and TinyOS). To fully benefit from platform independent modeling additional platforms should be included. Ideally, existing applications for these platforms can then be abstracted to platform specific models and later to platform independent models with reverse engineering (which is not yet sufficiently solved in any existing tools). A first step would be to rather transform between meta-models at the same level of abstraction (e.g., PSM to PSM). Thereby we could tackle fast technical developments by adapting existing models to new platforms or new versions of platform specific languages (e.g., TinyOS 1.x to TinyOS 2.x). Precondition for the mentioned enhancements is an extensible development environment, in which new platforms can be integrated easily. An abstract textual syntax as alternative to the graphical syntax should be included in the modeling environment to alleviate known problems of graphical programming, like representing large-scaled models (Schiffer, 1998). The benefits of platform independent modeling could be exploited on a global level. Our vision is to provide some sort of modeling artifact market place, in which developers can share their pervasive healthcare application building blocks to speed up development.

On a conceptual level pervasive healthcare applications may need to evolve into situation-aware systems: the envisioned pervasive healthcare applications produce a huge amount of raw sensor data, features, and low-level context. "The problem with today's systems is not a lack of information, but finding what is needed when it is needed" (Endsley, 2000, p. 4). She describes situation

awareness as "the perception of the elements in the environment within a volume of time and space, the comprehension of their meaning and the projection of their status in the near future" (p. 5), which we agree to be a possible solution to this problem. To be beneficial and applicable to situation awareness the low-level context derived by machine learning algorithms must adhere to a formal model in order to relate and assess current situations, but also to predict future developments. Baumgartner & Retschitzegger (2006) propose the use of upper ontologies as modeling constructs for situation awareness in road traffic management, as they could permit the integration of information about perceived objects, identify situations, and share knowledge. Wang, Gu, Zhang, & Pung (2004) additionally name the possibility of logic inference and knowledge reuse as major reasons for using ontologies. Numerous ontologies already exist in the pervasive computing domain: Baumgartner & Retschitzegger (2006), Krummenacher & Strang (2007), and Strang & Linnhoff-Popien (2004) present surveys on ontologies for situation awareness and context modeling. Baumgartner, Retschitzegger, Schwinger, Kotsis, & Schwietering (2007) elaborate the basic ideas (deriving additional meaning by reasoning about situations) towards prediction of future developments in the road traffic management domain. We consider these concepts also to be relevant and beneficial in pervasive healthcare systems and other pervasive environments. A common shortcoming we found among all described models is missing tracing information. Medical data typically needs to be available in raw format for detailed inspection by medical staff; thus, trace links from derived high-level context and low-level context to raw data must be preserved to allow medical staff to quickly navigate to relevant data. Additionally, modeling situation awareness should be included in the development tools. The described tool currently supports modeling the Acquisition Layer, the Data Layer and the Representation Layer but misses Aggregation Layer as well as Inference Layer.

## CONCLUSION

Pervasive healthcare applications aim at improving elderly and handicapped persons' habitability by assisting them in living autonomously. But the distributed nature of such highly interconnected pervasive healthcare applications leads to an increased system complexity. The discussion of several related projects revealed the necessity of a reference architecture. The amount of data delivered by the heterogeneous wireless sensor network platforms and their attached sensors lead to the discussion of context-awareness and machine learning algorithms to derive low-level context (semantics) and thereby reduce the amount of information for higher processing layers (towards situation inference). Deriving low-level context from raw data usually requires extensive prototyping work, which must be supported with tools. Therefore we presented a model-driven software development approach as well as a tool, which supports platform-independent modeling, transforming these models to platform-specific models and lust but not least generating platform specific code. The current implementation of the tool focuses on data acquisition and deriving low-level context. The challenge now is to aggregate information from different sources into a common ontology and to thereby enable situation- and action-awareness. These high level concepts again demand modeling support, possibly represented in the form of Computation Independent Models (CIM).

## REFERENCES

Ailisto, H., Alahuhta, P., Haataja, V., Kyllönen, V., & Lindholm, M. (2002). Five-Layer Model and Example Case. In *Proceedings of Ubicomp 2002, Concepts and Models for Ubiqutious Computing Workshop*. Structuring Context Aware Applications.

Baldauf, M., Dustdar, S., & Rosenberg, F. (2004). A Survey on Context-Aware Systems. *International Journal of Ad Hoc and Ubiquitous Computing* .

Balfanz, D., Klein, M., Schmidt, A., & Santi, M. (2008). Participatory development of a middleware for AAL solutions: requirements and approach - the case of SOPRANO. *GMS Medizinische Informatik, Biometrie und Epidemiologie, 4*(3).

Bannach, D., Amft, O., & Lukowicz, P. (2008). Rapid Prototyping of Activity Recognition Applications. *IEEE Pervasive Computing / IEEE Computer Society [and] IEEE Communications Society, 7*, 22–31. doi:10.1109/MPRV.2008.36

Baumgartner, N., & Retschitzegger, W. (2006). A Survey of Upper Ontologies for Situation Awareness. In *Proceedings of the International Conference on Knowledge Sharing and Collaborative Engineering.*

Baumgartner, N., & Retschitzegger, W. (2007). Towards a Situation Awareness Framework Based on Primitive Relations. In *Proceedings of the Conference on Information Decision and Control*, Adelaide, Australia.

Baumgartner, N., Retschitzegger, W., & Schwinger, W. (2007). Lost in Space and Time and Meaning - An Ontology-Based Approach to Road Traffic Situation Awareness. In *Proceedings of the 3rd Workshop on Context Awareness for Proactive Systems*, Guildford, UK.

Baumgartner, N., Retschitzegger, W., Schwinger, W., Kotsis, G., & Schwietering, C. (2007). Of Situations and Their Neighbors: Evolution and Similarity in Ontology-Based Approaches to Situation Awareness. In *Proceedings of the 6th International and Interdisciplinary Conference on Modeling and Using Context*, Roskilde, Denmark.

Becker, M. (2008). *Software Architecture Trends and Promising Technology for Ambient Assisted Living Systems. Assisted Living Systems - Models, Architectures and Engineering Approaches. Dagstuhl Seminar Proceedings*. Dagstuhl, Germany: Internationales Begegnungs- und Forschungszentrum für Informatik, Schloss Dagstuhl.

Bézivin, J. (2005). On the Unification Power of Models. *Journal on Software and Systems Modeling, 4*(2).

Bourke, A. K., & Lyons, G. M. (2008). A threshold-based fall-detection algorithm using a bi-axial gyroscope sensor. *Medical Engineering & Physics, 30*, 84–90. doi:10.1016/j.medengphy.2006.12.001

Budinsky, F., Steinberg, D., Merks, E., Ellersick, R., & Grose, T. J. (2004). *Eclipse Modeling Framework*. Reading, MA: Addison Wesley.

Buschmann, F., Henney, K., & Schmidt, D. C. (2007). *Pattern-Oriented Software Architecture 4: A Pattern Language for Distributed Computing*. New York: John Wiley & Sons Inc.

Chazko, Z., & Ahmad, F. (2005). Wireless Sensor Network Based System for Fire Endangered Areas. In *Proceedings of the Third Intl. Conf. on Information Technology and Applications (ICITA'05) Volume 2* (pp. 203-207). Washington DC: IEEE Computer Society.

Crossbow Technology, Inc. (2008). *MICAz Datasheet*. Retrieved January 29, 2009, from http://www.xbow.com/Products/Product_pdf_files/Wireless_pdf/MICAz_Datasheet.pdf

Czarnecki, K., & Helsen, S. (2006). Feature-based survey of model transformation approaches. *IBM Systems Journal, 45*(3), 621–645.

Dalal, S., Alwan, M., Seifrafi, R., Kell, S., & Brown, D. (2005). A Rule-Based Approach to the Analysis of Elders' Activity Data: Detection of Health and Possible Emergency Conditions. In *Proceedings of the AAAI 2005 Symposium, Workshop on Caring Machines: AI in Eldercare*.

Demiris, G., Parker Oliver, D., Dickey, G., Skubic, M., & Rantz, M. (2008, April). Findings from a participatory evaluation of a smart home application for older adults. *Journal of Technology and Health Care, 16*(2), 111–118.

Dey, A. K., Salber, D., & Abowd, G. D. (2001). A Conceptual Framework and a Toolkit Supporting the Rapid Prototyping of Context-Aware Applications. *Human-Computer Interaction Journal, 16*(2-4), 97–166. doi:10.1207/S15327051HCI16234_02

Duda, R. O., Hart, P. E., & Stork, D. G. (2001). *Pattern Classification (Vol. 2)*. New York: John Wiley & Sons, Inc.

*Eclipse Modeling project*. (2009). Retrieved January 23, 2009, from http://www.eclipse.org/modeling/

Endsley, M. R. (2000). Theoretical Underpinnings of Situation Awareness: A Critical Review. In M. R. Endsley, & D. J. Garland, Situation Awareness Analysis and Measurement (pp. 3-32). Mahwah, NJ: Lawrence Erlbaum Associates.

Ferscha, A. (2007). Informative Art Display Metaphors. In *Proceedings of the 4th International Conference on Universal Access in Human-Computer Interaction (UAHCI 2007)*, (pp. 82-92). Beijing, China: Springer LNCS.

France, R., & Rumpe, B. (2007). Model-driven Development of Complex Software: A Research Roadmap. In *Proceedings of 29th Inernational Conference on Software Engineering*. Washington, DC: IEEE Computer Society.

Hill, J., Szewczyk, R., Woo, A., Hollar, S., Culler, D., & Pister, K. (2000). System architecture directions for networked sensors. *Proceedings of the 9th Intl. Conf. on Architectural Support for Programming Languages and Operating Systems.* Cambridge, MA: ACM Press.

Intanagonwiwat, C., Govindan, R., & Estrin, D. (2000). Directed diffusion: A scalable and robust communication paradigm for sensor networks. In *Proceedings of 6th Annual Intl. Conf. on Mobile Computing and Networking.* Boston.

Jouault, F., & Kurtev, I. (2005). Transforming Models with ATL. In Proceedings of Model Transformations in Practice Workshop of MODELS'05.

Karl, H., & Willig, A. (2005). *Protocols and Architectures for Wireless Sensor Networks.* New York: Wiley. doi:10.1002/0470095121

Karp, B., & Kung, H. T. (2000). *GPSR: greedy perimeter stateless routing for wireless networks* (pp. 243–254). MOBICOM.

Klein, M., Schmidt, A., & Lauer, R. (2007). Ontology-Centred Design of an Ambient Middleware for Assisted Living: The Case of SOPRANO. In T. Kirste, B. König-Ries, & R. Salomon (Ed.), *Towards Ambient Intelligence: Methods for Cooperating Ensembles in Ubiquitous Environments (AIM-CU), Proceedings of the 30th Annual German Conference on Artificial Intelligence (KI 2007).* Osnabrück.

Köngis, A. (2005). Model Transformation with Triple Graph Grammars. *In Proceedings of Model Transformations in Practice Workshop at MoDELS Conference.* Montego Bay, Jamaica.

Krummenacher, R., & Strang, T. (2007). Ontology-Based Context Modeling. In *Proceedings of Context Awareness for Proactive Systems (CAPS 2007),* Guildford, UK.

Kuhn, T., Gotzhein, R., & Webel, C. (2006). Model-Driven Development with SDL - Process, Tools, and Experiences. In O. Nierstrasz, J. Whittle, D. Harel, & G. Reggio (Ed.), *Proceedings of the 9th Intl. Conf. on Model Driven Engineering Languages and Systems.* (LNCS, pp. 83-97). Berlin: Springer Verlag.

Kühner, J. (2008). *Expert. NET Micro Framework.* New York: APRESS.

Kulik, J., Heinzelman, W., & Balakrishnan, H. (2002). Negotiation-based protocols for disseminating information in wireless sensor networks. [New York: ACM.]. *Wireless Networks,* 169–185. doi:10.1023/A:1013715909417

Kurschl, W., Mitsch, S., Schönböck, J., & Beer, W. (2008). Modeling Wireless Sensor Networks based Context-Aware Emergency Coordination Systems. In *Proceedings of the 10th Intl. Conf. on Information Integration and Web-based Applications & Services (iiWAS2008)* (pp. 117-122). Linz, Austria: ACM Press.

Levis, P., Madden, S., Polastre, J., Szewczyk, R., Whitehouse, K., & Woo, A. (2005). TinyOS: An Operating System for Wireless Sensor Networks. In Weber, W., Rabaey, J., & Aarts, E. (Eds.), *Ambient Intelligence.* doi:10.1007/3-540-27139-2_7

Lewis, F. L. (2005). Wireless Sensor Networks. In Cook, D. J., & Das, S. K. (Eds.), *Smart Environments - Technology, Protocols, and Applications* (pp. 13–46). Mahwah, NJ: John Wiley & Sons.

Losilla, F., Vicente-Chicote, C., Alvarez, B., Iborra, A., & Sanchez, P. (2007). Wireless Sensor Network Application Development: An Architecture Centric MDE Approach. In *Proceedings of the First European Conference on Software Architecture* (S. 179-194). Madrid, Spain: Springer.

*mediniQVT.* (2009). Retrieved January 21, 2009, from ikv++ technologies AG: http://projects.ikv.de/qvt

Miller, J., & Mukerji, J. (2006, March). *MDA Guide Version 1.0.1*. Retrieved January 21, 2009, from http://www.omg.org/docs/omg/03-06-01.pdf

Mini, R. A., Loureiro, A., & Nath, B. (2005). A State-Based Energy Dissipation Model for Wireless Sensor Nodes. In *Proceedings of the 10th IEEE Conference on Emerging Technologies in Factory Automation*. Catania, Italy: IEEE Computer Society.

Muras, J., Cahill, V., & Stokes, E. (2006). A taxonomy of pervasive healthcare systems. In *Pervasive Health Conference and Workshops*, (pp. 1-10).

Nehmer, J., Becker, M., Karshmer, A. I., & Lamm, R. (2006). Living Assistance Systems - An Ambient Intelligence Approach. In *Proceedings of the 28th Intl. Conf. on Software Engineering* (pp. 43-50). Shanghai, China: ACM Press.

Nick, M., & Becker, M. (2007). A Hybrid Approach to Intelligent Living Assistance. In *Proceedings of the 7th Intl. Conf. on Hybrid Intelligent Systems* (pp. 283-289). Washington, DC: IEEE Computer Society.

Pomberger, G., & Weinreich, R. (1994). The role of prototyping in software development. In *Proceedings of the 13th Intl. Conf. on Technology of Object-Oriented Languages and Systems*. Versailles, France: Prentice Hall.

QVT. (2008, April). Retrieved January 23, 2009, from Meta Object Facility (MOF) 2.0 Query/View/Transformation Specification: http://www.omg.org/docs/formal/08-04-03.pdf

Rantz, M. J., Marek, K. D., Aud, M., Tyrer, H. W., Skubic, M., & Demiris, G. (2005). A Technology and Nursing Collaboration to Help Older Adults Age in Place. *Nursing Outlook, 53*(1), 40–45. doi:10.1016/j.outlook.2004.05.004

Rantz, M. J., Skubic, M., Miller, S. J., & Krampe, J. (2008). Using Technology to Enhance Aging in Place. In *Proceedings of the International Conference on Smart Home and Health Telematics* (pp. 169-176). Berlin: Springer-Verlag.

Ratnasamy, S., Karp, B., Yin, L., Yu, F., Estrin, D., Govindan, R., et al. (2002). GHT: A geographic Hash Table for Data-Centric Storage. In *Proceedings of the First ACM Intl. Workshop on Wireless Sensor Networks and Applications* (pp. 78-87). Atlanta, GA: ACM.

Reiter, T. (2008). *T.R.O.P.I.C.: Transformations On Petri Nets In Color*. PhD Thesis, Johannes Kepler University, Faculty of Bioinformatics, Linz.

Römer, K. (2005). *Time Synchronization and Localization in Sensor Networks*. Phd Thesis, Swiss Federal Institute of Technology Zürich (ETH Zürich), Zürich, Schweiz.

Schauerhuber, A., Schwinger, W., Retschitzegger, W., Wimmer, M., & Kappl, G. (2007). *A Survey on Web Modeling Approaches for Ubiquitous Web Applications*. Vienna: Vienna University of Technology.

Schiffer, S. (1998). *Visuelle Programmierung*. Phd Thesis, Johannes Kepler University, Linz.

Schwinger, W., Grün, C., Pröll, B., & Retschitzegger, W. (2008). Context-Awareness in Mobile Tourism Guides. In Khalil-Ibrahim, I. (Ed.), *Handbook of Research in Mobile Multimedia*. Hershey, PA: IGI Global.

Sentilla Corporation. (2009). *Sentilla Developer Community*. Retrieved January 29, 2009, from http://www.sentilla.com/developer.html

Shnayder, V., Chen, B.-R., Lorincz, K., Fulford-Jones, T. R., & Welsh, M. (2005). *Sensor Networks for Medical Care*. Harvard University, Division of Engineering and Applied Sciences.

SOPRANO Consortium. (2007). *Review state-of-the-art and market analysis.* Deliverable D1.1.2.

Stahl, T., Völter, M., Efftinge, S., & Haase, A. (2007). Modellgetriebene Softwareentwicklung (Vol. 2). Heidelberg, Germany: dpunkt.verlag.

Stankovic, J. A., Lee, I., Mok, A., & Rajkumar, R. (2005, November). Opportunities and Obligations for Physical Computing Systems. *IEEE Computer, 38*(11), 23–31.

Strang, T., & Linnhoff-Popien, C. (2004). A Context Modeling Survey. *Proceedings of the 1st Intl. Workshop on Advanced Context Modelling, Reasoning And Management at UbiComp.* Nottingham, England.

Taentzer, G. (2004). *AGG: A Graph Transformation Environment for Modeling and Validation of Software in Application of Graph Transformations with Industrial Relevance. In 2nd Intl. Workshop of AGTIVE.* Charlottesville, NC: Springer.

Tyrer, H. W., Alwan, M., Demiris, G., He, Z., Keller, J., Skubic, M., et al. (2006). Technology for Successful Aging. In *Proceedings of the 28th Intl. Conf. of the IEEE Engineering in Medicine and Biology Society (EMBS),* (pp. 3290-3293). New York: IEEE Computer Society.

Tyrer, H. W., Aud, M. A., Alexander, G., Skubic, M., & Rantz, M. (2007). Early Detection of Health Changes in Older Adults. In *Proceedings of the 29th Intl. Conf. of the IEEE EMBS* (pp. 4045-4048). Lyon, France: IEEE Computer Society.

Varginadis, Y., Gouvas, P., Bouras, T., & Mentzas, G. (2008). Conceptual Modeling of Service-Oriented Prgrammable Smart Assistive Environments. In F. Makedon, & L. Baillie (Ed.), *Proceedings of the 1st ACM Intl. Conf. on Pervasive Technologies Related to Assistive Environments, PETRA,* Athens, Greece.

Virone, G., Wood, A., Selavo, L., Cao, Q., Fang, L., Doan, T., et al. (2006). An Assisted Living Oriented Information System Based on a Residential Wireless Sensor Network. In *Proceedings of the 1st Transdisciplinary Conf. on Distributed Diagnosis and Home Healthcare,* (pp. 95-100). Arlington, VA: IEEE Computer Society.

Völter, M., Haase, A., Efftinge, S., & Kolb, B. (2006). Graphical Modeling Framework. *iX, 12,* 17.

Wang, X. H., Gu, T., Zhang, D. Q., & Pung, H. K. (2004). Ontology Based Context Modeling and Reasoning using OWL. In *Proceedings of the Intl. Conf. on Pervasive Computing and Communication* (pp. 18-22). Washington, DC: IEEE Computer Society.

Wolf, P., Schmidt, A., & Klein, M. (2008). SOPRANO - An extensible, open AAL platform for elderly people based on semantical contracts. In *Proceedings of the 3rd Workshop on Artificial Intelligence Techniques for Ambient Intelligence,* Patras, Greece.

Wood, A., Virone, G., Doan, T., Cao, Q., Selavo, L., & Wu, Y. (2006). *ALARM-NET: Wireless Sensor Networks for Assisted-Living and Residential Monitoring.* USA: University of Virginia, Department of Computer Science.

Wu, C. W., & Tay, Y. C. (1999). A Multicast Protocol for Ad hoc Wireless Networks. In *IEEE MILCOM'99.* AMRIS.

Zhang, D., Gu, T., & Wang, X. (2005). Enabling context-aware Smart Home with Semantic Web Technologies. *International Journal of Human-friendly Welfare Robotic Systems, 4*(6).

Zhao, F., & Guibas, L. (2004). *Wireless Sensor Networks - An Information Processing Approach.* San Francisco: Morgan Kaufmann.

# Chapter 13
# Designing Pervasive Healthcare Applications in the Home

**Toshiyo Tamura**
*Chiba University Japan*

**Isao Mizukura**
*Chiba University Japan*

**Yutaka Kimura**
*Kansai Medical Univeristy Japan*

**Haruyuki Tatsumi**
*Sapporo Medical University Japan*

## ABSTRACT

*The authors propose a new home health care system for the acquisition and transmission of data from ordinary home health care appliances, such as blood pressure monitors and weight balances. In this chapter, they briefly explain a standard protocol for data collection and a simple interface to accommodate different monitoring systems that make use of different data protocols. The system provides for one-way data transmission, thus saving power and extending to CCITT. Their standardized protocol was verified during a 1-year field test involving 20 households in Japan. Data transmission errors between home health care devices and the home gateway were 4.21/day with their newly developed standard protocol. Over a 1-year period, they collected and analyzed data from 241,000 separate sources associated with both healthy, home-based patients and chronically ill, clinic-based patients, the latter with physician intervention. They evaluated some possible applications for collecting daily health care data and introduce some of their findings, relating primarily to body weight and blood pressure monitoring for elderly subjects in their own homes.*

## INTRODUCTION

Health promotion is a critical process that enables people to increase control over and to improve their health and health determinants. Currently, this capability is provided via assistive technology through information communication technology (ICT), which supports medical and health care services such as electronic healthcare and telemedicine. Us-

DOI: 10.4018/978-1-61520-765-7.ch013

ing ICT tools for health informatics can prevent disease and promote optimal health. Furthermore, mobile-health (m-health) applications deliver mobile communication and network technology for health care systems to improve a patient's quality of life. Finally, personalized health care will improve the safety, quality, and effectiveness of health care for individuals. Health care promotion enables people to become more involved in their own wellness, and the interoperability of several monitoring techniques assists in maintaining and improving health conditions for individuals.

New criteria in ISO/IEEE 11073 standards for medical device communication have led to the proposal of new health promotion goals to enable plug-and-play interoperability for personal health devices. These new ISO/IEEE 11073 standards address transport-independent applications and information profiles between personal telehealth devices and monitors. Current research has culminated in several proposals (Brennan et al., 2007; Chadwick, 2007; Galarraga et al., 2007a, b; Laakko et al., 2008; Martinez et al., 2008) although very little work has been conducted on the actual settings (Yao and Warren, 2005; Yao et al., 2005).

Recently, home health care users have been motivated to maintain their health and to avoid metabolic syndrome; in this endeavor, many people buy several home health care devices, such as blood pressure monitors, body scales, and pedometers.

Metabolic syndrome encompasses a wide range of medical disorders often associated with increased weight and obesity, which increase the risk of cardiovascular disease, stroke, and diabetes. The term "metabolic" refers to biochemical processes, some of which are readily monitored, that are involved in the body's normal functioning. Metabolic and behavioral risk factors are conditions that increase the probability of disease, and these risk factors are generally high in the elderly. Thus, we propose a new home health care system

to monitor such risk factors, maintain good health, and reduce disease in the elderly.

Home health care and home-based primary care have been commercialized for reasons of cost and convenience. Patients with chronic conditions are heavy users of the health care system, and ideally, considerable cost savings and improvements in health care can be achieved if patients maintain their health and continue to live in their homes. Home telecare and telemonitoring systems have been demonstrated, but are not yet satisfactory. Inadequate health monitoring has been associated with adverse outcomes, including increased emergency department visits and hospitalization, and decreased caregiver well-being.

Previously, some systems for data acquisition and transmission have been used to reduce disease, and some automated systems have also been developed, but high costs have prevented their general implementation (Tamura et al., 1998, 2007). Established automated systems include ECG monitoring during sleep and bathing, and monitoring for routine health care is generally an underdeveloped area. In this chapter, we propose a new health care system to monitor data from ordinary home health care appliances, such as blood pressure monitors and body weight scales. We also discuss some of the potential applications of this new system for elderly home-based patients.

## BACKGROUND

A system for automatic health monitoring in the home has been considered for health management and disease prevention. The onset of lifestyle diseases, such as hypertension, arteriosclerosis, and diabetes, is highly correlated with daily activities, such as physical exercise, sleep, and nutrition. Daily monitoring is important in preventing such diseases and in achieving a healthier quality of life. Although the monitoring of daily activities is not well established in evidence-based health care, many attempts have been made at installing sensors and transducers to monitor daily home life.

We have attempted smart house projects, which have been established at Georgia Tech (the Aware Home Research Initiative). The first development involved computer interfaces for the elderly. Primarily, the smart house projects concerned memory assistance and physical assistance devices to improve quality of life. Then, our group developed physiological monitoring at the smart house (Tamura et al., 1998). Problems in the smart house project include cost-effectiveness, regulation, physician involvement in preventative medicine, and intervention.

When the government and local agencies support the project, the system works well, but presently it cannot work properly without subsidization. A simpler and lower-cost system is required that does not depend on the support of government and local agencies.

One solution to generalizing the home health care system is a data transmission protocol. The ISO/IEEE 11073 standards for medical device communications define a family of standards providing interconnection and interoperability of medical devices and computerized health care information systems. Medical devices include a broad range of clinical monitoring, diagnostic, and therapeutic equipment. Computerized health care information systems similarly include a broad range of clinical data management systems, patient care systems, and hospital information systems. The ISO/IEEE 11073 standards, originally defined for acute care applications in bedside environments, are easily amenable to frequent network reconfigurations. Additionally, ISO/IEEE 11073 standards offer clinician-friendly plug-and-play operation, and provide robust, safe, and reliable communication for the critical application and association of a device with a specific patient. The IEEE 11073 criteria, prepared by the IEEE 1073 Committee of the IEEE Engineering in Medicine and Biology Society, was the first American National Standards Institute (ANSI) set of standards developed specifically for health care informatics. The physical layer and transport profiles were approved as ANSI standards in August 1995. The first hospital trial for ISO/IEEE 11073 was conducted at the McKay-Dee Hospital Center in Ogden, Utah, USA, in January 1997.

Personal telehealth systems, including remote patient monitoring and management devices, are being increasingly recognized as having the potential to help overcome this challenge of personalizing health care. By introducing wireless technology, cumbersome cables can be eliminated, enabling greater physical mobility and rendering the system less obtrusive and more ubiquitous for the patient. To establish a wireless link at the patient's bedside, the technologies being considered range from enabling a simple cable replacement to allowing real networking of vital-sign measurement devices, as in the context of body sensor networks (BSNs).

An overall definition of the IEEE 1073 family of standards is provided, describing mainly the interconnection and interoperation of wireless network with computerized health care information systems in a manner suitable for the clinical environment. In reality, data collection and transmission are rather complex. It is easy if only one device is used and data are collected on a computer. However, in home health care, subjects typically buy different health care devices from different manufacturers. Knowledge of the relationships among various physiological parameters, such as walking step counts, sleeping time, and blood pressure, is most important in assessing and promoting health. Thus, we compared data with the same time stamp. We propose a simple application protocol to collect more than two data sets easily. We explain our proposed network protocol and also show a similar study with HL7.

Finally, research in evidence-based health care has found some correlation between daily activity monitoring and the onset of disease, and identifying risk factors is a major subject of epidemiology. In general, this requires conducting interviews with or administering questionnaires to a large study population to evaluate the details of their daily routine, including daily food intake. More reliable and objective data could be obtained if an automatic monitoring system were available.

## METHOD

In this chapter, we propose standardized application-layer protocols for communication between home health care measurement devices and a home gateway, and we evaluate the performance of these protocols in a field test. We examine some possible uses of daily home health care data and present major findings, based on an analysis of our data.

## SYSTEM CONFIGURATION

The system consists of three parts. The first is a data acquisition system connecting the health care monitoring devices for health care data measurements and an interface for data collection. The second is the data transmission system, connecting the interface and center server via the Internet. The third part is a Web-based system connecting the Internet server to the subjects' personal computers and the terminals of health care professionals, including doctors, administrative dieticians, and physical trainers, if such intervention is permitted and authorized by the home subjects.

### Data Acquisition System

For the field test, the timing of data acquisition was carefully considered with regard to the behavioral patterns and daily routines of each subject. For blood pressure and body weight data, the measurements and data acquisition were most conveniently carried out once in the morning and once at night. Urine sugar was measured and transmitted after each acquisition. The step

counter data were acquired and transmitted at the end of each day.

The blood pressure monitor, the scale for body weight, and the urine sugar have an identifier button for the subjects to identify themselves prior to taking their individual measurements. Each device can accommodate up to four personal IDs for assignment to family or household members. The IDs were registered to the monitoring device or the interface, with appropriate attributes for each subject. Each device, except the scale for body weight, transmits the data automatically after the measurements are completed. Body weight is transmitted only after patient approval, with the push of a button. The system allows for the continuous or intermittent transmission of small or large data sets at specific times or intervals, as may be convenient or required.

### Data Transmission Protocol

A standard protocol for interfacing the monitoring devices and the interface are important aspects of this project. In general, each commercial home gateway has a unique communication system and users must purchase different communication adaptors accordingly. Additionally, combining or analyzing data from different instruments is difficult because each instrument has it own data format. For example, problems arise when trying to plot the data for body weight and blood pressure at the same time on a display. Combining and analyzing data from different appliances is also problematic because each instrument has its own data format and time stamp method. We modified the application, presentation, and session layers in the OSI model. We did not modify the layers assigned to controlling the wireless technology, which is still advancing and remains part of the present protocol.

The basic requirements of the communication protocols between the monitoring devices and the data collection interfaces are as follows:

*Figure 1. System configuration*

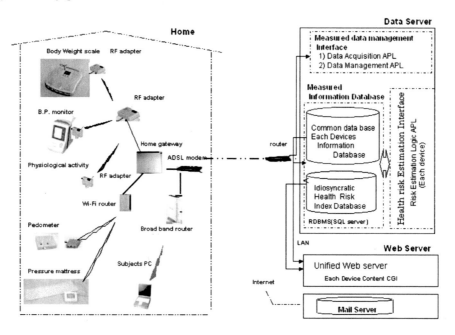

1. Data measured by several monitoring devices can be transmitted.
2. Newly developed monitoring devices and parameters can establish communication with the interface readily.
3. Both the monitoring device and the interface can inquire about health care information with each other.
4. Lightweight communication software is needed, considering often limited CPU and battery power.
5. The protocol defines the upper three layers of communication in the OSI layer model.
6. Monitoring parameters can be multi-informational, including, for example, English names, units, and scales.

In home health care, the transmission line covers data from multiple devices. Thus, the amount of data in the transmission line increases, as does the collision rate. The data capacity is increased more than 100-fold when only limited data, such as blood pressure, are transmitted. Because of the increase in collision rate and transmission capac-

ity, common unsynchronized data transmission, such as CCIV 21 or 23, cannot be used for a home health care network. The main issue is minimizing the amount of data traveling between the home health monitoring device and the gateway.

Generally, health care data contain a parameter name, unit, and scale information in every data transaction. We adopted a byte name (BN) code to reduce the amount of traveling data. The protocol between the monitoring device and the gateway was designed to minimize the total data transmission, accept new devices into the system, and exchange the byte name, registration of communication data information, and definitions for reserved words with the monitoring devices. The BN allocation table of each device was registered, and then data were transferred.

We uniquely standardized the registration and communication information formats based on BN codes. Each manufacturer registered the device code and device communication code to the gateway and then communication between device and gateway could occur. The manufacturer provides this program embedded in the software, wireless

*Figure 2. Summary of physiological parameters and data transmission times*

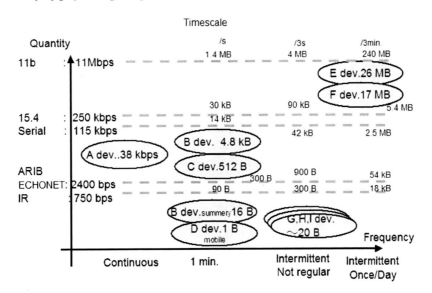

## WEB SYSTEM

registration, and an installation program on a CD-ROM. Thus, any manufacturer can participate in this program.

In the transmission of data, we have four services and three communication procedures. The sequence of data communication is as follows. First, device registration serves to declare the manufacturer name or product name of the home health monitoring devices. Second, information registration serves to declare code values to compress the data. Then, data communication serves to communicate the data using the BN code. Finally, inquiry communication serves to inquire about the information required for measurement with the BN code. Three types of communication, data indication without acknowledgment, data indication with acknowledgment, and the data request and response, are uniquely determined by the device. For example, for low-power battery devices, we accept one-way data communication, with data indication without acknowledgment.

To establish a field test system, we chose either IEEE 802 11b or ARIB STD-T67 and set the serial interface specifications between the application protocols and the radio communication adapter of home health care devices.

Collected data were transferred to the center server via the Internet using the secure communication protocol, SSL. The center server creates a database for each subject and plots the data graphically for display using the Web server.

To monitor a subject's health condition, a gateway that acquires data from the monitoring device is installed in the home of the subject. Collected data are then transferred to the center server via the Internet using a secure communication protocol. The center server creates the database and Web pages for each subject.

Subjects can check only their own vital data through the Web pages, after personal authentication by ID number and passwords. Figure 3 shows 1 month of data for blood pressure, body weight, and walking steps. It links to each device page by clicking. The clients can consider their health condition by checking multiple vital data points through a 1-day, 1-week, or 1-month view.

*Figure 3. One-month view of blood pressure, body weight, and walking steps*

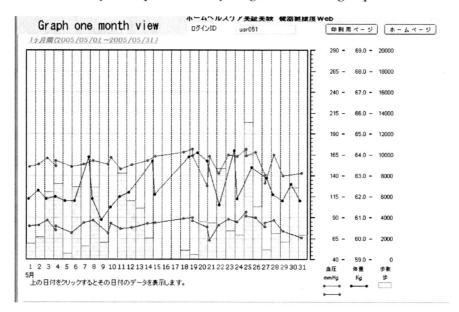

## Experimental Procedure in the Field Test

The subjects selected for the field test were patients at the hospital of Kansai Medical University and the procedure was approved by the ethics committee of the institute. We obtained written informed consent from all members of the 20 families, including both normal and borderline-type patients before participation. Subjects received no monetary compensation for this field test, with the exception of the reimbursement for the appropriate Internet service provider fee and electricity charges.

The conceptual design and operation of the first stage of unified communication protocols between the monitoring devices and the interfaces were executed from December 2004 to August/October 2005. We received no monetary compensation for the field test.

## Results

Overall, we automatically acquired and analyzed 241,000 individual data transmission packets for the monitored subject health care parameters during approximately 1 year of field testing. A typical example of the graphical data presentation method for 39 individual subjects from 20 families (1.95 individuals/family) demonstrated the overall trend in the body weight parameter over a 10-month period. The level of involvement for each subject was determined through physician intervention.

## A. Error Rate

Transmission errors are due to collisions of radiowaves, electromagnetic interference, and the power of the radiowave communication driver. To verify the performance of the protocol, we used the same radiowave driver and the same allocation of the repeater for radiowaves in-house. The outcome of the error rate between the monitoring device and the interface was 4.21 times/day.

## B. Feasibility of the System

Through extensive patient parameter monitoring in the field test, we observed several data trends that provide some interesting medical insights.

1. **Seasonal variation in body weight.** The subjects could observe their own changes in body weight and effectively monitor themselves with respect to causal factors, such as festive overeating, holiday binges, and responses to job stress. Our intervention staff changed the intervention cycle from biweekly to weekly in the event of overeating.

2. **Predictive information for the appearance of disease.** Data were gathered in real time, but the prediction of disease is much more difficult. Figure 5 shows trends in systolic and diastolic pressure. In the middle of July 2005, the subject measured his/her blood pressure in the morning and in the evening. After measuring blood pressure twice a day, systolic and diastolic pressures were diverse before an attack of transient cerebral ischemia. After observing this trend, we could estimate abnormalities in blood pressure. In such a case, we may be able to predict disease by the trend in blood pressure.

3. **Blood pressure changes by day and season.** Figure 6 shows the time course of systolic and diastolic blood pressure changes. These data show that systolic pressure gradually increased, while diastolic pressures remained about constant. The blood pressure in the right half of the panel shows the risk of disease. Additionally, Figure 5 shows risk identification from the daily blood pressure data. After increasing systolic pressure in the morning and in the evening, a transient cerebral ischemia attack occurred.

## DISCUSSION

A home health care network was successfully implemented. The data were transmitted smoothly from private houses to the data collection center. When various kinds of health care appliances in private homes were connected to a data collection interface, we could obtain several kinds of health care data simultaneously.

The proposed system has at least three advantages. One advantage is the altered role of the gateway. Current ISO/IEEE 11073 is normally a one-way data transmission from the gateway to the monitoring devices. Thus, the peripheral home health care monitor devices are burdened by carrying a large data load compared to that carried by the gateway. We improved the one-way communication by reducing the load on peripheral devices with a new application protocol. A second advantage of our system is that it reduces the data size and length. The volumes of stored data were huge and types of data were different: some were continuous functions and others were intermittent values. We solved this problem by reducing the large amount of data transmitted using a BN allocation code. The application of the BN code shortened the monitoring device code and the data length. Therefore, the total data volume was less than an ordinary data transmission.

The final advantage of our system is that the monitoring device can send the data with a predetermined sampling rate. Thus, the monitoring device does not always wait for the calling signal to arrive from the gateway. Yao et al. (2005) studied a similar setup with the Bluetooth module, but the operating time was only 10 h. The reason for this is the use of interactive two-way transmission. The monitoring device always works in the standby mode to receive the call signal from the gateway. For home health care, the battery-type monitoring device must operate for a full year on the same battery.

*Figure 4. Body weight changes by season*

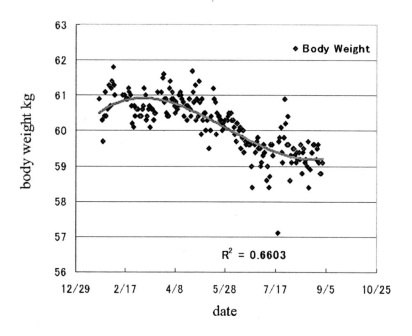

*Figure 5. The possibility of predicting heart attacks*

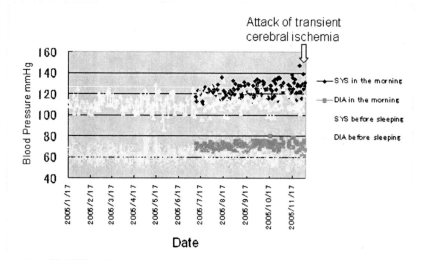

Furthermore, we can use the monitoring devices with different sampling rates. In our system, blood pressure was measured twice a day, while the pedometer monitored walking steps during the daytime. We could establish the plug-and-play solution with the proposed new application layer.

In addition, the intervention staff had to revise the measurement protocols several times. Nevertheless, the staff members were aware of the vari-

*Figure 6. Trends in systolic and diastolic blood pressure*

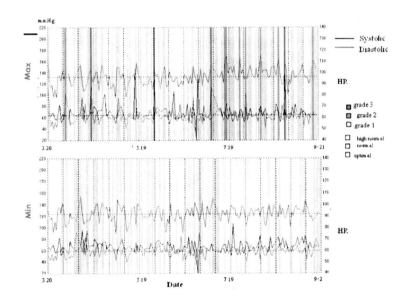

ous types of data, allowing precise intervention. The number and variety of interventions interfered with the subjects' lifestyles, and thus the subjects sought to avoid the risk by developing their own strategies in this regard. Further studies are needed to address the reduction or prevention of disease with long-tern data acquisition.

## FUTURE RESEARCH DIRECTIONS

Our proposal aimed to create a personal telehealth ecosystem with interoperability. Device connectivity to enterprise services is currently proprietary. In an effort to develop interoperability guidelines for the emerging personal telehealth ecosystem, the Continua Health Alliance (www.continuaalliance.org), an international alliance of more than 133 companies, has been formed (Schmitt et al., 2007a, b) The guidelines will be based on a comprehensive set of industry standards, which will serve as a blueprint for integrating a product into the ecosystem.

Continua aims to enable the alignment of different vendors and domains, focusing on

- disease management: managing a chronic disease outside the clinical setting,
- aging independently: using technology and services to enable patients to live in their own homes longer, and
- health and fitness: expanding personal health and wellness to where people live and play.

Within the context of the ISO/IEEE 11073 family of standards for device communication, this standard defines a common framework for making an abstract model of personal health data available in transport-independent transfer syntax required to establish logical connections between systems and to provide presentation capabilities and services needed to perform communication tasks. The protocol is optimized to personal health usage requirements and leverages commonly used methods and tools when possible.

## CONCLUSION

We propose a new home health care network system based on ordinary home health care appliances, including blood pressure monitors and weight scales. Data were successfully obtained with the new protocol using commercially available home health care devices.

Patients and family caregivers indicated a need for intelligent self-care technology, which supports early diagnoses of health changes, intervention enablement, and improvement of communication quality between patients and the health care system. Of these, only intervention enablement was commonly found in the home health technology items identified. An opportunity exists to meet consumer self-care needs through increased research and development in intelligent self-care technology.

Furthermore, home care involves more than simply transferring a particular technology from the hospital to the home. It requires transferring knowledge and skills to laypeople, and making sure that the home and social environments enable a safe, effective, appropriate, and personally satisfying use of technology. Otherwise, ineffective, potentially hazardous, and socially compromising treatments may be disseminated. Policies aimed at increasing the provision of home care must carefully integrate principles and resources that support the appropriate use of technology, and close monitoring of patients must be part of all technology-enhanced home care programs.

Finally, further studies are needed to address the prediction and prevention of diseases based on data obtained from home health care monitoring. The goals of home health care are prediction, prevention, personalization, and participation.

This research was conducted in close collaboration with the developers of the equipment used by the home health care model verification project. The authors thank the Technology Association of Medical and Welfare Apparatus (TRAMWA) for cooperation in a development committee composed members from academia and industry.

## ACKNOWLEDGMENT

The English in this document has been checked by at least two professional editors, both native speakers of English. For a certificate, see: http://www.textcheck.com/certificate/ZUBBgX

## REFERENCES

*Aware Home Research Initiative, The.* (n.d.). Retrieved February 1, 2009 from http://www.awarehome.gatech.edu/news/index.html

Brennan, P. F., Downs, S., Casper, G., & Kenron, D. (2007). *Project Health Design: Stimulating the Next Generation of Personal Health Records AMIA Annu Symp Proc. 2007*, (pp. 70–74).

Chadwick, P. E. (2007). Regulations and Standards for Wireless applications. In *eHealth 29th Annual International Conference of the IEEE Engineering in Medicine and Biology Society, EMBS 2007*, (pp. 6170 - 6173).

Galarraga, M., Martínez, I., Serrano, L., de Toledo, P., Escayola, J., Fernández, J., et al. (2007a) Proposal of an ISO/IEEE11073 platform for healthcare telemonitoring: plug-and-play solution with new use cases. 29th Annual International Conference of the IEEE EMBS. Cité Internationale, Lyon, France, pp. 6711–6712.

GalarragaM.SerranoL.MartinezI.de ToledoP.ReynoldsM.,(2007b).

*ISO/IEEE 11073 Committee.* (n.d.). Available at http://www.ieee1073.org

Laakko, T., Leppänen, J., Lähteenmäki, J., & Nummiaho, A. (2008)... *Mobile Health and Wellness Application Framework Methods of Information in Medicine, 47*(3), 217–222.

Martinez, I., Escayola, J., Fernandez de Boba-dilla, I., Martinez-Espronceda, M., Serrano, L., Trigo, J., et al. (2008). Optimization proposal of a standard-based patient monitoring platform for ubiquitous environments. In *30th Annual International Conference of the IEEE Engineering in Medicine and Biology Society, EMBC2008*, (pp. 1813 – 1816).

Schmitt, L., Falck, T., Wartena, F., & Simons, D. (2007a). *Towards plug-and-play interoperability for wireless personal telehealth systems. In* IF-MBE Proceedings of the 4ᵗʰ Interim Workshop on Wearable and Implantable Body Sensor Networks, *(pp. 257–263).*

Schmitt, L., Falck, T., Wartena, F., & Simons, D. (2007b) Novel ISO/IEEE 11073 standards for personal telehealth systems interoperability. In *2007 Joint Workshop on High Confidence Medical Devices, Software, and Systems and Medical Device Plug-and-Play Interoperability*, (pp. 146–148).

Tamura, T., Kawarada, A., Nambu, M., Tsukada, A., Sasaki, K., & Yamakoshi, K. (2007). E-Health-care at an experimental welfare techno house in Japan. *The Open Medical Informatics Journal, 1*, 1–7. doi:10.2174/1874431100701010001

Tamura, T., Togawa, T., Ogawa, M., & Yoda, M. (1998). Fully automated health monitoring system in the home. *Medical Engineering & Physics, 20*(8), 573–579. doi:10.1016/S1350-4533(98)00064-2

Telemonitoring, S. I. C. An Updated Review of the Applicability of ISO/IEEE 11073 Standards for Interoperability in Telemonitoring. In *29th Annual International Conference of the IEEE Engineering in Medicine and Biology Society, 2007. EMBC 2007*, (pp. 6161 – 6165).

Yao, J., Shmitz, R., & Warren, S. (2005). A wearable point-of-care system for home use that incorporates plug-and-play and wireless standards. *IEEE Transactions on Information Technology in Biomedicine, 9*(3), 363–371. doi:10.1109/TITB.2005.854507

Yao, J., & Warren, S. (2005). Applying the ISO/IEEE 11073 standards to wearable home health monitoring systems. *Journal of Clinical Monitoring and Computing, 19*(6), 427–436. doi:10.1007/s10877-005-2033-7

## ADDITIONAL READING

Carroll, R., Cnossen, R., Schnell, M., & Simons, D. (2007). Continua: an interoperable personal healthcare ecosystem. *IEEE Pervasive Computing / IEEE Computer Society [and] IEEE Communications Society, 6*(4), 90–94. doi:10.1109/MPRV.2007.72

Chronaki, C. E., & Chiarugi, F. (2005). Interoperability as a quality label for portable & wearable health monitoring systems. In Nugent, C., McCullagh, P., McAdams, E., & Lymberis, A. (Eds.), *Personalized Health Management Systems: The Integration of Innovative Sensing, Textile, Information and Communication Technologies* (pp. 108–116). IOP Press.

Galarraga, M., Serrano, L., Martinez, I., & de Toledo, P. (2006). Standards for medical device communication: X73 PoC-MDC. *Studies in Health Technology and Informatics, 121*, 242–256.

Horwitz, C. M., Mueller, M., Wiley, D., Tentler, A., Bocko, M., & Chen, L. (2008). Is home health technology adequate for proactive self-care? *Methods of Information in Medicine, 47*(1), 58–62.

IEEE 11073 Standard Committee (2008) Health Informatics – Personal Health Device Communication – Part 20601: Application Profile – Optimized Exchange Protocol.

IEEE Standard for Medical Device Communication (1996) – Overview and Framework: ISO/IEEE 11073 Committee.

Health Informatics (1998) – Point-of-Care Medical Device Communication – Device Specialization – ECG Component.: ISO/IEEE 11073 Committee.

Health Informatics (1999) – Point-of-Care Medical Device Communication – Device Specialization – Pulse Oximeter: ISO/IEEE 11073 Committee.

Health Informatics (2004) – Point-of-Care Medical Device Communication – Application Profiles – Base Standard: ISO/IEEE 11073 Committee.

Kennelly, R. J., & Gardner, R. M. (1997). Perspectives on development of IEEE 1073: 'The Medical Information Bus.'. *International Journal of Clinical Monitoring and Computing, 14*, 143–149. doi:10.1023/A:1016930319825

Lehoux, P. (2004). Patients' perspectives on high-tech home care: a qualitative inquiry into the user-friendliness of four technologies. *BMC Health Services Research, 4*(1), 28. doi:10.1186/1472-6963-4-28

Nijland, N., van Gemert-Pijnen, J. E., Boer, H., Steehouder, M. F., & Seydel, E. R. (2008). Evaluation of Internet-based technology for supporting self-care: problems encountered by patients and caregivers when using self-care applications. *Journal of Medical Internet Research, 10*(2), e13. Available at http://www.jmir.org/2008/2/13/. doi:10.2196/jmir.957

Personal Health Devices, P. H. D. IEEE Standards Association Web page: http://standards.ieee.org/, accessed on February 21, 2009.

Shabot, M. M. (1989). Standardized acquisition of bedside data: the IEEE P1073 medical information bus. *International Journal of Clinical Monitoring and Computing, 6*, 197–204. doi:10.1007/BF01733623

Standard for Medical Device Communications (1994) – Transport Profile – Connection Mode: ISO/IEEE 11073 Committee.

VandenBos, G., Knapp, S., & Doe, J. (2001). Role of reference elements in the selection of resources by psychology undergraduates. *Journal of Bibliographic Research 5*, pp. 117–123. Retrieved October 13, 2001, from http://jbr.org/articles.html.

Zhao, X., Fei, D.-Y., Doarn, C. R., Harnett, B., & Merrell, R. A. (2004, November 1). Telemedicine system for wireless home healthcare based on Bluetooth and the Internet Web site. *Telemedicine Journal and e-Health, 10*(Supplement 2), S-110–S-116. doi:10.1089/tmj.2004.10.S-110

# Chapter 14
# TUM-AgeTech:
## A New Framework for Pervasive Medical Devices

**Tim C. Lueth**
*Technical University Munich, Germany*

**Lorenzo T. D'Angelo**
*Technical University Munich, Germany*

**Axel Czabke**
*Technical University Munich, Germany*

## ABSTRACT

*In this chapter, the program of the Technical University Munich regarding implementation of technologies for an aging society is introduced. Various departments from the faculties of both technology and medicine are working jointly to actualize a technological basis for the development of assistance devices. Industrialized countries such as Japan and Germany will be facing an extreme demographic shift over the next 15 years. More than half of the population will be over 50 years of age. Belief in technological progress – initiated by the innovations of computer and the Internet – harbors the risk that the time required for necessary technological advancements is being significantly underestimated. This chapter describes the motivation and the concept of hardware architecture for implementation of assistance devices and for integration of pre-existing (or concurrently developed) sensors and concepts.*

DOI: 10.4018/978-1-61520-765-7.ch014

## INTRODUCTION

## Demographic Change

### Aging

Aging of the population and its respective challenges are impacting numerous industrialized countries, Japan and Germany in particular. In Germany, for example, the rate of aging for the society, according to the Federal Statistical Office, will achieve its most extreme velocity over the next few decades. They have attributed the reasons for this to the so-called "second demographic transition". This is characterized by a considerable decline in the birthrate in the years from 1965 and 1975, which came after the high-birthrate years of the 50s and 60s (baby-boom generation), which led to the emergence of a demographic wave in age distribution (Figure 1).

### Time Line

The demographic wave in age distribution will manifest itself, over time, in an ever-increasing average age. In the year 2030, when the baby-boom-generation reaches retirement age, society's aging process will have reached the highest level. The old-age dependency rate (the ratio between individuals of an employable age and those of retirement age) at this time will be 100:50. This is in contrast to the current 100:33. Every third individual will be 65 years old or older (Figure 2).

Even if the rate of birth and/or the rate of immigration were to immediately and drastically increase, this process could no longer be avoided today (Dorbritz et al., 2008b; Radermacher, 2007).

### Costs

In light of the proportion of individuals needing care (care quota), we can anticipate, for an aging society, an increase in the costs for such care. This care quota indicates what percentage of individuals in an age group is in need of care. It rises with an increase in age; for example, 82% of those in need of care in Germany in 2005 were 65 years old or older (Figure 3).

Based on the projected development of the population and the current care quota, one has to expect an increase of 37% in the number of individuals in need of care by the year 2020 and of 58% by the year 2030 (Dorbritz et al., 2008a).

Alone due to the registration of admissions into nursing home lists for services covered by care insurance (the German equivalent of Medicare nursing-care insurance, "Pflegeversicherung"), their respective expenditures grew by 16% from 1997 to 2003. This amounted to EUR 17.5 billion in 2003. Full-care in a residential facility, at 47%, represented the most significant item of expenditure from this total (Lange & Ziese, 2006).

### Productivity

From an economic point of view for the employable population, potential losses accompanied by work incapacity, disability and early death are not taken into consideration for the directly-assessed costs of illness. A feature of these losses is irretrievable years of employment, which amounted to 4.2 million in 2004. In comparison to 2002, this corresponded to a decline of 296000, which is principally attributed to a decline in injuries and poisonings, the most common cause for irretrievable years of employment. The second-most common cause for irretrievable years of employment is to be found in mental and behavioral disorders such as depression and schizophrenia, which increased by 13.7% in comparison to 2002. Back disorders also play a significant role, in that they result in half of the irretrievable years of employment caused by impairments to muscles, bones and/or connective tissue (Böhm et al., 2006).

*Figure 1. Age distribution of the population in the EU-nations (© 2008 European Communities. Used with permission)*

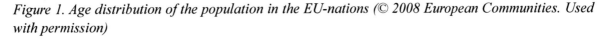

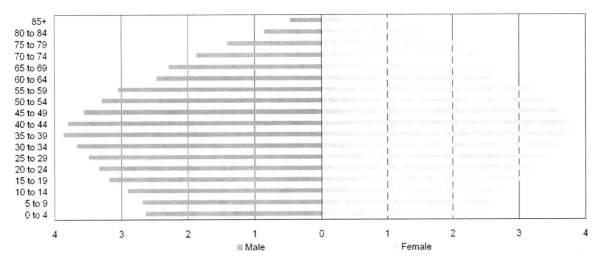

*Figure 2. Age distribution of the population in the EU-Nations 2030.(© 2008 European Communities. Used with permission.)*

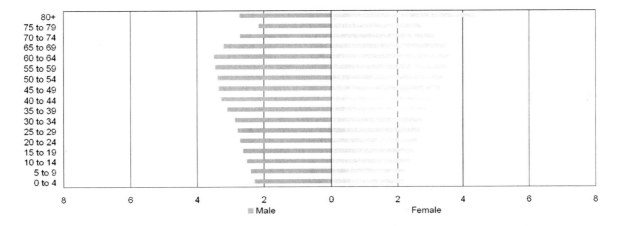

## Need for a Basic Framework

Due to this aging of the population, what awaits the German society and individuals for the near feature are considerable economic and physical encumbrances, which will be difficult to manage in the context of hitherto existing resources. New technologies for elderly care can contribute not only to an avoidance of the formation of such age-related challenges, but to a reduction in previously-formed challenges as well. By means of medical monitoring that is constantly on-hand (pervasive health systems), the appearance of age-specific maladies can be recognized early on and the duration for in-patient treatments can be reduced. And last but not least, individuals are thus able to lead an independent style of life, for as long as possible, within their familiar environment.

In order to achieve these goals at the necessary rate of development and the necessary scope, a

*Figure 3. Care quotas according to age and gender in Germany, 2005. (© 2008 Bundesinstitut für Bevölkerungsforschung und Statistisches Bundesamt. Used with permission.)*

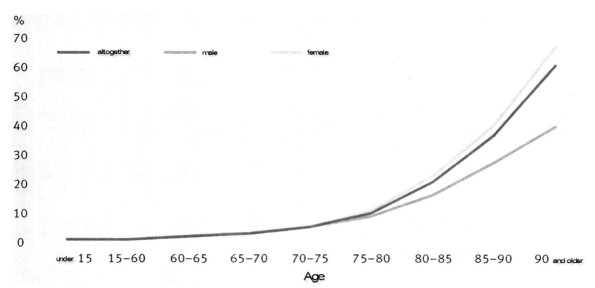

## Concepts to Use for a Mass Product

In order to assure that the developed solutions would actually be distributed and implemented among the population, it is important to evaluate the current state of the market and to understand, through what mechanisms today's mass products have been developed. It is equally important not to neglect pre-existing platforms; due to the rapid distribution of tech-products such as iPhone, iPod and Nintendo DS, millions of users today already own a portable calculation and communication unit that does not have to be newly developed and that has computing power, which was not even imaginable just a few years ago. Products such as the Nintendo Wii are also available in many households and illustrate how a rudimentary alteration to a product concept can incorporate entirely new target groups and get them excited about new issues.

common technological basis is necessary that would provide for the development of solutions for specific problems and create the respective substructure.

## Demand and Fields of Application

### Medical View

An individual reaches his/her highest level of performance efficiency at the age of 35, on average. He/she begins to physically deteriorate and mentally degrade thereafter. This is typically a gradual process, which leads at some point to either abnormal or normal limitations. These have been classified into physical, cognitive and vegetative impairments.

Physical limitations are widely prevalent in aging individuals and easiest to detect. A reduction in physical efficiency is a consequence of the normal aging process and does not necessarily have to lead to severe problems. Early detection and support of physical limitations are most often helpful, in order to keep everyday complications in check. Examples for physical limitations are: diminishment of muscle strength, limitations in the flexibility of joints and a drop in sensory faculties (sight and hearing in particular).

Mental efficiency also decreases with age. Even individuals who are in perfect physical shape can develop cognitive deficits. Early support for such individuals can assure that daily life within their familiar environment can continue to be possible, thereby avoiding an abatement of cognitive and physical capacities. The corresponding supervision is, however, connected with either considerable imposition for the family structure or high costs for care personnel.

The spectrum of cognitive efficiency losses spans from diminished learning capacity to the well-known symptoms of low, medium or high-level dementia. Some examples for this are the slowing-down of cognitive processes, reduction in memory capacity, and extensive loss of spatial and temporal orientation and/or communication skills.

"Vegetative limitations" refers to the degradation of the body's own self-regulatory system of vital functions. These can emerge separate from physical or mental disruptions. The most common are illnesses of the cardio-vascular system. By means of early recognition and corresponding adjustment in one's lifestyle, severe consequences can, for the most part, be decidedly protracted, or even completely avoided. Depending on the specificity of the vegetative limitation, it can occur that affected individuals perceive a decreased sensation of thirst, subsequently causing them not to drink enough. This can lead to dangerous dehydration conditions, which can have cognitive disruptions as a consequence. By the same token, the sensation of hunger as well as the need to empty the bowels and/or bladder can be lost. Such problems can be solved on the one hand by means of monitoring and reminding functions, which are carried out by the nursing-home staff in a nursing home. Or, on the other hand, these problems can be solved through technology. Self-monitoring by patients is another possibility, but is not always dependable – especially when an additional and (possibly) non-recognized dementia situation exists.

## Technical View

Innovative technologies for a society that is aging must be able to solve concrete, age-related medical problems in order to support people in terms of elderly care. The International Classification of Functioning, Disability and Health (ICF) of the World Health Organization offers a standard tool for the classification of health conditions, and this tool draws on the ability to solve certain tasks as an evaluation criterion (ICF, 2001).

One classification tailor-made for age-related problems has been utilized for many years in gerontology: the Katz Basic Activities of Daily Living (ADL) scale (Katz et al., 1963) and the Lawton Instrumental Activities of Daily Living (IADL) scale (Lawton & Brody, 1969). They ascertain the individual's health condition similar to the ICF concerning the ability to execute certain tasks in everyday life. In this context the ADL scale evaluates simple tasks such as continence or the ability to ingest meals, while the IADL scale evaluates complex tasks such as using the telephone or preparing a meal. These scales are quite suitable, through the definition of a problem to be solved, for ascertaining the demands made upon a technical system. Depending on the application scenario, technical assistance devices can be subdivided into several operational spheres. Based on human beings, they describe a continuously-increasing radius of action, thereby enabling a continuously-higher degree of independence. The spheres are grouped into body area network, home environment, local environment and mobility.

Technical support by pervasive health systems begins with the human body. A body area network is a network of sensors, actors and intelligent units that are worn directly on the body. The sensors are able to collect information such as body data, movement and activities concerning the individual, whereas actors such as monitors or loudspeakers can affect/influence the individual.

In this manner the individual can be interpreted as a system, according to a classic control point of view and, supported by recognition of departures from the nominal condition, can then re-establish this nominal condition.

The system worn on the body then becomes a constant companion and central element of the technical support. With this system, it is possible to monitor bodily functions, to detect accidents and, in critical situations, to sound an alarm. Problems can be solved in this context, which can be settled prior to the safety aspect of the ADL scale. Furthermore, activity profiles can be generated with this technology and movements or positions that are adverse to health can be detected.

Over and above the monitoring of vital functions, it is important to enable the individual to have an independent life for as long as possible in his familiar environment. It is necessary to this end that the tasks listed in the ADL and IADL scales can be completed. Through interaction of the body area network with sensors and actors that are installed in the house, many of these tasks are alleviated. By means of monitoring of the movements and activities within the house, illness-related modifications in behavior can be detected early on, and habits that are detrimental to health can be corrected. Equally, assistance with the orientation within the house, with communication with relatives and/or medical personnel can be provided.

After technical support in the house, assistance with the immediate surroundings represents the next step on the path to longer independence within the familiar living environment. Mobility within a tight periphery can often times suffice to carry out complex tasks such as daily shopping, visits to the doctor and clarification of financial matters at the bank. Through monitoring of the habits and the connection of classic mobility aids with the body area network, help with orientation can be offered and individuals can be provided with a sense of safety and independence. Finally, these systems are also meant to motivate the individual to a sufficient level of movement.

Use of public transport or a vehicle enables a far-reaching field of mobility and represents the final component for complete independence. Technical aids can support individuals in this regard as well, e.g. in the selection of the correct ticket or in the search for the parked automobile. Moreover, being able to use modes of transportation can motivate the individual to more physical activity. The time spent in the car can, for example, be used to carry out periodic, automatic health checkups by a sensor system integrated into it.

In Figure 4, the spheres relevant to an independent lifestyle – body area network, home environment, local environment and mobility – are illustrated. A selection of corresponding medical necessities and possible technical aids are also represented.

## Support Classification

Support is divided into the areas of monitoring, training, compensation and replacement. The first area can function as both care for as well as control of the progress of the disease. The last three areas are based on the assumption that a physical, cognitive or vegetative limitation has been previously diagnosed. From the moment of diagnosis, the highest priority is to stabilize the health condition and to delay its further degradation for as long as possible. This represents the only strategy for many age-related limitations, since, contrary to a normal illness, there are no expectations for either a complete cure or a complete regression of symptoms.

Monitoring describes the targeted observing of certain body parameters, performance data and patterns of behavior. The information attained in this manner is compared with previously known general comparative values and/or older values for the same individual. In this manner, these can be, on the one hand, divided into normal (healthy) raised values or values that are too low, and on

*Figure 4. Matrix of the technical and medical challenges associated to an independent lifestyle, depending on the sphere*

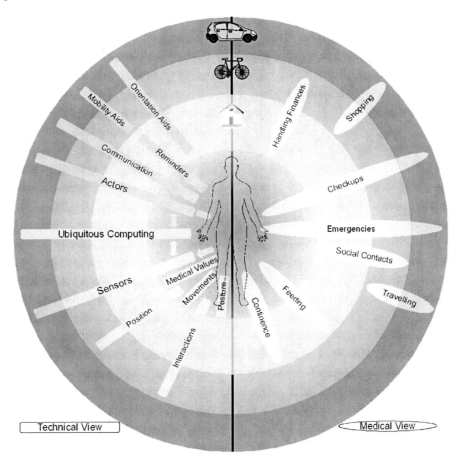

the other hand, trends can be identified starting at a determined value quantity. Monitoring represents the basis for medical diagnoses and can be executed by means of either a single measurement, or over a longer period of time. Well-known examples are

- Measurement of blood pressure
- Measurement of blood-sugar level
- Long-term / short-term ECG
- Exertion tests

The area of training refers to efforts to exert a desired effect upon the organism by means of targeted measures. In this manner, the individual's performance efficiency can be increased, main-

tained or re-established. A decrease in age-related performance can thus be decelerated and postponed. Training can include all areas of daily life. The most important area is physical and mental skills. A few examples of these are:

- Physiotherapeutic exercises for rehabilitation after injuries
- Movement training as a preventative measure
- Solving riddles as a form of memory training
- Brain-jogging as a form of training for logical reasoning powers

Compensation measures are targeted at equalization of existing deficits by means of technical aids. The tasks to be performed can thus be executed in a familiar or similar manner, without having to completely replace a detected weak point. Depending on the limitations of the user, these can constitute considerable assistance. Examples of compensation are:

- Walking aids for compensation of muscle strength
- Adjustments in the house infrastructure and furniture, e.g. stairway escalators for compensation of mobility limitations
- Seeing aids for compensation of eye weakness
- Small household aids for compensation of various limitations, e.g. swivel latches

Solutions are ideally found in order to completely equalize existing deficits, so that a life without further aids and in the familiar form is possible. If this is not possible, the next step is to completely replace weaknesses with technical aids, thus enabling retention of a relatively high level of independence. However, a few replacement measures can exert considerable impact upon the living conditions, e.g. dialysis. Examples for replacement are:

- Artificial retina implants (replacement of the retina)
- Endoprosthesis (replacement of joints)
- Exoprosthesis (replacement of limbs)
- Dialysis (replacement of kidney function)

## BACKGROUND

### Basic Concepts

The term "ubiquitous computing" is used a lot in recent research projects. But the concept of ubiquitous computing is much older than most people think. In fact it was coined by Wiser (1991) at the end of the 80s. This concept designates a model for human-machine interaction that follows that of the desktop computer. With ubiquitous computing interaction does not take place through an individual apparatus, rather through several intelligent objects embedded in the user's environment. The interaction ensues parallel to normal activities, and the user is not necessarily aware of it.

Ambient intelligence refers to an intelligent environment, which emerges through the embedding of such unperceived and functioning intelligent units. This forms the foundation for technologies for an aging society, since it provides the opportunity, for the first time, to observe an individual, his activities and bio-medical parameters 24 hours a day, enabling one to detect changes and, if necessary, to intervene with support. Weber et al. (2005) have summarized the experiences of numerous groups with a focus on the topic of ambient intelligence. In the first section, various applications and scenarios are introduced, beginning with the general social, ethical and economic implications of ubiquitous computing. The second section describes the basic required components and technologies for a low-cost, energy-saving and small-dimension network of communication and calculation nodes, and illuminates issues such as program surroundings, energy supply, data protection and security, compression procedures and algorithms for various applications. The last section describes the basically needed components and technologies for an affordable, energy saving and small dimensioned network of communication and computation nodes and illuminates questions like programming environment, energy supply, privacy, security as well as compression procedures and algorithms for several applications.

Becker et al. (2006) introduce a new approach in the form of Home Care Systems, which is meant to overcome the existing disadvantages of the newly developed Home Care Systems through the use of ambient intelligence with characteristics as described by (Weber et al., 2005). The most significant disadvantages are: an extreme focus on technology with disregard for the usability, "portable" systems that are too large, and a lack of awareness of context for most systems. The three basic functions of a Home Care System are considered here to be: treatment of accidents, an increase in independence and functions of comfort. However, the concept Home Care is used variably: the German medical technology enterprises understand this to be a continuation of and supplement for therapies at home, mainly in order to shorten the length of stay in the hospital ("Homecare", 2007).

Intelligent textiles play an important role for the body area network: the goal of intelligent textiles is to embed functions in articles of clothing, so that these do not have to be carried as an apparatus; rather they can be worn. Their beginnings originate with GeorgiaTech Wearable Motherboard or the SmartShirt (Gopalsamy et al., 1999). The next level of miniaturization includes implantable micro-systems, which carry out their functions directly within the body.

## Conferences

As the number of conferences related to pervasive technologies for healthcare is growing steadily it is very difficult to offer a complete list containing all of them. Thus the following section is to be seen as a selection of conferences that are considered to be of significant relevance to the topic.

The conference for the *IEEE Engineering in Medicine and Biology Society (EMBC)* covers a broad spectrum of topics, and many of these topics are relevant to the area of technologies for aging human-beings. A large portion of the scholarly contributions in this area are presented here. This includes the handling of medical signals, sensors, intelligent textiles, rehabilitation systems, apparatus and technologies for diagnosis and therapy, health information systems, telemedicine and commercialization of technology.

The *IEEE International Conference on Pervasive Computing and Communications (PerCom)* was assembled for the first time in 2003 as a forum for both researchers from the sectors of industry and commerce, as well as for developers who are involved with applications and technologies for Pervasive Computing. The conference includes all areas of Pervasive Computing and has clearly evidenced, every year since its foundation, continued development regarding the factors of diversity and quality of technical programs. It is considered by many universities and organizations today to be a first-class conference.

A relatively new conference is the *IEEE Pervasive Computing Technologies for Healthcare (Pervasive Health)*. Research is introduced here that can solve health problems, especially with solutions from the pervasive computing area. Treated topics are intelligent textiles, sensor networks, mobile-systems and wireless systems, network support, patient portals and data security issues, patient needs and usability.

The *IEEE Transactions on Information Technology in Biomedicine (TITB)* focuses on global information technology advances in medicine and biology and thus addresses the implementation and management of the broad spectrum of health care innovations arising from these developments.

Research results from German and European-funded projects regarding the topic ambient assisted living are presented at the (also) new conference *VDI/VDE/IT AAL Deutschland*.

The *Med-e-Tel* is a newly recognized conference, by the European Accreditation Council for Continuing Medical Education (EACCME), which concerns itself with the topics of e-health and telemedicine, such as further applications at the interface between informatics, communication and medicine, which should lead to an improvement in treatment quality, efficiency and availability, as well as lower costs for treatment.

To be presented at the *IFESS* are the most innovative advancements in the fields of functional electro-stimulation, neuro-engineering, neuro-sciences and neurological treatment.

The *IEEE European Conference on Smart Sensing and Context (EuroSSC)* has been taking place every year since 2006 in the European area. This comprises treatment of technology, architecture, algorithms, protocols, as well as user aspects of intelligent environments, objects and their applications.

Last but not least, the *Wearable Technologies Conference* under the auspices of the ISPO offers the opportunity, in addition to presentations regarding the topic "intelligent textiles", to introduce new demonstrators and their technologies in a special exhibition.

## International Research Teams

The same situation described for conferences above, of course, also applies to international research teams. Thus this section is meant to offer an overview of the different fields of research related to pervasive technologies for healthcare by introducing a selection of well known research groups.

Several groups have, in the context of their quest for an intelligent living environment that enables an independent and, if possible, longer life, equipped experimental living quarters for research purposes. These have the advantage of being able to test embedded sensors and actors in a laboratory-like environment with test persons, in order to integrate them early on into the development process (Henkemans et al., 2007). Well-known representatives are the GeorgiaTech Aware Home (Mynatt et al., 2000), the PlaceLab of MIT (Intille et al., 2005), the SmartHouse project (Barger et al., 2005), the Experience Labs of the University of Delft and the Home&Care Lab of Philips. A few of the approaches funded by Intel are introduced in Dishman (2004). The focus is put on sensor networks and embedded computers, and the largest challenges recognized are technological implementation, preservation

of the private sphere and demands made on usability. The Ubiquitous Home of Yamazaki (2006) is equipped with cameras, microphones, binary pressure sensors in the floor, infra-red sensors, RFID systems and acceleration sensors in each room. A room is reserved for technical control, and for human-machine interactions, Ubiquitous Home Robots will be used. It also includes context-sensitive functions such as TV channel recommendations, cooking recipe display, and an RFID-based system to remind an individual of objects that should not be left behind. Their vision includes the next step: the Ubiquitous City. Two living quarters were equipped with infra-red sensors and magnet-contacts in the Health Smart Home, in order to record the occupants' times of movement and immobility (Le et al., 2007). Wilken et al. (2009) present an approach that ascertains the behavior and activities of the occupants solely based on the use of electrical equipment, thereby enabling an evaluation of electrical-current usage within the living quarters.

Other challenges are faced by groups that are developing portable equipment. These can serve human-machine interaction in intelligent environments, but are often times developed as autonomous body-systems with their own functions. Fulford-Jones et al. (2004) have presented, as a part of the CodeBlue-Project, an apparatus for the recording and wireless transmission of pulse oximeter data and ECG signals. The MICA2 by Crossbow serves as a platform, TinyOS has been deployed as the software basis and two AA batteries are used as an electrical power supply. The MyHeart Project has adopted the crusade against cardio-vascular diseases with prevention and early recognition as its goal, whereby they have developed a device with which ECG data can be logged and transmitted via a PDA and Bluetooth to a doctor. Textile electrodes are deployed for recording (Villalba et al., 2006). The system by (Borromeo et al., 2007) records ECG data with normal electrodes, digitalizes it with a PIC and transmits it via Bluetooth to a Java-compatible end-unit. Through changes in the Bluetooth-protocol, it was possible to lower power consumption for data transmission from 35 to 17 mA. The system developed by Shah et al. (2007) fulfills a similar function: the EG1000 from the Firm MedLab is used as a sensor, while MICAz Motes are deployed for data transmission. Maitland et al. (2006) have developed a software-based activity logger that runs on a mobile telephone. This activity logger can differentiate between immobility, activity and car driving from the varying differences in signal intensity. Recognition of the recording of these conditions and the reciprocal comparison were in themselves enough to motivate test persons to increase their movement. The ActiBelt developed by Daumer et al. (2007) is deployed for the recognition of activity through acceleration sensors. By analyzing the movement data, it is possible to count steps and differentiate between running, walking, laying down, standing still and sitting. The system developed by Beckmann et al. (2009), integrated into textiles, deploys bio-impedance spectroscopy, in order to record information concerning the water level of an individual, enabling early detection of dehydration. For the detection of falls, Lüder et al. (2009) have introduced a system that combines both acceleration and pressure sensors.

Implantable micro-systems make very high demands on miniaturization and bio-compatibility; nevertheless they can offer the opportunity to compensate for missing or weakened bodily functions right within the body. Stieglitz et al. (2005) have introduced a concept for manufacturing nerve-prostheses as a bio-medical micro-system. This involves the manufacturing of flexible electrodes and substrata as well as chip-connection with the Microflex Interconnection Technology and the concept of modular, flexible micro-implants. Electrode-tubes with multiplexers, Siebel-electrodes with channel selection and the retinal sight prosthesis serve as examples for applications. In Schanze et al. (2007) the development and manufacturing of such a single-channel stimulation implant for the retina is described in detail. This implant is optically supplied with power through photo-diodes and stimulates nerve endings, which are connected to cells in the retina. With a considerably higher quantity and concentration of electrodes, a regeneration of sight information would be quite realizable for a case in which retina cells had died, but the optic nerve was still intact. The implant is produced with BioMEMS-technology and cast in bio-compatible silicon. Three implants have been tested in vivo on cats.

Numerous works were concerned exclusively with data transmission, for which a low level of energy consumption and high data security, in particular, had to be taken into consideration. As mentioned in previous works, motes from the MICA series of the Firm Crossbow are often times used in combination with the software TinyOS. Another approach is described by Falck et al. (2007) who have developed a system for data transmission over the human body. Due to the low data rate, however, only IDs are exchanged, which enable data security in the wireless transmission for all devices worn on the body. Another method for securing wireless transmission in a body area network is described in Venkatasubramanian & Gupta (2006): body parameters, which are measured by all network components, are used as a basis for computing a coding key. Juels (2006) provides an overview of the research in problems with data security in RFID systems. For the monitoring of activity, these are often times deployed in combination with sensor networks: the system presented by Ho et al. (2005) serves as a support for medication intake at home. In the aggregation of medical data from different producers, proprietary transmission protocols become an obstacle, which the Continua Health Alliance has attempted to overcome (Caroll et al., 2007). This integration of 133 international producers was established in order to create a standard (ISO/IEEE 11073) for transmission of medical data and to execute the certification thereof. Some exemplary working groups are involved in a general protocol, a protocol for cable-less transmission via Bluetooth and cable-connected transmission via USB.

For improvement of mobility, several groups are engaged in integration of additional functions in classic aid devices. Tashiro & Murakami (2008) thus describe a motor-operated wheel chair that is equipped with torque and pitch sensors, in order to control and exact exertion of strength by the user and to monitor the negotiation of a threshold. Chan & Green (2008) are also working on an intelligent walking frame: sensors were installed to gauge all of the following: distance and speed, acceleration, strength in the grips, utilization of the seat and oximetry.

## THE AGETECH FRAMEWORK

### Scope and Differentiation

The field of pervasive technologies and telemedicine for an aging society is quite broad and is currently being developed by numerous groups. The group AgeTech of the Chair for Micro-Technology and Medical Device Technology at the Technical University Munich is placing emphasis on the use of a common approach to the solution of several concrete problems. The focus of the group concerns the recording, assessment and use of information regarding the human body as well as activities and movements of human beings. With the aid of this information, improvements in diagnostics, cognitive support and detection of accidents can be achieved. It has been shown that usability and security of the private sphere constitute the decisive points in the development of such assistance home care devices. Regarding usability, the design of the user interface, size of the devices, economical management of energy, and minimization of the changes within said user environment are highly significant. Regarding security of the private sphere, the focus concerns the type of data transmission and data use.

## Approach and Architecture

### Team Structure in Munich

The team AgeTech of the Chair for Micro-Technologies and Medical Equipment Technologies of the Technical University Munich is structured in a way that corresponds to the various levels in the composition of an assistance device. These levels consist of:

- Development of the hardware platform based on motes and programming of basic functionalities of the software (data logging, communication)
- Integration of sensors and respective software interfaces on the mote (sensor integration)
- Integration of actors and software for the implementation of functionalities (actor integration)
- Implementation of hardware and software interfaces for integration into systems (system integration)

By means of modular erection of the basic architecture, various functionalities in the domains of sensors, actors and system operability can be simply integrated:

- Sensor integration
  - Acceleration: recording of movements and body position
  - RFID: recording of local positions and interactions
  - GPS: recording of the global position
  - Vital parameters: recording of the pulse rate, ECG, respiration, skin temperature
  - ANT communication: recording of data from devices that use the ANT interface

*Table 1. AgeTech team structure and projects overview*

|  | OFSETH | Fit4Mobility | Fit4Life |
|---|---|---|---|
| Mote | Communication, recording and processing of sensor data | Communication, registration of vital functions | Communication, recording of body parameters and behavioral info |
| Sensor integration | In textiles | Commercial sensors | Portable, on the body and in home surroundings |
| Function implementation | Monitoring of respiration | Vital function monitoring, mobile check-ups, adjustment of music and climate to the body condition | Activity recording, control of home technologies |
| System integration | Into portable device | Mobility unit | HomeCare-Unit |

- Bluetooth communication: connection with portable devices, use of the GSM network
- Actor integration
  - Loudspeakers, LEDs: simple reminders by means of optical or acoustic signals
  - Display: visually clear representation of complex information and reminders
  - Television: display through familiar, trusted and already-available devices
  - Laser: projection of instructions into the user's immediate field of vision
  - Communication: transmission of emergency calls, integration and simplification of communication
  - Household technologies: automatic adjustment of the surroundings to the individual's needs
- System integration
  - Home-Care Unit: Central memory and control centers within the house
  - Portable devices, such as iPod: Display and communication through existing technologies, mobile data storage
  - Vehicle: Mobile data recording and display

  - Mobility aids: Orientation assistance for local surroundings, support and motivation for more movement

The contents of the individual projects are briefly described in the following text.

## Architectural Basis

The hardware architecture used in the group to develop sensor networks is based on the application of motes. Motes are very small modules, which consist of a micro-controller and a radio unit for communication. These modules are deployed to record sensor data, to process it in an initial step and to relay it. Through the use of the sensor data made available, functionalities for the solution of concrete problems are developed.

## Hardware

A common component in all developed systems is the mote (Figure 5a). This serves to facilitate recording and initial processing of sensor signals and for communication. It essentially consists of a Microcontroller with digital and analogue inputs and outputs, and a communication chip.

Sensors are connected with the mote. These include acceleration sensors, GPS sensors, RFID reading devices as well as complex, commercially

*Figure 5. a) Hardware structure used. Based on this structure, various functions can be realized through the utilization of desired sensors and actors. b) Illustration of the integration of a few sensors and actors into the body area network and the house*

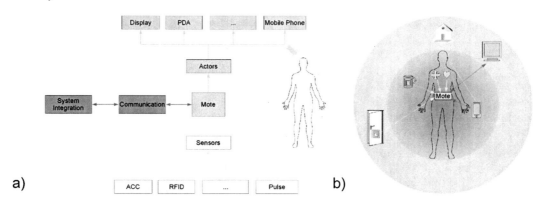

a)                                                                    b)

available sensors for the measurement of body parameters, for example pulse, $SpO_2$, ECG, etc.

In order to make relevant information available to the user, the unit consisting of sensor and mote is connected to suitable actors (Figure 5b). These can be, for example, output units such as monitors or signal LEDs. Additional communication units such as Bluetooth-modules can also be integrated for the implementation of functions on devices such as mobile telephones or PDAs.

## Architecture Integration

For the implementation of a function, the necessary sensors and actors are connected to the mote. The resulting device can be used either independently, or integrated into an existing system.

In Figure 6, this is represented through the example of a system to be integrated into an automobile from the project Fit4Mobility (which will be described in more detail later). The signals used comprise, in the context of a vehicle, measured bio-signals, vehicle signals and vehicle information. These are then recorded, pre-processed and transmitted to the display of the on-board computer for the implementation of various functions, for example to adapt the volume of music to the stress level of the driver.

## Exemplary Applications in Selected Projects

### OFSETH

The project Optical Fibre Sensors Embedded into technical Textile for Healthcare monitoring (OFSETH) is funded by the European Union. It has set as its goal the development of portable pervasive health systems to monitor vital parameters such as respiration and pulse oximetry. As opposed to previous approaches, which are based on the integration of electrical sensors into textiles, optical sensors are deployed with OFSETH. This approach offers the advantage of being able to use the textiles even in places where electrical wires would be of disturbance, e.g. during an MRI scan in a hospital.

The challenges are in the development and embedding of sensors into textiles and thus making it an intelligent textile. In the context of the project, a t-shirt with an embedded sensor and a portable module for data processing and transmission is developed, with which the gauging of respiratory activities is possible (D'Angelo et al., 2008).

The intelligent textile system is able to collect and transmit data about the wearer's breathing frequency and amplitude and consists of a T-shirt and a measuring unit with a wireless communica-

*Figure 6. The integration of architecture using the example of the Fit4Mobility project. Body signals are recorded and used in the vehicle, in order to enable independent mobility for as long as possible*

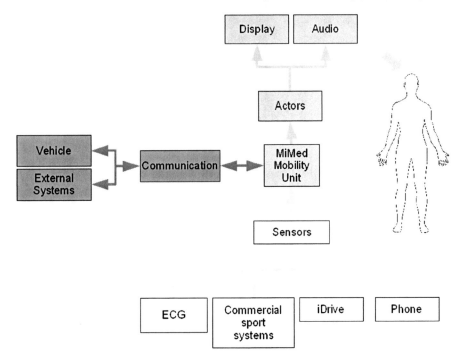

tion link. The T-shirt is worn like a normal piece of clothing, containing optical fibers. These fibers are stitched on it in a sinusoidal shape consisting of curves with small radii that attenuate the passing light according to the actual radius of the curvature (Figure 7a). The underlying measuring principle is the attenuation of intensity of laser light (Fabry-Perot, $\lambda$=1300 nm) passing through the embedded optical fiber (Corning SMF28e, 900μm tight buffer) due to macro-bending effects in the bent fiber parts. By analyzing the bending of these fibers it is possible to recognize the breathing movements of the wearer's upper body part. To measure the bending, the fibers are connected to a wearable measuring unit which will be located inside a bag on the T-shirt's side (Figure 7b). This unit contains a laser source to generate the optical signal passing through the fibers and two photo diodes, driven by two electrical circuits operating both the laser and the diodes. The first diode receives the signal directly coming from the laser

through an optical 50:50 coupler (reference path) in order to detect intensity changes of the light source due to temperature and other disturbing effects, while the second diode collects the light after it passed through the sinusoidal fiber sensor inside the T-shirt (measuring path). Both diodes generate a voltage proportional to the intensity of the collected light. An analogue to digital converter (ATMega128) is used to digitalize the output voltages. To transmit the collected data, a radio chip (CC1000) is connected to the analogue to digital converter. A similar device, connected to a serial to USB converter, receives the data and can be plugged to the USB slot of a monitoring PC. Thus, the only external cable the system needs is the power supply cable, which will be replaced by a mobile power supply in the next developing step. Using software designed for this purpose, data acquired by the wireless USB receiver can be processed and visualized on a PC's monitor,

*Figure 7. a) Sensor design of respiratory motion detection system. b) Module for processing data*

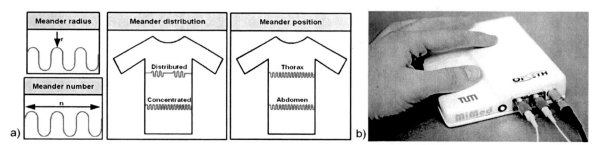

showing the current respiratory rate and warning on detection of apnea.

## Fit4Mobility

Fit4Mobility is a subject area of the project Fit4Age funded by the Bavarian Research Foundation and is concerned with the topic mobility as an essential and basic requirement for an independent life in old age. The goal of the subject area consists of providing technological foundations for an improved mobility for individuals of all ages. Human beings are hereby analyzed throughout their total life span, so that innovative technologies and products that support mobility can be respectively and broadly deployed.

The field "vehicle mobility" the group is working on focuses on the car as an essential mobility symbol of society. Many people spend a considerable amount of their time in the car. Therefore, this time should be used as efficiently as possible. It is the goal of this project to integrate unobtrusive bio-sensors into the car in order to enable monitoring of the individual's body signals while driving. Thus it will be possible to use the time in the car for health checks and to adapt the driver's environment to his/her state.

In order to evaluate whether integrated sensors in the car are able to record vital functions just as consistently as those sensors worn on the body, an experiment was carried out in a driving simulator with the company BMW AG. Furthermore, an assessment was made regarding whether or

not correlations between the recorded data and the driving situation are recognizable. For this purpose, sensors were placed to measure skin conductance, skin temperature, pulse rate and arterial oxygen saturation. In this manner the simulator data were recorded to illustrate the driving situation. While the measurements were being made, several driving scenarios were simulated, which diversified the stress-level of the driving situations through combinations of various levels of traffic density, dynamics of external traffic and additional mental tasks. The body signals were registered prior to, during and after the driving scenarios. Between the individual scenarios, questionnaires were filled out by the test persons in order to record the subjective impressions of stress-levels and condition of health. A stabile reading of the body signals throughout the whole measuring period was possible (sensors recorded valid data 98% of the time). An increase in the pulse rate was often times identified during critical situations. The skin conductance rose in many cases as well, but with a higher time delay and at a lower level. In one scenario, test persons were confronted with an additional mental burden in the form of a calculation task while driving. Overall, a higher pulse rate was observed during these tests. All test persons stated that the sensors represented either minimal or no distraction while driving. On average, the situation involving peripheral tasks induced statistically significant higher pulse rates than the other situations (T-test for paired random samples according to Fisher, and α-adjustment according to Bonferoni), in both absolute values as well as in observation of the difference when compared to the baseline. A few seconds after a critical situation (sudden merging or braking by other drivers), a slight increase in pulse rate can be relatively consistently observed. This effect did not, however, always occur and also indicates considerable variance. Several effects that occurred in connection with critical situations were not able to be recorded, since even normal situations for the driver, under certain conditions, were recognized by the simulator as being critical and were logged as such. A comparison between the baseline measurement prior to the experiment and the baseline measurement after the experiment showed no significant effects. Skin temperature, skin conductance as well as oxygen saturation indicated no discernable effects in reference to various scenarios. In consideration of the results from this experiment, the following applications were identified as being reasonable:

1. Registration and display of vital parameters in the car. The most important parameters for evaluation of the health condition are pulse rate, oxygen saturation and skin conductance. Blood pressure and ECG are equally significant parameters. For non-invasive, continual blood-pressure measurement, there are however no dependable systems available. Measurement by means of ECG demands a number of specifically located measuring points on the body, which is contradictory to a simple application of sensors integrated into the vehicle.
2. Adjustment of the driver's surroundings separate from the recorded situation.
3. Data export is possible with mobile equipment.

In the course of determining the desired applications, the required interfaces of a mobility-unit were developed and sensors for the recording of body signals were integrated into the steering wheel (Figure 8). The sensors record skin conductance and skin temperature, as well as heart rate through a pair of electrodes. The values ascertained are sent to the mobility unit, which then makes them visible to the driver through an interface to the vehicle display. The mobility unit is equally connected to the CAN-BUS of the vehicle computer, so that input data can be recorded in the vehicle data system and used to guide the system.

## Fit4Life

Fit4Life is a subject area of the Fit4Age project funded by the Bavarian Research Foundation. It is the goal of the subject area Fit4Life to lower the quota for age-related care, i.e. to enable, in a simple manner, older individuals to live longer and more self-determined within the four walls of their home. It is information technologies in particular, which have heretofore been primarily targeted at improvement of medical care within clinics, which must be used in the future to significantly improve and lengthen the self-determined life period within the domestic environment. In order to avoid problems of acceptance and the subsequent insufficient application of support systems, particular care should be taken that the technology is optimally adjusted to its user, easy to use, thereby securing the social connection of the older tier of the population. The technologies developed by the group AgeTech within the topic Fit4Life are meant to integrate modern technologies, through a central control system, for the gauging and assessment of vital parameters into the routines of domestic life. The "HomeCare-Unit" is meant to be capable of automatically recording data and displaying it at any time according to need in the form of a movement or activity analysis, in order to enable feedback concerning the condition of health of the occupant. For example, a portable device "Motionlogger" able to measure and interpret accelerations was developed to col-

*Figure 8. a) Integration of a pulse sensor in a steering wheel. b) Displaying of heart frequency through the car monitor*

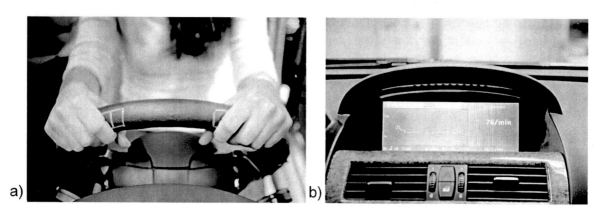

a)    b)

lect information about the user's movements and behaviors (Figure 9) (Czabke et al., 2009).

The overall system can be divided into a portable unit for the recording and documentation of activity conditions (the Motionlogger) and a user surface to display the recorded movement information. In the following the make-up of the Motionlogger is described. A 3D acceleration sensor from the firm Bosch serves to measure movements. This is read out by a micro-controller made by Atmel. The micro-controller processes the accelerator data and stores relevant information (activity situation and time) on an external flash-memory. The Motionlogger itself contains no user interface. Therefore, the stored information must be exported for display. In a current project status, the data are transferred to a PC for evaluation. This is accomplished through a USB connection. An SUB converter in the Motionlogger converts the signals from the USB to UART-signals processable for the μC. The USB interface is also used, in addition to the data communication, to charge the rechargeable batteries.

A simple window-algorithm runs in the micro-controller and this algorithm differentiates, on the basis of threshold levels, between the activity levels of inactive, active and very active (and/ or inactive, walking and running). To facilitate

*Figure 9. a) "Motionlogger" system for measuring of accelerations. b) Hardware structure of the Motionlogger*

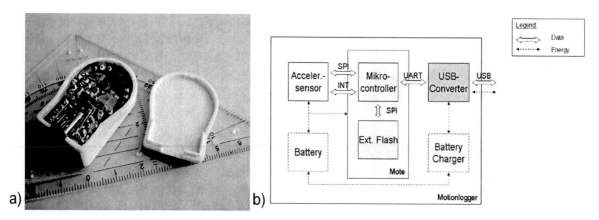

a)    b)

separate functioning of this classification vis-à-vis alignment of the Motionlogger on the body, the value of the resulting vectors is calculated from the three axes of the acceleration sensor as follows:

$$\left|\vec{a}(t)\right|$$

$$\left|\vec{a}(t)\right| = \sqrt{a(t)_x^2 + a(t)_y^2 + a(t)_z^2}$$

In the inactive phase is always equal to 1 g. The acceleration sensor is set to a value range of ± 2g and is read by µC with a frequency of 50 Hz. A window of time amounting to five seconds (250 values) is always observed, for which a status classification is given by the µC. This occurs in a fashion that is dependent upon the frequency at which the thresholds ascertained in the laboratory experiment are surpassed in the time window. In order to save resources, the ascertained activity statuses are not displayed on the flash memory every five seconds. Only when the µC recognizes a change in comparison to the status attained in the previous time window, does it store the new status together with a time stamp on the external flash memory of the Motionlogger. The data of the flash memory can be graphically represented, analyzed and stored with a simple program on the PC.

After the Motionlogger was developed as a hardware platform and the individual components were checked regarding their functionality, an initial simple algorithm was implemented to determine the statuses of inactivity, walking and running. In order to determine the precision of this simple algorithm, trials with five different test persons were carried out. In this way, the frequency of the correct status determinations was to be indicated by the Motionlogger over a time period of 10 minutes. Execution of the experiment was carried out in a double-blind comparative trial. A comparison of the trial protocol conducted by an observer with the movement status ascertained by the Motionlogger indicated mid-level precision of 85% as regards recognition of the status.

For ascertainment of activities and, most of all, interactions with objects, RFID technology, in addition to acceleration sensors, is also quite suitable. It offers the possibility to detect any contact with marked objects, and subsequently to document them. In order to make an RFID detection process possible, objects of interest must be furnished with a so-called transponder (tag). The tags do not require their own energy source; rather they are supplied with the necessary energy from the reading device via wireless connection. As opposed to other units, they can thus be used over many years without having to be charged at all. Moreover, the low cost for tags make this technology attractive for application in Ubiquitous Computing. Obviously, physical limitations exist concerning the maximum detection range. This depends primarily on the chosen frequency band, the size of the antennae and the transmission power of the reading unit. Subsequently, a compromise must always be found between size, detection range and rechargeable battery strength of the reading device, which is why the RFID technology is dependent upon further technical developments, before it can find everyday use in every private household. In order to evaluate the various technologies available, an RFID reading device made by Skyetek (13.56 MHz) was integrated into the applied mote platform. Since the size of a device represents a crucial factor regarding its use, considerable effort was made to make sure that the antennae, despite the minimal size of the device, was configured as efficiently as possible.

The resulting unit measures only 62 x 30 x 8.5 mm and contains flash-memory and a Bluetooth module as well (Figure 10a). Once a tag is detected, the unit stores its ID number together with the time on the flash-memory. As soon as the unit recognizes the basis tag with a specific ID number, it then begins to independently transmit the stored information, by means of the Blu-

*Figure 10. a) tagged door with RFID reader. b) Representation of the patterns of movement on the PCr*

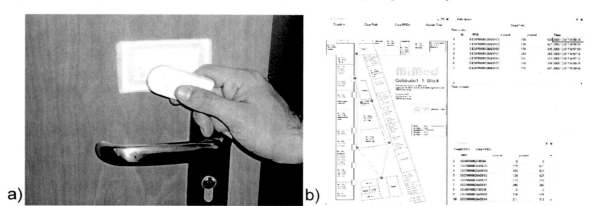

a)                                                                                                       b)

etooth, to a previously determined receiver. For this purpose a special PC program was written, which represents the patterns of movement of a test person upon any chosen map from day to day, and the information regarding tag ID, time of contact and duration of stay was then entered into a table (Figure 10b). As a trial, several individuals were equipped with the reading device and their movement patterns were mapped for half of a day. If the reading device is worn on the wrist similar to a watch, the reading detection range is not sufficient to reliably register tagged objects in the context of every contact. Therefore, the test persons were instructed to make sure that the reading device signaled, during every contact with tagged objects, detection of these tagged objects through the illumination of an LED. As a result, the tag contacts and, respectively, the patterns of movement of the test persons could be compared to one another.

## MART

It is the goal of the project Muscle Activity Recorder and Transceiver (MART) to develop an implantable system for the recording of muscle activity and further processing of collected data. Such a system could be used to measure activity habits, to control prostheses or other technical devices. The biggest challenges in this regard

are with the miniaturization of the system, the selection of bio-compatible materials, the radio communication and the power supply.

In order to evaluate the functionality, a system has been developed that can be attached externally to a person's leg, enabling the transmission of movement data through MICA2DOT motes and the software TinyOS to a receiving station.

The system consists of a combination measuring and transmitting unit, a receiver with USB interface and the evaluation system (PC). Found within the evaluation system are functions for memory and signal processing as well as graphic evaluation functions. The sending unit is worn by test persons, the measuring electrodes are fastened directly to the skin. The measuring unit picks up the EMG signal by means of bi-polar discharge technology and is able to guarantee a precise and secure detection of movement with a sampling rate of only 64 Hz. Such a low sampling rate is in contrast to the EMG sampling rate of more than 1 kHz. The low sampling rate enables implementation of very small, energy-saving micro-processors with a narrow communication band-width. This EMG signal is transmitted in the measuring and transmitting unit to the receiver, with a resolution of 8 bit digitalized, in real-time and via wireless. The signal is then processed at the PC as follows: First of all, signal alignment is carried out. Then the signal edges are submitted to an actively regulated damping process and finally, signal smoothing is applied by means of low-pass filtration. The EMG signal surpasses, whenever there is a muscle contraction, a pre-defined threshold level. For differentiation between walking status and stopping status, an additional time criterion is inserted. Muscle activity can be easily divided into the two conditions active and inactive with this principle. The system was experimentally implemented in its first application as a monitor for the analysis of walking activity of test persons. For this purpose, two electrodes are placed on the (calf) lower leg and a reference electrode on the front of the leg. The EMG activity of the calf muscles during the walking phase of the leg was analyzed and used as a characteristic for differentiating between the walking status and the stopping status. It was possible thereby to measure and analyze the walking activity of test persons in the course of a day.

After successful evaluation of the system, another system with low dimensions and molded in silicon was developed to evaluate the feasibility of an implant. This system can be charged wireless using an induction loop and the silicon housing is bio-compatible. The components that are presently available, however, are not yet sufficient for the miniaturization of the system required for implantation with sufficient power-supply.

## FUTURE RESEARCH DIRECTIONS

### Movement Sweater

A movement and acceleration-measurement system was integrated into a sweater, which can three-dimensionally record and evaluate the movements of the upper extremities and the upper body in all joints. Precise spatial and temporal analyses of complex patterns of movement are thereby enabled. The system will be implemented in order to optimize series of movements as they appear in sports or gymnastic exercises. Furthermore,

it offers the possibility to permanently record patterns of movement. It would be possible to measure, for example, whether an individual is sleeping soundly, is moving, or has left the bed and is wandering around the living quarters. Another important function is the possibility to develop a textile with integrated fall-detection that is able to independently carry out a distress call in the event of a detected fall.

### Work-Desk Exercises

Many people sit at a work station at a desk and work with their computers. They do not move during this time and do nothing for their health. Contemporary equipment for work-desk exercise makes it possible to use a treadmill while seated, in order to assimilate bicycle-riding motion. It is, however, a problem that movement of the legs begins to diminish during periods of increased concentration on the work at hand, while exercise activity that is too energetic usually leads to a decrease in cognitive output. Within the department Chair, a feedback system will be developed that uses a work-desk exercise unit to enable an individual to observe (in a display) his actual performance on the unit and to receive a reminder once the quantity of revolutions surpasses or falls below a certain pre-determined range.

### Networking

The long-term goal in this endeavor is to create solutions for concrete problems for a large number of people. The examples presented above can indeed provide assistance, but will only be able to provide the highest level of usefulness once they are intelligently networked with one another. In this regard, successfully evaluated partial functionalities are to be joined together into a modular formation of an overall system in the not too distant future. The key here lies in the creation of trouble-free interoperability among individual devices, and sensible utilization of the data obtained. The last point in particular signifies a considerable challenge for future development yet to be accomplished. For this vision of intelligent assistance devices can only become reality once the enormous quantities of data, generated by means of an uninterrupted record of various sensor values, are able to be securely mastered and evaluated.

## CONCLUSION

In the not too distant future, the social structures of many industrialized nations will be significantly changed. A demographic transition is approaching which can presently no longer be avoided. The corresponding impact upon health and care systems represents one of the biggest challenges for the future. A promising opportunity to confront society's approaching problems is offered by the development of novel assistance devices. If, through their implementation, it does in fact become possible to offer a longer life to a majority of the population, independent of third parties and within their own four walls, enormous sums for health and care costs could be saved. However, the pathway to that target is long. There do indeed exist a few promising approaches, but the expenditure of time and money involved in transforming a solution from a laboratory environment into a completed mass production product should not be underestimated. It is therefore important to transfer, as soon as possible, system approaches into a product status that can be operated not only by scientists, but by average users, thereby enabling evaluation of their suitability under real-life conditions. Subdivision into the separate categories body area network, home environment, local environment and mobility is a very helpful aid for being able to precisely determine the demands made on such systems. Moreover, it is also very important to know what kind of support the system should offer. For this purpose, the catego-

rizations of monitoring, training, compensation und replacement have been offered.

The group AgeTech of the Technical University Munich is working on the development of various systems, which are meant to support older individuals in their independence. The systems are developed in such a way that the areas from body network to mobility can thus be covered. The emphasis of the systems lies in the area of monitoring and training (i.e. motivation to train, if necessary). This foundation forms a modular construction based on motes, which enables a simple integration of various sensors and actors. The focus in this context lies on very small devices, which can hardly be noticed by the user and do not inhibit his activities. This is the case with, for example, intelligent textiles as developed in the OFSETH project involving t-shirts, or the vehicle with integrated sensors in the Fit4Mobility project. This should enable consistent and uninterrupted monitoring of important body parameters, through which disease-related changes can be detected early on. The earlier health deficits are recognized, the more successfully these can receive appropriate therapy. Ideally, the formation of severe bodily and/or cognitive limitations can thus be avoided through early diagnosis and therapy. If this can occur through the implementation of technical assistance devices, these will have been able to then achieve their goal of helping to support, as long as possible, a long and independent style of living.

## ACKNOWLEDGMENT

All of the works described here are carried out within the Chair MiMed and at the Central Institute for Medical Technology (IMETUM) of the TU Munich under the guidance of Prof. Dr. Tim C. Lüth. The projects Fit4Life and Fit4Mobility are supported by the Bavarian Research Foundation. The project OFSETH is supported by the European Union under the contract number IST-

2004-027869 in the context of the 6th Framework Program.

## REFERENCES

Barger, T. S., Brown, D. E., & Alwan, M. (2005). Health-status monitoring through analysis of behavioral patterns. *Systems, Man and Cybernetics, Part A, IEEE Transactions on, 35*, 22-27.

Becker, M., Werkman, E., Anastasopoulos, M., & Kleinberger, T. (2006). Approaching Ambient Intelligent Home Care Systems. *Pervasive Health Conference and Workshops*, 2006, 1-10.

Beckmann, L., Kim, S., Jungebecker, N., Leonhardt, S., & Ingerl, G. (2009). Entwicklung intelligenter Textilien für die Überwachung des Ernährungs- und Wasserhaushalts. In *Proceedings of 2nd German AAL congress*.

Böhm, K., Cordes, M., Afentakis, A., Müller, M., & Nöthen, M. (2006). *Krankheitskosten 2004.* Wiesbaden, Germany: Statistisches Bundesamt.

Borromeo, S., Rodriguez-Sanchez, C., Machado, F., Hernandez-Tamames, J. A., & de la Prieta, R. (2007). A Reconfigurable, Wearable, Wireless ECG System. *Engineering in Medicine and Biology Society, 2007.EMBS 2007.29th Annual International Conference of the IEEE*, (pp. 1659-1662).

Carroll, R., Cnossen, R., Schnell, M., & Simons, D. (2007). *Continua: An Interoperable Personal Healthcare Ecosystem* (pp. 90–94). IEEE PERVASIVE COMPUTING.

Chan, A. D. C., & Green, J. R. (2008). Smart Rollator Prototype. Medical Measurements and Applications. *MeMeA 2008.IEEE International Workshop on*, (pp. 97-100).

Czabke, A., D'Angelo, L. T., Niazmand, K., & Lüth, T. C. (2009). Ein kompaktes System zur Erfassung und Dokumentation von Bewegungsgewohnheiten. In *Proceedings of 2nd German AAL congress*.

D'Angelo, L., Weber, S., Honda, Y., Thiel, T., Narbonneau, F., & Lüth, T. C. (2008). A system for respiratory motion detection using optical fibers embedded into textiles. In *Engineering in Medicine and Biology Society, 2008.EMBS 2008.30th Annual International Conference of the IEEE*, (pp. 3694-3697).

Daumer, M., Thaler, K., Kruis, E., Feneberg, W., Staude, G., & Scholz, M. (2007). Steps towards a miniaturized, robust and autonomous measurement device for the long-term monitoring of patient activity: ActiBelt. *Biomedizinische Technik, 52*, 149–155. doi:10.1515/BMT.2007.028

Dishman, E. (2004). *Inventing Wellness Systems for Aging in Place.*

Dorbritz, J., Ette, A., Gärtner, K., Grünheid, E., Mai, R., Micheel, F. et al. (2008). *Bevölkerung: Daten, Fakten, Trends zum demographischen Wandel in Deutschland.* Wiesbaden, Germany: Bundesinstitut für Bevölkerungsforschung und Statistisches Bundesamt.

Falck, T., Baldus, H., Espina, J., & Klabunde, K. (2007). Plug æn Play Simplicity for Wireless Medical Body Sensors. *Mobile Networks and Applications, 12*, 143–153. doi:10.1007/s11036-007-0016-2

Fulford-Jones, T. R. F., Wei, G. Y., & Welsh, M. (2004). A portable, low-power, wireless two-lead EKG system. *Engineering in Medicine and Biology Society, 2004.EMBC 2004.Conference Proceedings.26th Annual International Conference of the*, 1.

Gopalsamy, C., Park, S., Rajamanickam, R., & Jayaraman, S. (1999). The Wearable Motherboard: The first generation of adaptive and responsive textile structures (ARTS) for medical applications. *Virtual Reality (Waltham Cross), 4*, 152–168. doi:10.1007/BF01418152

Henkemans, O. A. B., Caine, K. E., Rogers, W. A., Fisk, A. D., Neerinx, M. A., & de Ruyter, B. (2007) Medical Monitoring for Independent Living: User-Centered Design of Smart Home Technologies for Older Adults. In *Proceedings of the 2007 Med-e-Tel conference for eHealth.*

Ho, L., Moh, M., Walker, Z., Hamada, T., & Su, C. F. (2005). *A prototype on RFID and sensor networks for elder healthcare: progress report* (pp. 70–75). Applications, Technologies, Architectures, and Protocols for Computer Communication.

Homecare. (2007). *Berlin: Bundesverband Medizintechnologie e.V.*

International Classification of Functioning. Disability and Health (ICF). (2001) Geneva: World Health Organization (W.H.O.).

Intille, S. S., Larson, K., Beaudin, J. S., Nawyn, J., Tapia, E. M., & Kaushik, P. (2005). A living laboratory for the design and evaluation of ubiquitous computing technologies. In ACM New York (pp. 1941-1944)

Juels, A. (2006). RFID security and privacy: a research survey. *IEEE Journal on Selected Areas in Communications, 24*, 381–394. doi:10.1109/JSAC.2005.861395

Katz, S., Ford, A. B., Moskowitz, R. W., Jackson, B. A., & Jaffe, M. W. (1963). Studies of Illness in the aged. The Index of ADL: a Standardized Measure of Biological and Psychosocial Function. *Journal of the American Medical Association, 185*, 914–919.

Lange, C., & Ziese, T. (2006). *Gesundheit in Deutschland*. Berlin: Robert Koch-Institut.

Lawton, M. P., & Brody, E. M. (1969). Assessment of Older People: Self-Mantaining and Instrumental Activities of Daily Living. *The Gerontologist, 9*(3), 179–186.

Le, X. H. B., Di Mascolo, M., Gouin, A., & Noury, N. (2007). Health Smart Home-Towards an assistant tool for automatic assessment of the dependence of elders. *Engineering in Medicine and Biology Society, 2007.EMBS 2007.29th Annual International Conference of the IEEE*, 3806-3809.

Lüder, M., Salomon, R., & Bieber, G. (2009). StairMaster: A New Online Fall Detection Device. *Proceedings of 2nd German AAL congress.*

Maitland, J., Sherwood, S., Barkhuus, L., Anderson, I., Hall, M., Brown, B. et al. (2006). Increasing the Awareness of Daily Activity Levels with Pervasive Computing. *Proceedings of Pervasive Health, 6.*

Mynatt, E. D., Essa, I., & Rogers, W. (2000). Increasing the opportunities for aging in place. *Proceedings of the 2000 conference on Universal Usability*, 65-71.

Radermacher, W. (2007). *Demografischer Wandel in Deutschland*. Wiesbaden: Statistisches Bundesamt.

Schäfer, G., Baryn, M., Fritz, M., Augier, A. J., & Wieland, U. (2008). *Europe in Figures - Eurostat yearbook 2008*. Statistical Office of the European Communities.

Schanze, T., Hesse, L., Lau, C., Greve, N., Haberer, W., & Kammer, S. (2007). An Optically Powered Single-Channel Stimulation Implant as Test System for Chronic Biocompatibility and Biostability of Miniaturized Retinal Vision Prostheses. *Biomedical Engineering. IEEE Transactions on, 54*, 983–992.

Shah, P. J., Aroul, P., Hande, A., & Bhatia, D. (2007). Remote Cardiac Activity Monitoring Using Multi-Hop Wireless Sensor Networks. *Engineering in Medicine and Biology Workshop, 2007 IEEE Dallas*, 142-145.

Stieglitz, T., Schuetter, M., & Koch, K. P. (2005). Implantable biomedical microsystems for neural prostheses. *Engineering in Medicine and Biology Magazine, IEEE, 24*, 58–65. doi:10.1109/MEMB.2005.1511501

Tashiro, S., & Murakami, T. (2008). Step Passage Control of a Power-Assisted Wheelchair for a Caregiver. *Industrial Electronics. IEEE Transactions on, 55*, 1715–1721.

Venkatasubramanian, K. K., & Gupta, S. K. S. (2006). Security for Pervasive Health Monitoring Sensor Applications. *Intelligent Sensing and Information Processing, 2006. ICISIP 2006. Fourth International Conference on*, 197-202.

Villalba, E., Ottaviano, M., Arredondo, M. T., Martinez, A., & Guillen, S. (2006). Wearable Monitoring System for Heart Failure Assessment in Mobile Environment. *Computers in Cardiology, 33*, 237–240.

Weber, W., Rabaey, J. M., & Aarts, E. H. L. (2005). *Ambient Intelligence*. Berlin: Springer. doi:10.1007/b138670

Wilken, O., Huelsmann, N., & Hein, A. (2009). Bestimmung von Verhaltensmustern basierend auf der Nutzung elektrischer Geräte. *Proceedings of 2nd German AAL congress.*

Wiser, M. (1991). The Computer of the twenty-first century. *Scientific American*, 94–110.

Yamazaki, T. (2006). Beyond the Smart Home. *Proceedings of the 2006 International Conference on Hybrid Information Technology-Volume 02*, 350-355.

## ADDITIONAL READING

Barger, T. S., Brown, D. E., & Alwan, M. (2005). Health-status monitoring through analysis of behavioral patterns. *Systems, Man and Cybernetics, Part A, IEEE Transactions on, 35*, 22-27.

Becker, M., Werkman, E., Anastasopoulos, M., & Kleinberger, T. (2006). Approaching Ambient Intelligent Home Care Systems. *Pervasive Health Conference and Workshops*, 2006, 1-10.

Beckmann, L., Kim, S., Jungebecker, N., Leonhardt, S., & Ingerl, G. (2009). Entwicklung intelligenter Textilien für die Überwachung des Ernährungs- und Wasserhaushalts. In *Proceedings of 2nd German AAL congress.*

Böhm, K., Cordes, M., Afentakis, A., Müller, M., & Nöthen, M. (2006). *Krankheitskosten 2004*. Wiesbaden: Statistisches Bundesamt.

Borromeo, S., Rodriguez-Sanchez, C., Machado, F., Hernandez-Tamames, J. A., & de la Prieta, R. (2007). A Reconfigurable, Wearable, Wireless ECG System. *Engineering in Medicine and Biology Society, 2007. EMBS 2007. 29th Annual International Conference of the IEEE*, 1659-1662.

Carroll, R., Cnossen, R., Schnell, M., & Simons, D. (2007). Continua: An Interoperable Personal Healthcare Ecosystem. *IEEE PERVASIVE COMPUTING*, 90-94.

Chan, A. D. C., & Green, J. R. (2008). Smart Rollator Prototype. Medical Measurements and Applications. *MeMeA 2008. IEEE International Workshop on*, 97-100.

Czabke, A., D'Angelo, L. T., Niazmand, K., & Lüth, T. C. (2009). Ein kompaktes System zur Erfassung und Dokumentation von Bewegungsgewohnheiten. In *Proceedings of 2nd German AAL congress.*

D'Angelo, L., Weber, S., Honda, Y., Thiel, T., Narbonneau, F., & Lüth, T. C. (2008). A system for respiratory motion detection using optical fibers embedded into textiles. In *Engineering in Medicine and Biology Society, 2008. EMBS 2008. 30th Annual International Conference of the IEEE* (pp. 3694-3697).

Daumer, M., Thaler, K., Kruis, E., Feneberg, W., Staude, G., & Scholz, M. (2007). Steps towards a miniaturized, robust and autonomous measurement device for the long-term monitoring of patient activity: ActiBelt. *Biomedizinische Technik, 52*, 149–155. doi:10.1515/BMT.2007.028

Dishman, E. (2004). Inventing Wellness Systems for Aging in Place.

Dorbritz, J., Ette, A., Gärtner, K., Grünheid, E., Mai, R., Micheel, F. et al. (2008). Bevölkerung: Daten, Fakten, Trends zum demographischen Wandel in Deutschland. *Wiesbaden: Bundesinstitut für Bevölkerungsforschung und Statistisches Bundesamt.*

Falck, T., Baldus, H., Espina, J., & Klabunde, K. (2007). Plug æn Play Simplicity for Wireless Medical Body Sensors. *Mobile Networks and Applications, 12*, 143–153. doi:10.1007/s11036-007-0016-2

Fulford-Jones, T. R. F., Wei, G. Y., & Welsh, M. (2004). A portable, low-power, wireless two-lead EKG system. *Engineering in Medicine and Biology Society, 2004. EMBC 2004. Conference Proceedings. 26th Annual International Conference of the,* 1.

Gopalsamy, C., Park, S., Rajamanickam, R., & Jayaraman, S. (1999). The Wearable Motherboard: The first generation of adaptive and responsive textile structures (ARTS) for medical applications. *Virtual Reality (Waltham Cross), 4*, 152–168. doi:10.1007/BF01418152

Henkemans, O. A. B., Caine, K. E., Rogers, W. A., Fisk, A. D., Neerinx, M. A., & de Ruyter, B. (2007) Medical Monitoring for Independent Living: User-Centered Design of Smart Home Technologies for Older Adults. *Proceedings of the 2007 Med-e-Tel conference for eHealth*

Ho, L., Moh, M., Walker, Z., Hamada, T., & Su, C. F. (2005). A prototype on RFID and sensor networks for elder healthcare: progress report. *Applications, Technologies, Architectures, and Protocols for Computer Communication*, 70-75.

Homecare. (2007). *Berlin: Bundesverband Medizintechnologie e.V.*

International Classification of Functioning. Disability and Health (ICF). (2001) Geneva: World Health Organization (W.H.O.).

Intille, S. S., Larson, K., Beaudin, J. S., Nawyn, J., Tapia, E. M., & Kaushik, P. (2005). A living laboratory for the design and evaluation of ubiquitous computing technologies. In ACM New York (pp. 1941-1944)

Juels, A. (2006). RFID security and privacy: a research survey. *IEEE Journal on Selected Areas in Communications, 24*, 381–394. doi:10.1109/JSAC.2005.861395

Katz, S., Ford, A. B., Moskowitz, R. W., Jackson, B. A., & Jaffe, M. W. (1963). Studies of Illness in the aged. The Index of ADL: a Standardized Measure of Biological and Psychosocial Function. *Journal of the American Medical Association, 185*, 914–919.

Lange, C., & Ziese, T. (2006). *Gesundheit in Deutschland.* Berlin: Robert Koch-Institut.

Lawton, M. P., & Brody, E. M. (1969). Assessment of Older People: Self-Mantaining and Instrumental Activities of Daily Living. *The Gerontologist, 9*(3), 179–186.

Le, X. H. B., Di Mascolo, M., Gouin, A., & Noury, N. (2007). Health Smart Home-Towards an assistant tool for automatic assessment of the dependence of elders. *Engineering in Medicine and Biology Society, 2007.EMBS 2007.29th Annual International Conference of the IEEE*, 3806-3809.

Lüder, M., Salomon, R., & Bieber, G. (2009). StairMaster: A New Online Fall Detection Device. *Proceedings of 2nd German AAL congress.*

Maitland, J., Sherwood, S., Barkhuus, L., Anderson, I., Hall, M., Brown, B. et al. (2006). Increasing the Awareness of Daily Activity Levels with Pervasive Computing. *Proceedings of Pervasive Health*, 6.

Mynatt, E. D., Essa, I., & Rogers, W. (2000). Increasing the opportunities for aging in place. *Proceedings of the 2000 conference on Universal Usability*, 65-71.

Radermacher, W. (2007). *Demografischer Wandel in Deutschland*. Wiesbaden: Statistisches Bundesamt.

Schäfer, G., Baryn, M., Fritz, M., Augier, A. J., & Wieland, U. (2008). *Europe in Figures - Eurostat yearbook 2008*. Statistical Office of the European Communities.

Schanze, T., Hesse, L., Lau, C., Greve, N., Haberer, W., & Kammer, S. (2007). An Optically Powered Single-Channel Stimulation Implant as Test System for Chronic Biocompatibility and Biostability of Miniaturized Retinal Vision Prostheses. *Biomedical Engineering. IEEE Transactions on, 54*, 983–992.

Shah, P. J., Aroul, P., Hande, A., & Bhatia, D. (2007). Remote Cardiac Activity Monitoring Using Multi-Hop Wireless Sensor Networks. *Engineering in Medicine and Biology Workshop, 2007 IEEE Dallas*, 142-145.

Stieglitz, T., Schuetter, M., & Koch, K. P. (2005). Implantable biomedical microsystems for neural prostheses. *Engineering in Medicine and Biology Magazine, IEEE, 24*, 58–65. doi:10.1109/MEMB.2005.1511501

Tashiro, S., & Murakami, T. (2008). Step Passage Control of a Power-Assisted Wheelchair for a Caregiver. *Industrial Electronics. IEEE Transactions on, 55*, 1715–1721.

Venkatasubramanian, K. K., & Gupta, S. K. S. (2006). Security for Pervasive Health Monitoring Sensor Applications. *Intelligent Sensing and Information Processing, 2006. ICISIP 2006. Fourth International Conference on*, 197-202.

Villalba, E., Ottaviano, M., Arredondo, M. T., Martinez, A., & Guillen, S. (2006). Wearable Monitoring System for Heart Failure Assessment in Mobile Environment. *Computers in Cardiology, 33*, 237–240.

Weber, W., Rabaey, J. M., & Aarts, E. H. L. (2005). *Ambient Intelligence*. Berlin: Springer. doi:10.1007/b138670

Wilken, O., Huelsmann, N., & Hein, A. (2009). Bestimmung von Verhaltensmustern basierend auf der Nutzung elektrischer Geräte. *Proceedings of 2nd German AAL congress.*

Wiser, M. (1991). The Computer of the twenty-first century. *Scientific American*, 94–110.

Yamazaki, T. (2006). Beyond the Smart Home. *Proceedings of the 2006 International Conference on Hybrid Information Technology-Volume 02*, 350-355.

# Chapter 15
# Economic and Organizational Factors in the Future of Telemedicine and Home Care

**Giuseppe Turchetti**
*Scuola Superiore Sant'Anna, Italy*

**Elie Geisler**
*Illinois Institute of Technology, USA*

## ABSTRACT

*The chapter reviews the state of the art of telemedicine and remote care in the home and the economic and organizational factors that impinge on its future success. Because of the constraints of distance, costs, and availability of providers (doctors and nurses) in specific areas of medical specialties, the model of treating patients in the general hospital is losing its luster in favor of dedicated clinics dispersed in the community and remote care in the home. Such a trend of decentralization of medical services has been in existence for some time. Yet, although technologies are quickly evolving and the need for telemedicine and home care is increasing, the progress of this mode of delivery of medical services has not kept up with the demand. The chapter attempts to review the economic and organizational factors which act as facilitators and barriers to the rapid diffusion of telemedicine and home care. In particular, the chapter explores the case of chronic diseases, and also offers a valuable comparison between two systems of national healthcare: the Italian and the American.*

## INTRODUCTION

This chapter reviews the state of telemedicine and home remote care. We focus on the economic and organizational factors that impinge upon the adoption and implementation of these technologies by healthcare delivery organizations. Growing challenges to the healthcare delivery system include issues of constantly increasing costs, limited access, and the quality of care. In addition, there is a demographic shift in the United States and Western Europe, whereby the population is aging, thus requiring additional care. Such care is also increasingly being directed to home care (Park, 2008).

Due to constraints of distance, costs, and the availability of providers (doctors and nurses) in specific medical specialties, the traditional model of treating patients in a general hospital is losing

DOI: 10.4018/978-1-61520-765-7.ch015

its appeal in favor of dedicated clinics dispersed throughout the community and the remote care in the home. Together, all these trends are making a strong case for the application of telemedicine technologies to service the emerging needs of delivering care over distances. The progress of this mode of delivery of medical services has not kept up with the demand. We therefore review the economic and organizational factors impinging upon the rapid diffusion and utilization of telemedicine technologies and home care (Wickramasinghe and Geisler, 2008).

## THE SCOPE OF TELEMEDICINE

Telemedicine or telehealth is broadly defined as the practice of medicine over a distance. This means providing care remotely in the next room or across the globe (Institute of Medicine, 1995). There are two general modes of telemedicine. The first is remote monitoring, communication, and access to data. In this mode caregivers can monitor vital signs of patients, read and interpret test results, and access patient records and other databases from anywhere in the hospital or the world (Blount et al., 2007; Darkins and Cary, 2000).

The second mode is the practice of remote clinical services. Caregivers can order the administration of medications, and even conduct surgery, via robotic instruments or by providing real-time instructions to other caregivers who are on the scene in direct contact with the patient (Martinez and Gomez, 2008; Norris, 2007).

Telemedicine includes several clinical specialties that to varying degrees lend themselves to remote practice. Among the early specialties to make use of the technologies was radiology in the form of technology. With the introduction of Picture Archiving and Communication Systems (PACS), clinicians are able to store, access, and read x-ray tests without the need for costly films. These systems also allow for remote access of other tests, such as MRI (Magnetic Resonance Imaging),

from anywhere in the world with increasingly acceptable levels of clarity and precision of the images (Fraunholtz ad Unnithan, 2007; Krizner, 2008; Kumar and Krupinski, 2008).

Other clinical specialties in telemedicine are telecardiology, telesurgery, telepathology, teleopthalmology, and teledermatology (Geisler and Wickramasinghe, 2009; Wickramasinghe and Geisler, 2008). As imaging and telecommunication technologies continually improve, more clinical specialties will be inducted into the realm of telemedicine. The growing ubiquity of the global Internet network allows for access to images and databases from any corner of the world. Real-time consultation and interface among clinicians across wide distances are becoming more commonplace as the technologies of transmission and communications continue to improve.

## APPLICATIONS AND BENEFITS FROM TELEMEDICINE AND HOME CARE

The combination of the aging population, the prevalence of chronic diseases, and the emergence of telemedicine technologies have been instrumental in ushering home care as a viable alternative to the traditional in-patient model of care (American Medical Association, 2001; Davies et al., 2009). Home care has long been recognized as a less expensive mode of provision of care (Hayes, 2008). Some estimates suggest that the savings are in the range of 50-70 percent of in-patient costs for certain diseases such as chronic diabetes, cardio-pulmonary, and arthritis (Kvedar et al., 2006; Geisler and Wickramasinghe, 2009).

The categories of applications of telemedicine in home care are the two modes of telehealth: monitoring and administration of clinical service. The monitoring category includes routine collection of vital signs and specific tests for certain chronic diseases, such as levels of blood glucose for patients with diabetes. Administration of

*Table 1. Barriers and facilitators to the application of telemedicine in home care*

| CATEGORY OF FACTORS | ACTING AS BARRIERS | ACTING AS FACILITATORS |
|---|---|---|
| **Technology:**<br>• Connectivity<br>• Level of sophistication<br>• Set-up & training<br>• Lack of universal platform & standards | Technology is evolving, lacking ease of use and connectivity—hence HC providers are reluctant to adopt. | Technology in some specialties is already ubiquitous and easy to adopt by savvy users. |
| **Human Behavior:**<br>• Fear of innovation<br>• Comfort level with the technology<br>• Distrust of remote care<br>• Data security & privacy | Providers & patients are weary of innovations, have little trust in remote care, and are worried about privacy. | As comfort levels with telemedicine increase, past successes alleviate fears & improve rate of adoption. |
| **Organizational/Managerial:**<br>• Integration with traditional care structures<br>• Issues of change management<br>• Need for training & special skills<br>• Pressures of short-term problems | Short-term problems and fighting immediate fires are added to problems in the integration of telemedicine with existing hospital structures. | As more caregivers experience telemedicine and acquire needed skills, adoption will be facilitated. |
| **Economic**<br>• Cost savings<br>• Cost effectiveness<br>• Freeing resources for other improvements | Cost of set-up & training & lack of quantitative success metrics may hinder applications. | Measures of economic benefits & actual cases may help to stimulate applications. |

clinical services includes remote instructions for medications at prescribed intervals and remote examinations in such specialties as teledermatology, telepedagogy, teleradiology, and telepsychiatry (Nesbit et al., 2006).

Telemedicine applications in home care offer benefits beyond cost savings. They are a key resource for healthcare delivery to rural populations by providing them access to major medical centers usually located in large metropolitan areas. Such access includes virtual visits with highly skilled clinicians in medical specialties hitherto inaccessible to these remotely located patients. Savings are also achieved by centralizing key testing facilities, such as MRI, in fewer locations. Patients in rural and remote areas need not travel far to large cities. The nearest testing facility can be in contact with any medical center in the country, or the world (Tan, 2008).

The development of telemedicine in home care is also instrumental in preventing skilled clinical caregivers from leaving remote, rural areas and small towns for the lure of larger and more advanced medical centers in big cities. Rather, these caregivers are now able to stay current in

the latest clinical developments and to practice in conjunction with the most sophisticated facilities and clinicians in their country.

## FACTORS IMPINGING UPON THE APPLICATION OF TELEMEDICINE AND HOME CARE

There are four major categories of factors which may act as facilitators or barriers to the successful implementation of telemedicine in home care: (1) technological factors; (2) human behavioral factors; (3) organizational and managerial factors; and (4) economic factors. Table 1 shows these factors in their roles on barriers or facilitators.

### Technological Factors

The application of telemedicine in home care depends on the impacts of the technology embedded in remote care. The issue of connectivity is an important facet of the technology. There is the need to connect telecare systems to the existing systems in the medical facility and in the home.

Connectivity involves such systems as PACS, pharmacy, and patient records.

Another technology factor is the level of sophistication of telemedicine and the need for complicated set-up procedures. As these improve, the technological barriers may be overcome. But, presently telemedicine technologies lack a universal platform and standards. Clinicians, information technology managers, and hospital administrators are therefore reluctant to fully embrace these technologies until these issues are resolved (Jennett and Watanabe, 2006).

## Human Behavior Factors

Organizational members are generally reluctant to adopt new systems, procedures, and technologies. They may feel threatened by change, concerned with the magnitude and difficulties with new technologies, and they tend to perceive innovations as creating more problems than bringing about positive outcomes.

In the area of home care and telemedicine, some caregivers harbor distrust of remote care. They prefer direct personal contact with patients. The combination of aversion to technological change and the virtual nature of remote care tend to act as barriers to the adoption and implementation of telemedicine. Additionally, issues of the security of patient information and threats to patient privacy also contribute to the reluctance of caregivers to fully embrace telemedicine (Doan, 2008).

As the comfort level that caregivers have with telemedicine increases, the barriers to its application may be overcome. An important element in elevating the comfort level is the accumulation of actual cases of successful implementation of telemedicine and home care. Such stories of positive outcomes and measurable benefits help to dispel some of the sentiments of threat that are felt by caregivers (Nesbit et al., 2006).

## Organizational and Managerial Factors

The first of these factors is the integration of telemedicine and remote care with traditional in-patient care structures and procedures (Davies et al., 2009). In the case of teleradiology, the implementation of the Picture Archiving and Communication System (PACS) has met with a host of difficulties in the effort to integrate PACS with the existing computer and manual systems in the hospital. This case illustrates the barriers embedded in the effort to integrate remote care (and its specialized systems) with the traditional clinical and administrative system in the care facility (Kumar and Krupinski, 2008).

A different factor is the set of issues involving change management. Hospital administrators are heavily engaged in the resolution of short-term problems and immediate crises. They are reluctant to undertake change programs, and even when such programs are enacted, there are problems embedded in the management of change. Many organizations (including healthcare delivery entities) are poorly trained in change management. They lack the managerial and human relations skills to effectively institute successful change programs.

Finally, the implementation of telemedicine and remote care requires specialized training of clinical and administrative personnel (Jennett and Watanabe, 2006). Healthcare delivery organizations consider added training of their already over-stretched clinical staff to be a burden. These organizations would need a good case made for the benefits from remote care before they are willing to support programs of remote care that require investments in the time and skills of their clinical care-givers (Mango and Riefberg, 2008).

## Economic Factors

A crucial factor in the adoption and implementation of telemedicine and home care is the cost of such applications (Hayes, 2008; Nesbit et al., 2006). The notion that moving away from the in-patient model of care to the outpatient and home care model can produce major savings in the cost of care delivery has been widely accepted in many quarters (Brownlee, 2008).

The costs of implementing telemedicine and home care include, in addition to the technology itself, the costs of set-up (in the home and the hospital) and the training of specialized staff. To be cost-effective, remote care also requires changes in the culture of care, particularly in those segments of patient populations that are in most need of telemedicine: rural patients and those in urban centers who are underserved.

Telemedicine and home care are designed to replace the use of emergency departments in hospitals and lengthy hospital stays in the preferred modes of care. When, however, patients who receive remote care continue nevertheless to crowd emergency services in the hospitals, any cost-savings embedded in remote care are doomed to evaporate (Geisler and Wickramasinghe, 2009). Thus, in order to maintain the viability of cost-savings in telemedicine, there is a need for intensive enculturation of the target population of patients.

To be counted as facilitators in the process of implementation of telemedicine, cost savings and cost-effectiveness measures must be developed. Such metrics and cases of successful applications are necessary to tell the story of telemedicine as a program that generates indisputable economic benefits (Baker, Atlas, and Afendulis, 2008).

The economic implications of telemedicine and home care extend beyond cost-savings. In the climate of spiraling costs of healthcare delivery, cost-savings due to telemedicine allow healthcare providers to free sorely needed resources and target them towards, for example, improvements in quality of care and improved access to hitherto underserved populations of patients, particularly those with chronic diseases (Geisler and Wickramasinge, 2009). In economic terms, the applications of telemedicine and home care evolve into an activity in which everyone wins (McKinsey & Company, 2008).

## THE ROLE OF NATIONAL HEALTH SYSTEMS IN THE FUTURE OF TELEMEDICINE

The nature of the national health system has far-reaching implications for the future of telemedicine and home care. The mode of financing of the healthcare system, its organization, and the influence of political forces in a centralized or decentralized fashion, all have an effort on how well, how fast, and how successful the implementation of telemedicine and home care will be in each country.

In this chapter we review the cases of the U.S. national system of health care and the Italian system. We show the key variables in each system (economics, organization, and politics) and how they impinge—differently—on the future of telemedicine. We recognize that the main distinction between the two national systems is the role played by the government. In the United States, the government is a large payer, responsible for almost half of the expenditures for healthcare delivery. But, with the exception of the military healthcare system, the government is not in the position to manage the operations of health care for the majority of the American citizenry. In the Italian case, there is a larger role that the government—at all levels—plays in the funding, organization, and politics of the healthcare delivery system.

### The Case of the European/Italian System

The development of the eHealth market, particularly telemedicine and home care, is driven by a number of variables such as the aging of the population (between 2010 and 2030, 40% of the European population will be aged over

65 years), the increasing demand for health and social services, the changes in diseases patterns, the expectations of citizens-patients, patient's empowerment (i.e. that patients want to be more involved in the management of their own health and lifestyle) and, finally, the demand for increased efficiency in healthcare provision. According to these factors, there are at least two orders of issues—the *demographic structure of the Italian population and its epidemiological features* and the *organization of the national healthcare system* (Servizio Sanitario Nazionale—SSN) *and its financial sustainability problems*—that would lead Italy to benefit very much from the eHealth applications of telemedicine and home care (Andreassen et al., 2007).

Italy is the European country most invested by the phenomenon of the aging of the population. In 2008, the old age index of the Italian population, calculated as the ratio between the population aged 65 years or more and the population aged less than 15 years, was estimated to be equal to 142.6 percent, with a steady increase compared to previous years.

Chronic-degenerative diseases are more frequent in older age groups: 57% of subjects aged between 55 and 59 years suffer these pathologies and the population reaches 86.9% of those aged 75 years and over. Co-morbidity, defined as the coexistence of two or more chronic diseases, is observed in 68.3% of subjects over 75 years (ISTAT, Annuario Statistico Italiano, 2008).

In addition, the changes in the family structure, from an extended family to a mononuclear model, may be added to the effects of aging and the increasing incidence of chronic-degenerative diseases. In such context, telemedicine and home care could facilitate the access of elder, sick, and living-alone citizens to health assistance and could increase their quality of life, making them feel included in and protected by the community. The most accredited Italian and European economic and statistical Institutes have sent warnings to Italy because of the serious concerns that the expense projections pose on the financial sustainability of the healthcare system in the near future.

The national health expenditure continues to increase faster than the national gross domestic product (GDP), due to the development of healthcare technologies, the aging of the population, and the increasing expectations from the community. In 2007 the total health expenditure on GDP was 8.9 per cent, composed by 1.8 per cent on GDP of private and 7.1 per cent on GDP of public health expenditure.

National and regional administrations are working on strategies and measures that could help in controlling the upward trend of healthcare costs. Examples are the closing of small rural hospitals (as the majority of these perform a limited amount of healthcare procedures and very often constitute, improperly, long term care residencies for elder citizens) and the promotion of de-hospitalization, favoring a rapid transfer of the patients from the hospital setting to territorial health and socio-health structures and, more frequently, to their homes.

## The Role of the National System in the Development of Telemedicine

In addition to the above-mentioned demographic, epidemiological, economical, and social reasons, the presence of a health-care system that guarantees uniform provision of comprehensive care throughout the country and characterized by vertically integrated organizations (from the central government that shares responsibility with the 20 regions to the local health authorities, providing a wide range of hospital and community healthcare services) should represent a very favorable environment that may favor the design, the implementation, and the management of wide and complex eHealth projects in Italy. However, in spite of all these aspects, eHealth is not adequately widespread in the country.

eHealth is the result of an increased use of advanced Information and Communication Technologies (ICT) such as the Internet, telephone lines, video-conferencing, and the need to provide to healthcare professionals and patients more efficient healthcare services.

In 2008, the ICT total expenditure of the Italian regional Administrations amounted to 1.124.975.000€, the 18.58% of these was represented by the ICT healthcare expenditure (Netics, 2008). Focusing on IT only, the costs for healthcare sustained by Regional Administrative Authorities were 298.354.000€; if we include also the IT expense for health care sustained by Local Health Authorities, the estimation for 2008 is of about 806 million Euros. The IT healthcare expenditure was 5€ per capita at the national level (versus the amount of 17,136€ per capita as far as the total IT expenditure is concerned).

There are other barriers for the ICT healthcare development due to technical issues, such as infrastructure, interoperability, quality of transmission, organization, lack of awareness, training, and the lack of strong evidence of cost-effectiveness and regulatory issues, accreditation, and authorization of telemedicine activities, and medical liability (see Table 1).

Evidence of the ICT diffusion among the Italian population and the healthcare providers show that the development of eHealth in Italy is not impeded by a lack of ICT culture: Italy is among the average eHealth performers in the EU27 as reported by the European Commission Survey on the ICT use among General Practitioners (GPs) in Europe. In terms of infrastructure, 86% of the Italian GP practices use a computer (EU27 average is 87%), 71% of GPs use an Internet connection (EU27 average is 69%), and 49% of practices use a broadband connection (EU27 average is 48%). Italian GPs frequently use eHealth applications, such as the electronic storage of patient data on medications (95% versus 90% of average EU27), on diagnoses (85% versus 90% average of EU27), and for retrieving analysis results (82% versus 75% of average EU27). The use of a computer during patients'

assessments is above the European mean (81% versus 66% of average EU27).

However, the positive propensity to ICT use by the Italian GPs is also associated with a delay in storing electronic radiological images (only 5% of Italian GPs compared to 34% of the average of EU27), and with a lack of electronic exchange of patient data via Internet or other dedicated networks. Only 8% of GP practices, in fact, use a network connection to receive results from laboratories while the European average is 40%; 7% of GP practices exchange data with other medical careers versus 10% of average EU27. Only 1% of GPs practice ePrescribing, as compared to 6% of the EU27 colleagues (Denmark 97%, Sweden 81%, and Netherlands 71%).

The low level of data transfer concerns not only medical data but also administrative patient data: only 3% of Italian GPs exchange administrative patient data with other careers (versus 10% of the average EU27).

## Other Key Barriers

Based on these trends and data, the following are the key barriers to the widespread development of eHealth, in general, and telemedicine and homecare, in particular, in Italy. The first are the costs related to eHealth projects, the selection of the appropriate technologies, the interoperability and standardization in eHealth technologies, and the capillary information and education of all the users – the healthcare professionals, the patients, and all types of careers -, the legal uncertainties related to liability of the professionals, the registration and licensing of technologies, the cross country operability, and the financing and reimbursement of eHealth technologies and services (Clark et al., 2007; Harrison and Lee, 2006).

eHealth investments and operational costs of healthcare supported by ICT are not considered an overriding investment by the national healthcare system, due to the limited resources available and cost reduction policies. The decisions regarding the implementation of e-Health concern three decisional levels: political, organizational, and clinical. The political decision to invest in a particular technology affects resource allocation at the organizational level and modifies clinical practice and health care professionals' activities (Sharma et al., 2006).

The lack of a joint effort by all healthcare professionals to exchange information for diagnosis, treatment, and prevention of disease and administrative data represent a barrier to the development of ICT. The use of regional/national health information networks and distributed electronic health record systems with associated services such as e-prescriptions or e-referrals could be facilitated by an appropriate training of medical personnel. An *ad hoc* curriculum of eHealth medical education for university students and a specific IT training for GPs could improve the sharing among all health actors of clinical and administrative information (Finch et al., 2008).

Apart from the described reasons, there are two more additional aspects that may represent a fatal limitation for the implementation of eHealth projects: the lack of an organized system for telemedicine and homecare and the lack of appropriate incentives for the proper functioning of the system. Both issues are at stake in Italy and must be adequately addressed (see Table 1).

Indeed, all the stakeholders - national and regional administrations, healthcare providers, specialists and general practitioners, ambulatories, laboratories, etc. - are linked and quite well organized for administrative and accounting purposes, but not enough for eHealth purposes. The Italian healthcare system has a structured hierarchical organization, but communications and information flow mainly along the vertical direction and not horizontally and/or circularly. A real network is missing (WHO, 2006; WHO, 2008).

The healthcare system presents different decisional levels (vertically- national, regional, local -, and horizontally - different health care providers), which could make it slow and expensive with different stakeholders having different incentive scheme structures. Very often we observe a lack of an adequate coordination among the incentive mechanisms of the several actors, which could impinge upon the successful implementation of telemedicine and home care. For example, the reward mechanism of Local Health Authorities (based on the capitation mechanism - quota capitaria), Hospital providers (based on the Diagnoses Related Groups system), and General Practitioners (based on the capitation mechanism - quota capitaria) are completely uncoordinated and can even act as obstacles for a correct functioning of telemedicine and/or homecare organization (Gagnon et al., 2008; Hailey et al., 2004).

## An Optimistic Forecast

Nevertheless, we can be optimistic for a stronger future development of telemedicine and home care in Italy. A clear political commitment and an ambitious national strategy orienting towards eHealth - the most important pre-requisites- in fact, are present. The Social and Healthcare Plans of most regions indicate several eHealth areas among the strategic fields in which to invest, such as telemedicine, second opinion, and teleconsulting. The development of Regional Social and Healthcare Information Systems include structuring of reports and sharing of information, e-procurement, and training for healthcare professionals (Jennett et al., 2003; Stroetmann et al., 2000).

The New Healthcare Information System of the Italian National Healthcare Plan 2006-2008 recognizes a shared database that will be useful in developing the evaluation activities of the Healthcare System. This Information System is integrated in a national strategy that monitors the balance between costs and quality of healthcare services. Several very interesting and promising eHealth experiences have been developed in many Italian regions, such as Veneto, Lombardia, and Emilia Romagna. The main strategic areas of intervention in medium and long term periods

emphasize, in particular, the definition and realization of online booking, the development of
telemedicine, the implementation of health cards,
and the reinforcement of the general practitioners
network (Stroetmann et al., 2000).

The ongoing *regionalization* of the organization and financing of the health system could help
to reduce the level of complexity of implementing
telemedicine and homecare programs. Regions
will probably move in different moments, as demonstrated by the gap on the IT healthcare expenditure between national geographical areas. Few
experiences of successful eHealth developments
related to health information networks, electronic
health records, telemedicine services, wearable
and portable monitoring systems, and health
portals are currently implemented in Italy.

The main access point for eHealth in Italy is
part of the official government portal "Italia.gov.
it" that has a dedicated section on health, "Vivere
in Salute". This is the most widely known eHealth
gateway for citizens in Italy, providing access to
information and services on general health issues
(Leff, 2009; Madden and Fox, 2006).

There is substantial evidence that eHealth, if
appropriately used, could improve the access of
citizens to health facilities, develop the quality
of care, efficiency, and productivity of healthcare
systems. eHealth would also promote prevention
plans for citizens as well as support the healthcare
professionals. Italy, as many of the industrialized
countries, has the resources, the competencies, and
the capabilities for developing eHealth projects
and for making telemedicine and homecare common modes of care.

## The Case of the American System

In the United States, national health expenditures
amounted to $2.3 trillion and the estimation for
2009 is $2.5 trillion. The projection for 2018
(unless major changes should occur) is for these
expenditures to reach $4.3 trillion (Sisko et al.,
2009). In terms of the gross national product,

healthcare spending amounted to 17.6% in 2009
(estimate) and is projected to top 20% in 2018.

There is, therefore, a valuable niche for telemedicine and home care to partake in efforts to
reduce the pressing burden of these expenditures
(Crowe, 1998). The market for telemedicine
devices and services is consistently growing. In
the American case the revenues to industry from
telemedicine are estimated to reach $2 billion
by 2012. Telecommunication companies such as
AT&T and Verizon make use of their wireline and
wireless capabilities in ventures with software and
equipment manufacturers and offer innovative
solutions for telemedicine and home care (Geisler
and Wickramasinghe, 2009).

But the rate of growth of telemedicine and
home care in the American healthcare sector
is consistently below expectations. Although
telemedicine has been applied in the majority
of medical specialties, there continues to exist a
host of barriers to its implementation. Globally,
the United States leads in the size of investments
in telemedicine, followed by Canada, Japan, the
United Kingdom, Australia, and the Scandinavian
countries. Several surveys in the United States
have shown that in the period 2000-2005, only
about 20% of hospitals (rural and urban) have
been practicing some form of telemedicine. Only
about 15% participate in any programs of effective
telehealth in home care. These data do not indicate
the lack of proven benefits of telemedicine and
home care. Rather, they can be attributed to the
factors shown in Table 1 above.

## The Role of Public Health Systems

In the United States health care is funded by both
private and public sources. In 2009 private funds
accounted for 52% of the total national health
expenditures (estimate). The projection for 2018
is for private funds to be reduced to 49% and the
share of *public* funding to increase from 48% in
2009 to 51% in 2018. By comparison, in 1993,
about the time when the Clinton initiative to re-

form health care was taking place, public funding of health care accounted for 44%. Expenses for Medicare (elderly care) more than tripled between 1993-2009, and payments for Medicaid (care for the poor) also tripled in this period.

Relative to the private health delivery sector, public hospitals, such as those of the Veterans Administration, have been more aggressive in their effort to implement telemedicine and home care for veterans. Faced with the demand from a very geographically dispersed population of patients and the influx of many wounded veterans since 2003, the Veterans Administration has grown its telecare programs by a rate twice as rapid as the private sector. The main reason may be the fact that its funding does not depend on the traditional public funding of healthcare services in the United States: Medicare and Medicaid. Although the Veterans Administration is effectively a trailblazer in the application of telemedicine together with the healthcare services of the active military branches, its impact on the private health sector in this regard has been minimal.

## Funding Telemedicine and Home Care

In 2008 expenditures for home health care in the United States reached $64 billion. For the period 2009-2018 the rate of growth of expenditures for home care are expected to be about 8% per year. The intersect of expenditures for telemedicine and home care is expected to rise by a similar annual percentage, but this rate of growth is about the same as the expected growth in total health expenditures for the same period. For our base year of 2008, spending for home care represented only 2.7% of the total national health expenditures in America. In the decade 2008-2018, total national expenditures are expected to rise by 87%, whereas telemedicine and home care are expected to rise by 80%.

The source of funding for home care is perhaps the key reason for the slow growth of this mode of health services, staying at just the rate of the natural growth in health expenditures. Public sources of funding are the main payer for home care through the government programs of Medicare and Medicaid. The private healthcare delivery system is more restrained in its investments in home care. Although the cost of treating patients in their home is substantially lower than that of inpatient care, private hospitals are more reluctant to embark on this road of long-term investments. These organizations are slow to adopt any innovations due to the few slack resources they possess. Before innovations in the delivery of care can be implemented by private providers, there is a need to clearly demonstrate that these innovations provide short-term clinical benefits (Table 1).

But the mode of funding is not the sole reason for the low rate of adoption of telemedicine and home care in the American healthcare system. The need to demonstrate benefits and a host of other managerial and behavioral factors are at play. Even the proof of benefits is not sufficient to encourage private and even public providers to fully support investments in the technology of telemedicine and home care. Sidorov (2006) has argued that electronic health records (EHR), for example, may not be a likely prospect for cost-reduction due to the nature of medical practice. As promising as it may be, the technology alone is not a guarantee that adoption by healthcare delivery organizations will be fully embraced by providers.

## Challenges to Implementation

In the American case, the barriers to the implementation and adoption of telemedicine are listed in Table 1. An overarching factor contributing to the reluctance to implement is the complexity of the American system. Evolved over six decades, this system has multiple payers, employer-supported insurance, and a host of stakeholders -including unions, government, employers, industry, special interest groups such as for specific diseases, and a complex array of medical providers. Any technology brought forth will meet diverse forces pushing and pulling in different, often opposing, directions (Sanders and Bashshur, 1995).

The category of human behavior in Table 1 includes factors that are characteristic of a complex system of different interests, distrust, and concerns with issues of privacy and the effects of new technologies. Healthcare managers are also challenged by economic considerations. Adopting a new technology would require its benefits to outweigh the investments in the technology, including training and changes the technology would engender in the clinical practice of the institutions. If providers are compelled to change the ways they practice, they will resist the technology-induced change unless unequivocally shown that there are substantial economic and clinical benefits as a result of the adoption. Telemedicine falls into this mold of economic and managerial reasoning (Masella and Zanaboni, 2008).

As a major payer in the American system, the federal government can act decisively to foster the adoption of health technologies. By channeling resources into electronic health records or telemedicine, the government helps to bring the topic of health technology to the forefront of the American public discourse and to establish a viable climate for broad adoption by the private sector. This process is currently underway by the Obama administration. Yet, the government's role in the American health system is confined to that of a major payer and a catalyst, by providing the leadership and workable incentives for the private sector to invest in these technologies.

## CONCLUSIONS: A COMPARATIVE ANALYSIS

There are similarities between the Italian and the American sets of factors that affect the implementation and adoption of telemedicine and home

care. The different modes of funding (single versus multiple payers) is a strong factor but not the only explanation to the pace of adoption or the characteristics of the telemedicine framework that is implemented in either country.

In both countries there is the specter of the upcoming demographic storm of the aging population. The increase in chronic diseases also dominates the forecasts on both sides of the Atlantic. In addition, the rising cost of healthcare delivery is a paramount consideration in both countries. These trends are shared by both Italy and the United States, and the host of barriers to implementation of telemedicine listed in Table 1 above is also common to both systems.

The lack of an organized system for telemedicine and the lack of a set of adequate incentives are present in both healthcare systems, regardless of the mode of funding. Even within the Italian system of a single payer, there are multiple stakeholders pushing in different directions for a slice of the limited resources allocated to healthcare delivery in the country. The case for eHealth as an innovative initiative is often diluted within the complex system of different actors at the regional and municipal levels, their diverse interests and the characteristics of their practice of medicine.

Similarly, in the American health system these obstacles are magnified. In addition to the existence of multiple payers, there is also a constant struggle for control of resources and the operational definitions of what constitutes quality delivery of care. As multiple actors vie for control, the outcomes are often a compromise, where innovation is sacrificed at the altar of solutions that create the least amount of change and noise in the system. Telemedicine and eHealth tend to fall into this category.

There are differences between the Italian and American health systems in the implementation and adoption of telemedicine and home care. Due to the Italian single payer system, the government has relatively more control and discretion over the allocation of resources for eHealth and home care.

Although there are competing interests within the Italian system, a concerted effort by government health agencies can - by fiat of the power of the centralized single payer - overcome resistance from providers.

Due to its complexity, the American healthcare system is much less flexible in allocating "top down" policies of preference to telemedicine and home care. Resistance by providers and other stakeholders is often anchored in the perception that such a mandated program is another attempt by the federal government to impose its own agenda on the healthcare delivery system - perhaps in opposition to the needs and preferences of employers, providers, and private insurers. Moreover, even when the government proposes programs such as increased investments in telemedicine, these initiatives are likely to be perceived by the various stakeholders as attempts to "transform" the system and as a threat to the cherished "status quo". These perceptions are hard to change. They tend to generate widespread resistance to such initiatives of the government. The American health care system lacks the cohesiveness that is present in the Italian system. The government in the United States is often perceived not only as a major payer and regulator, but also as a force that sometimes appears inimical to the smooth operation of the market-driven healthcare system of insurers, providers, patients, special disease-related organizations, and employers.

There is, however, a "silver cloud". In both countries there is hope for a more intensive acceptance of telemedicine and home care. As the government in Italy and major payers in the United States include eHealth in their planning and health resource allocation, many impediments to adoption can be overcome. The private health sector in the United State and the regional and hospital interests in Italy have several concerns in common, and these concerns have traditionally been translated into barriers to telemedicine. The factors listed in Table 1 are some of these concerns. They transcend political and economic boundaries

of the different modes of funding and different structures of the healthcare systems. Policies which will successfully focus on resolving the issues in Table 1 discussed in this paper will most likely enhance the adoption of eHealth, telemedicine, and home care in both countries.

In the United States these policies need to be embraced by the private health care delivery sector, as well as the public health agencies. In Italy, such policies need to be adopted by the central government as well as the regional and municipal organizations, all the way to the individual hospital. In both countries eHealth has shown to provide benefits and to have a very promising potential to helping resolve issues of cost, quality, and access to care. What is missing are policies that account for the various barriers impacting the adoption of eHealth.

## REFERENCES

American Medical Association. (2001). *American Medical Association Guide to Home Care*. New York: John Wiley & Sons.

Andreassen, H. K., Bujinowska-Fedak, M. M., Chronaki, C. E., Dumitru, R. U., Pudule, I., & Santana, S. (2007). European Citizens' Use of E-Health Services: A Study of Seven Countries. *BMC Public Health*, 7(147), 53. doi:10.1186/1471-2458-7-53

Baker, L., Atlas, S., & Afendulis, C. (2008). Expanded Use of Imaging Technology and the Challenge of Measuring Value. *Health Affairs*, 27(6), 1467–1478. doi:10.1377/hlthaff.27.6.1467

Blount, M. (2007). Remote Healthcare Monitoring Using Personal Care Connect. *IBM Systems Journal*, 46(1), 95–113.

Brownlee, S. (2008). *Overtreated: Why Too Much Medicine is Making US Sicker and Poorer*. London: Bloomsbury Publishers.

Clark, R. A., Inglis, S. C., McAlister, F. A., Cleland, J. G. F., & Steward, S. (2007). Telemonitoring or Structured Telephone Support Programmes for Patients with Chronic Heart Failure: Systematic Review and Meta-Analysis. *BMJ (Clinical Research Ed.)*, *334*, 942. doi:10.1136/bmj.39156.536968.55

Crowe, B. (1998). Cost-Effectiveness Analysis of Telemedicine. *Journal of Telemedicine and Telecare*, *4*(Supplement), 1, 14–17. doi:10.1258/1357633981931867

Darkins, A., & Cary, M. (2000). *Telemedicine and Telehealth: Principles, Policies, Performance and Pitfalls*. New York: Springer Publishing Company.

Davies, S., Froggatt, K., & Meyer, J. (Eds.). (2009). *Understanding Home Care: A Research and Development Perspective*. London: Jessica Kingsley Publishers.

Doam, C. (2008). The Last Challenges and Barriers to the Development of Telemedicine Programs. *Studies in Health Technology and Informatics*, *131*(1), 45–54.

Finch, T. L., Mort, M., Mair, F. S., & May, C. R. (2008). Future Patients? Telehealthcare, Roles, and Responsibilities. *Health & Social Care in the Community*, *16*(1), 86–95.

Fraunholz, B., & Unnithan, C. (2007). Potential of Telemedicines of Preliminary Evaluation Through the Inovation Diffusion Lens. *International Journal of Healthcare Technology and Management*, *8*(3/4), 315–332. doi:10.1504/IJHTM.2007.013166

Gagnon, M. P., Légaré, F., Fortin, J. P., Lamothe, L., Labrecquel, M., & Duplantie, J. (2008). An Integrated Strategy of Knowledge Application for Optimal e-Health Implementation: A Multimethod Study Protocol. *BMC Medical Informatics and Decision Making*, *8*, 17. doi:10.1186/1472-6947-8-17

Geisler, E., & Wickramasinghe, N. (2009). *The Role and Utilization of Wireless Technology in the Management and Monitoring of Chronic Diseases*. Washington, DC: IBM Center for the Business of Government.

Hailey, D., Ohinmaa, A., & Roine, R. (2004). Study Quality and Evidence of Benefit in Recent Assessments of Telemedicine. *Journal of Telemedicine and Telecare*, *10*(6), 318–324. doi:10.1258/1357633042602053

Harrison, J. P., & Lee, A. (2006, Nov-Dec). The Role of e-Health in the Changing Healthcare Environment. *Nurs. Econ.*, *24*(6), 2388, 279.

Hayes, H. (2008). *Home Health Monitoring Saves the Government Big Bucks*. Retrieved from http://www.govhealthit.com/print/4_21/features/350570-1.html

Institute of Medicine. (1996). *Telemedicine: A Guide to Assessing Telecommunications for Health Care*. Washington, DC: National Academy Press.

ISTAT. (2008). *Annuario Statistico Italiano*.

Jennett, P., & Watanabe, M. (2006). Healthcare and Telemedicine: Ongoing and Evolving Challenges. *Disease Management & Health Outcomes*, *14*(1), 9–13. doi:10.2165/00115677-200614001-00004

Jennett, P. A., Affleck Hall, L., Hailey, D., Ohinmaa, A., Andreson, C., & Thomas, R. (2003). The Socio-Economic Impact of Telehealth: A Systematic Review. *Telemed. Telecare*, *9*(6), 311–320. doi:10.1258/135763303771005207

Krizner, K. (2008). Digital Hospitals Aim to Document Better Outcomes. *Managed Healthcare Executive*, *18*(4), 28–30.

Kumar, S., & Krupinski, E. (Eds.). (2008). *Teleradiology*. New York: Springer Publishing Company. doi:10.1007/978-3-540-78871-3

Kvedar, J., Wootton, R., & Dimnick, S. (Eds.). (2006). *Home Telehealth: Connecting Care Within the Community*. London: Royal Society of Medicine Press.

Leff, B. (2009). Defining and Disseminating the Hospital-at-Home Model. *Canadian Medical Association Journal, 180*(2). doi:10.1503/cmaj.081891

Madden, M., & Fox, S. (2006). Finding Answers Online in Sickness and in Health. *Pew Internet & American Life Project Report*, May 2.

Mango, P., & Riefberg, V. (2008). Three Imperatives for Improving Health Care. *The McKinsey Quarterly*, (December): 2008.

Martinez, L., & Gomez, C. (Eds.). (2008). *Telemedicine in the 21st Century*. Hauppauge, NY: Nova Science Publishers.

Masella, C., & Zanaboni, P. (2008). Assessment Models for Telemedicine Services in National Health Systems. *International Journal of Healthcare Technology and Management, 9*(5/6), 446–472. doi:10.1504/IJHTM.2008.020198

McKinsey & Company. (2008). Why Americans Pay More for Health Care. *The McKinsey Quarterly*, (December): 2008.

Nesbit, T. (2006). Rural Outreach in Home Telehealth: Assessing Challenges and Reviewing Successes. *Telemedicine Journal and e-Health, 12*(2), 107–113. doi:10.1089/tmj.2006.12.107

Netics. (2008). *Le ICT nelle Regioni e Province Autonome. Rapporto 2008.*

Norris, A. (2002). *Essentials of Telemedicine and Telecare*. New York: John Wiley & Sons.

Park, A. (2008). America's Health Check-up. *Time Magazine, 172*(22), 41–49.

Sanders, J., & Bashshur, R. (1995). Challenges to the Implementation of Telemedicine. *Telemedicine Journal, 3*, 115–123.

Sharma, S. K., Xu, H., Wickramasinghe, N., & Ahmed, N. (2006). Electronic Healthcare: Issues and Challenges. *International Journal of Electronic Healthcare, 2*(1), 50–65. doi:10.1504/IJEH.2006.008693

Sidorov, J. (2006). It Ain't Necessarily So: The Electronic Health Record and the Unlikely Prospect of Reducing Healthcare Costs. *Health Affairs, 25*(4), 1079–1085. doi:10.1377/hlthaff.25.4.1079

Sisko, A., Truffer, C., & Smith, S. (2009). Health Spending Projections Through 2018: Recession Effects Add Uncertainty to Outlook. *Health Affairs, 24*(February), 346–357. doi:10.1377/hlthaff.28.2.w346

Stroetmann, K. A., Jones, T., Dobrev, A., & Stroetmann, V. N. (2006). eHealth is Worth It—The Economic Benefits of Implemented eHealth Solutions at Ten European Sites. *European Communities*.

Stroetmann, V. N., Cleland, J. G., Stroetmann, K. A. & Westerteicher, Ch. (2000). Evaluation Telehealth Homecare Services—The TEN-HMS Project: Medical, Quality of Life and Economic Efficiency Aspects. *Gesellschaft für Biomedizinische Technologien in Ulm e.V.*

Tan, J. (Ed.). (2008). *Healthcare Information Systems and Informatics: Research and Pratices*. Hershey, PA: IGI Global Publishers.

WHO. (2006). *Building FOUNDATIONS eHealth*.

WHO. (2008). *Home Care in Europe*.

Wickramasinghe, N., & Geisler, E. (Eds.). (2008). *Encyclopedia of Healthcare Information Systems*. Hershey, PA: IGI Global Publishers.

# Compilation of References

3GPP TR 25.896. (2004). *Feasibility Study for Enhanced Uplink for UTRA FDD, Release 6, v6.0.0.*

3GPP TS 25.308. (2004). *High Speed Downlink Packet Access; Overall Description; Stage 2, v6.3.0.*

*3rdGeneration Partnership Project.* (n.d.). Retrieved from www.3gpp.org

Abascal, J. (2004). Ambient Intelligence for people with disabilities and elderly people. *SIGCHI Workshop on Ambient Intelligence for Scienti_c Discovery (AISD). ACM 2004*, Vienna.

Ability Research Centre. (1999). *Environmental Control System for People with Spinal Injuries.* A report on Research Undertaken by the Ability Research Centre.

ABS. (2003). *Population Projections, Australia, 2002-2101, Cat. No. 3222.0.* Canberra, Australia: Australian Bureau of Statistics.

Ackerman, M., Craft, R., Ferrante, F., Kratz, M., Mandil, S., & Sapci, H. (2002). Telemedicine Technology. *Telemedicine Journal and e-Health, 8*(1), 71–78.

Active Endpoints. (n.d). *ActiveBPEL Open Source Engine Project.* Retrieved August 18, 2007, from http://www.activebpel.org/

*Activities.* (n.d.). Retrieved October 20, 2008, from http://www.hardingnh.com/

Adamodt, K. (2006). [Location Engine]. *Application Note, AN042,* CC2431.

Addlesee, M., Jones, A., Livesey, F., & Samaria, F. (1997). The ORL active floor [sensor system]. *IEEE Personal Communications, 4*(5), 35–41. doi:10.1109/98.626980

Agarawala, A., Greenberg, S., & Ho, G. (2004). The Context-Aware Pill Bottle and Medication Monitor. In *Video Proceedings and Proceedings Supplement of the UBICOM 2004 Conference*, Sept. 7-10, Nottingham, England.

Agrawal, R., Kiernan, J., Srikant, R., & Xu, Y. (2002). Hippocratic Databases. *Proceedings of VLDB'02 (pp. 143-154).*

AIHW. (2008). *Diabetes: Australian Facts 2008.* Canberra, Australia: Australian Institute of Health and Welfare.

Ailisto, H., Alahuhta, P., Haataja, V., Kyllönen, V., & Lindholm, M. (2002). Five-Layer Model and Example Case. In *Proceedings of Ubicomp 2002, Concepts and Models for Ubiquitous Computing Workshop.* Structuring Context Aware Applications.

*Akogrimo (Access to Knowledge through the Grid in a Mobile World).* (2007). Retrieved April 25, 2009, from http://www.akogrimo.org/modules.php?op=modload&name=AddFile&file=addfile&par=1& datei=scen_ehealth

Alexander, G. L. (2008). A Descriptive Analysis of a Nursing Home Clinical Information System with Decision Support. *Perspectives in Health Information Management / AHIMA, American Health Information Management Association, 5*(12).

Alhaqbani, B., & Fidge, C. J. (2007). Access Control Requirements for Processing Electronic Health Records Business. In Process Management Workshops, (pp. 371-382).

Alwan, M., Mack, D., Dalal, S., Kell, S., Turner, B., & Felder, R. (2006). Impact of Passive In-Home Health Status Monitoring Technology in Home Health: Outcome Pilot. In 1st Transdisciplinary Conference on Distributed Diagnosis and Home Healthcare ($D_2H_2$), 2-4 April 2006 (pp.79-82). Arlington, Virginia.

American Barcode and RFID. (n.d.). *Passive RFID Tags vs. Active RFID Tags.* Retrieved April 15, 2009, from http://www.abrfid.com/rfid/articles/passive-active-tags.aspx

American Health Information Management Association. (2005). *A road map for health IT in long-term care.* Chicago: Author.

*Analysis of the National Nursing Home Survey (NNHS)* (2004). AARP Public Policy Institute.

Anciaux, N., Benzine, M., Bouganim, L., Pucheral, P., & Shasha, D. (2007). GhostDB: querying visible and hidden data without leaks. In *ACM SIGMOD Conference* (pp. 677-688).

Anciaux, N., Bobineau, C., Bouganim, L., Pucheral, P., & Valduriez, P. (2001). PicoDBMS: Validation and Experience. In *International Conference on Very Large Data Bases (VLDB)* (pp. 709-710).

Anciaux, N., Bouganim, L., & Pucheral, P. (2006). Data Confidentiality: to which extent cryptography and secured hardware can help. *Annales des Télécommunications, 61*(3-4), 267–283.

Anciaux, N., Bouganim, L., & Pucheral, P. (2007). Future Trends in Secure Chip Data Management. *IEEE Data Eng. Bull., 30*(3), 49–57.

Anderson, R., Issel, L. M., & McDaniel, R. R. (2003). Nursing homes as complex adaptive systems: relationship between management practice and resident outcomes. *Nursing Research, 52*(1), 12–21. doi:10.1097/00006199-200301000-00003

Anderson, S., & Wittwer, W. (2004). Using bar-code point-of-care technology for patient safety. *Journal for Healthcare Quality, 26*(6), 5–11.

Andreassen, H. K., Bujinowska-Fedak, M. M., Chronaki, C. E., Dumitru, R. U., Pudule, I., & Santana, S. (2007). European Citizens' Use of E-Health Services: A Study of Seven Countries. *BMC Public Health, 7*(147), 53. doi:10.1186/1471-2458-7-53

Andreasson, J., Ekstrom, M., Fard, A., Castano, J. G., & Johnson, T. (2002). Remote system for patient monitoring using Bluetooth/spl trade. *IEEE Sensors, 1*, 304–307.

Andrews, J. (2009). Keeping record: long-term care may not deserve its reputation as a tech laggard. But more could be done to prepare for the electronic health record. (Information technology). *McKnight's Long-Term Care News, 30*(1), 42(43).

Arisoylu, M., Mishra, R., Rao, R., & Lenert, L. A. (2005). 802.11 wireless infrastructure to enhance medical response to disasters. In *AMIA Annual Symposium Proceedings*, (pp. 1-5).

Ashley, P., Hada, S., Karjoth, G., Powers, C., & Schunter, M. (2003). *Enterprise Privacy Authorization Language (EPAL 1.2). Technical report. IBM Tivoli Software.* IBM Research.

Assisted Living Facilities (ALF). (2007). Virginia Department of Social Services: Virginia.gov.

Augustin, I., Yamin, A. C., Da Silva, L. C., Real, R. A., Frainer, G., & Geyer, C. F. R. (2006). ISAMadapt: abstractions and tools for designing general-purpose pervasive applications. *Software, Practice & Experience, 36*, 1231–1256. doi:10.1002/spe.756

*Aware Home Research Initiative, The.* (n.d.). Retrieved February 1, 2009 from http://www.awarehome.gatech.edu/news/index.html

Aziz, O., Lo, B., Pansiot, J., Atallah, L., Yang, G.-Z., & Darzi, A. (2008, Oct). From computers to ubiquitous computing by 2010: Health Care. *Philosophical Transactions of the Royal Society A, 366*(1881), 3805-3811.

Bahl, P., & Padmanabhan, V. (2000). RADAR: an in-building RF-based user location and tracking system. In *INFOCOM 2000. Nineteenth Annual Joint Conference of the IEEE Computer and Communications Societies, 26-30 March 2001* (pp. 775-784).Tel Aviv, Israel: IEEE Computer Society.

Baker, L., Atlas, S., & Afendulis, C. (2008). Expanded Use of Imaging Technology and the Challenge of Measuring Value. *Health Affairs, 27*(6), 1467–1478. doi:10.1377/hlthaff.27.6.1467

Balas, E. A., Krishna, S., Kretschmer, R. A., Cheek, T. R., Lobach, D. F., & Boren, S. A. (2004). Computerized knowledge management in diabetes care. *Medical Care, 42*(6), 610–621. doi:10.1097/01.mlr.0000128008.12117.f8

Baldauf, M., Dustdar, S., & Rosenberg, F. (2004). A Survey on Context-Aware Systems. *International Journal of Ad Hoc and Ubiquitous Computing* .

Baldus, H., Klabunde, K., & Muesch, G. (2004). Reliable Set-Up of Medical Body-Sensor Networks. In *Proc. EWSN 2004*, Berlin, Germany.

Balfanz, D., Klein, M., Schmidt, A., & Santi, M. (2008). Participatory development of a middleware for AAL solutions: requirements and approach - the case of SO-PRANO. *GMS Medizinische Informatik, Biometrie und Epidemiologie, 4*(3).

Bannach, D., Amft, O., & Lukowicz, P. (2008). Rapid Prototyping of Activity Recognition Applications. *IEEE Pervasive Computing / IEEE Computer Society [and] IEEE Communications Society, 7*, 22–31. doi:10.1109/MPRV.2008.36

Bardram, J. E., & Christensen, H. B. (2007, Jan.-March). Pervasive computing support for hospitals: An overview of the activity-based computing project. *IEEE Pervasive Computing / IEEE Computer Society [and] IEEE Communications Society, 6*(1), 44–51. doi:10.1109/MPRV.2007.19

Bardram, J. E., Mihailidis, A., & Wan, D. (Eds.). (2007). *Pervasive Computing in Healthcare*. Boca Raton, FL: CRC Press.

Bardram, J., Hansen, T. R., Mogensen, M., & Soegaard, M. (2006). *Experiences from Real-World Deployment of Context-Aware Technologies in a Hospital Environment*. Paper presented at the Ubicomp, Orange County, CA, USA.

Barger, T. S., Brown, D. E., & Alwan, M. (2005). Health-status monitoring through analysis of behavioral patterns. *Systems, Man and Cybernetics, Part A, IEEE Transactions on, 35*, 22-27.

Baron, R. J., Fabens, E. L., Schiffman, M., & Wolf, E. (2005). Electronic health records: Just around the corner? Or over the cliff? *Annals of Internal Medicine, 143*(3), 222–226.

Barrick, A., & Rader, J. (2008). *Bathing without a battle: person-directed care of individuals with dementia*. New York: Springer Pub.

BASEscan. (n.d). *Accurate Patient Identification Using Encoded Driver License Information*. Retrieved May 12, 2009, from http://www.medibase.com/pdf/basescan.pdf

Bates, D. W., Cohen, M., Leape, L. L., Overhage, J. M., Shabot, M. M., & Sheridan, T. (2001). Reducing the frequency of errors in medicine using information technology. *Journal of the American Medical Informatics Association, 8*(4), 299–308.

Bates, D. W., Leape, L. L., Cullen, D. J., Laird, N., Petersen, L. A., & Teich, J. M. (1998). Effect of computerized physician order entry and a team intervention on prevention of serious medication errors. *Journal of the American Medical Association, 280*(15), 1311–1316. doi:10.1001/jama.280.15.1311

Bates, D. W., Teich, J. M., Lee, J., Seger, D., & Kuperman, G. J., Ma'Luf, N., et al. (1999). The impact of computerized physician order entry on medication error prevention. *Journal of the American Medical Informatics Association, 6*(4), 313–321.

Battlefield Medical Information System Tactical - Joint. (n.d.). *BMIST-J home page.* Retrieved 13 February 2009 from http://www.mc4.army.mil/AHLTA-Mobile_CBT. asp#, CleveMed. Cleveland Medical Devices Inc. (n.d.). home page. Retrieved 13 Feb 2009, from: http://www. clevemed.com/

Baumgartner, N., & Retschitzegger, W. (2006). A Survey of Upper Ontologies for Situation Awareness. In *Proceedings of the International Conference on Knowledge Sharing and Collaborative Engineering.*

Baumgartner, N., & Retschitzegger, W. (2007). Towards a Situation Awareness Framework Based on Primitive Relations. In *Proceedings of the Conference on Information Decision and Control,* Adelaide, Australia.

Baumgartner, N., Retschitzegger, W., & Schwinger, W. (2007). Lost in Space and Time and Meaning - An Ontology-Based Approach to Road Traffic Situation Awareness. In *Proceedings of the 3rd Workshop on Context Awareness for Proactive Systems,* Guildford, UK.

Baumgartner, N., Retschitzegger, W., Schwinger, W., Kotsis, G., & Schwietering, C. (2007). Of Situations and Their Neighbors: Evolution and Similarity in Ontology-Based Approaches to Situation Awareness. In *Proceedings of the 6th International and Interdisciplinary Conference on Modeling and Using Context,* Roskilde, Denmark.

Becker, M. (2008). *Software Architecture Trends and Promising Technology for Ambient Assisted Living Systems. Assisted Living Systems - Models, Architectures and Engineering Approaches. Dagstuhl Seminar Proceedings.* Dagstuhl, Germany: Internationales Begegnungs- und Forschungszentrum für Informatik, Schloss Dagstuhl.

Becker, M. Y., & Sewell, P. (2004). Flexible Trust Management, Applied to Electronic Health Records. In *Computer Security Foundations Workshop* (pp. 139–154). Cassandra.

Becker, M., Werkman, E., Anastasopoulos, M., & Kleinberger, T. (2006). Approaching Ambient Intelligent Home Care Systems. *Pervasive Health Conference and Workshops,* 2006, 1-10.

Beckmann, L., Kim, S., Jungebecker, N., Leonhardt, S., & Ingerl, G. (2009). Entwicklung intelligenter Textilien für die Überwachung des Ernährungs- und Wasserhaushalts. In *Proceedings of 2nd German AAL congress.*

Berger, L. (2006, January 13). Information technology feature: The IT payback. *McKnight's Long-Term Care News,* (pp. 34-37).

Bergeron, B. P. (2002). Enterprise digital assistants: the progression of wireless clinical computing. *The Journal of Medical Practice Management, 17,* 229–233.

Bézivin, J. (2005). On the Unification Power of Models. *Journal on Software and Systems Modeling, 4*(2).

Bias, R. (1991). Walkthroughs: Efficient collaborative testing. *IEEE Software, 8*(5), 94–95. doi:10.1109/52.84220

Bloom, B. (1970). Space/time tradeoffs in hash coding with allowable errors. *Communications of the ACM, 13*(7), 422–426. doi:10.1145/362686.362692

Blount, M. (2007). Remote Healthcare Monitoring Using Personal Care Connect. *IBM Systems Journal, 46*(1), 95–113.

Bodenheimer, T., Lorig, K., Holman, H., & Grumbach, K. (2002). Patient self-management of chronic disease in primary care. [JAMA]. *Journal of the American Medical Association, 288*(19), 2469–2475. doi:10.1001/jama.288.19.2469

Böhm, K., Cordes, M., Afentakis, A., Müller, M., & Nöthen, M. (2006). *Krankheitskosten 2004.* Wiesbaden, Germany: Statistisches Bundesamt.

Borromeo, S., Rodriguez-Sanchez, C., Machado, F., Hernandez-Tamames, J. A., & de la Prieta, R. (2007). A Reconfigurable, Wearable, Wireless ECG System. *Engineering in Medicine and Biology Society, 2007. EMBS 2007. 29th Annual International Conference of the IEEE,* (pp. 1659-1662).

Boumans, N., Berkhout, A., & Landeweerd, A. (2005). Efforts of resident-oriented care on quality of care, well-being and satisfaction with care. *Scandinavian Journal of Caring Sciences, 19*(3), 11–15. doi:10.1111/j.1471-6712.2005.00351.x

Bourke, A. K., & Lyons, G. M. (2008). A threshold-based fall-detection algorithm using a bi-axial gyroscope sensor. *Medical Engineering & Physics, 30*, 84–90. doi:10.1016/j.medengphy.2006.12.001

Bowie, L. (2000). *Smart Shirt Moves From Research to Market: Goal is to Ease Healthcare Monitoring.* Georgia Institute of Technology. Retrieved March 10, 2003 from http://www.news-info.gatech.edu/news_release/sensatex.html

Brady, M., & Rogers, M. (2002). DVB-RCS Background Book. Technical Report, Nera Broadband Satellite AS (NBS), Publication no. 102386.

Breen, G. M., & Matusitz, J. (2007). An interpersonal examination of telemedicine: Applying relevant communication theories. e-health. *International Journal (Toronto, Ont.), 3*(1), 187–192.

Breen, G., & Zhang, N. (2008). Theoretical Analysis of Improving Resident Care. *Journal of Medical Systems, 32*(2), 18–23. doi:10.1007/s10916-007-9121-9

Brennan, P. F., Downs, S., Casper, G., & Kenron, D. (2007). *Project Health Design: Stimulating the Next Generation of Personal Health Records AMIA Annu Symp Proc. 2007,* (pp. 70–74).

Breynaert, D. (2005). *2Way-Sat: A DVB-RCS Satellite Access Network. Technical Report, Newtec Cy N.V.* Belgium: NTC.

Britt, H., Miller, G. C., Charles, J., Pan, Y., Valenti, L., & Henderson, J. (2007). *General Practice Activity in Australia 2005-06, Cat. no. GEP 16.* Canberra, Australia: AIHW.

Brownlee, S. (2008). *Overtreated: Why Too Much Medicine is Making US Sicker and Poorer.* London: Bloomsbury Publishers.

Budinsky, F., Steinberg, D., Merks, E., Ellersick, R., & Grose, T. J. (2004). *Eclipse Modeling Framework.* Reading, MA: Addison Wesley.

Bui, F. M., & Hatzinakos, D. (2008). Biometric methods for secure communications in body sensor networks: resource-efficient key management and signal-level data scrambling. *EURASIP J. Adv. Signal Process, 8*(2), 1–16. doi:10.1155/2008/529879

Bults, R. (2004). Body Area Networks for Ambulant Patient Monitoring Over Next Generation Public Wireless Networks. In *Proceedings of the 13th IST Mobile and Wireless Communications Summit,* Lyon, France, (pp. 181-185).

Bundgaard, M., Hildebrandt, T., & Hojgaard, E. (2008, June). *Seamlessly Distributed & Mobile Workflow or: The right processes at the right places.* Paper presented at Programming Language Approaches to Concurrency and Communication-cEntric Software (PLACES), Oslo, Norway.

Burland, E. M. J. (2008). An Evaluation of a Fall Management Program in a Personal Care Home Population. *Healthcare Quaterly, 11*(3), 137–140.

Buschmann, F., Henney, K., & Schmidt, D. C. (2007). *Pattern-Oriented Software Architecture 4: A Pattern Language for Distributed Computing.* New York: John Wiley & Sons Inc.

Byun, J., & Li, N. (2008). Purpose based access control for privacy protection in relational database systems. *The VLDB Journal, 17,* 603–619. doi:10.1007/s00778-006-0023-0

*Caring for the Elderly: Is Adequate Long-Term Care Available.* (1998). Congressional Quarterly, Inc., CQ Researcher.

Caroll, J. (1995). Scenario-Based Design: Envisioning work and technology in system development. New York.

Carrasco, L. C. (1999). RDBMS's for Java Cards? What a Senseless Idea! White paper. *ISOL Corp.*

Carrillo, H., & Harrington, C. (2006). Cross the States 2006: Profiles of Long-Term Care and Independent Living. In AARP (Ed.).

Carroll, R., Cnossen, R., Schnell, M., & Simons, D. (2007). *Continua: An Interoperable Personal Healthcare Ecosystem* (pp. 90–94). IEEE PERVASIVE COMPUTING.

Carter, S., & Mankof, J. (2004). *Challenges for Ubicomp Evaluation*. EECS Department UC Berkeley.

Carter, S., & Mankoff, J. (2005). Momento: Early-Stage Prototyping and Evaluation for Mobile Applications. In n. o. C. a. Berkeley (Ed.).

Castle, N. G. (2008). Nursing Home Evacuation Plans. *American Journal of Public Health*, 98(7), 1235–1241. doi:10.2105/AJPH.2006.107532

Castro, L. A., & Favela, J. (2008). Reducing the Uncertainty on Location Estimation of Mobile Users to Support Hospital Work. *IEEE Transactions on systems, man and cybernetics--Part C: Applications and Reviews*.

Celler, B. G., Basilakis, J., Budge, M., & Lovell, N. H. (2006). A Clinical Monitoring and Management System for Residential Aged Care Facilities. In *Proceedings of the 28th IEEE EMBS Annual International Conference*, (pp. 3301).

Celler, B. G., Earnshaw, W., Ilsar, E. D., Betbeder-Matibet, L., Harris, M., & Clark, R. (1995). Remote monitoring of the elderly at home. A multidisciplinary project on aging at the University of New South Wales. *International Journal of Bio-Medical Computing*, 40, 147–155. doi:10.1016/0020-7101(95)01139-6

Celler, B. G., Hesketh, T., Earnshaw, W., & Ilsar, E. (1994). An instrumentation system for the remote monitoring of changes in functional health status of the elderly at home. In *Proceedings of the 16thAnnual International Conference of the IEEE EMBS*, (vol. 2, pp. 908–909).

Celler, B. G., Lovell, N. H., & Chan, D. K. Y. (1999). The potential impact of home telecare on clinical practice. *MJA*, 171, 518–521.

Chadwick, P. E. (2007). Regulations and Standards for Wireless applications. In *eHealth 29th Annual International Conference of the IEEE Engineering in Medicine and Biology Society, EMBS 2007*, (pp. 6170 - 6173).

Chambers, C. (2004). *Smart Home How Home Automation Works and what it can do.* http://islab.oregonstate.edu/koc/ece399/f04/explo/chambers.pdf

Chan, A. D. C., & Green, J. R. (2008). Smart Rollator Prototype. Medical Measurements and Applications. *MeMeA 2008.IEEE International Workshop on*, (pp. 97-100).

Chan, L. L., Celler, B. G., & Lovell, N. H. (2006). *Development of a Smart Health Monitoring and Evaluation System*. Paper presented at the TENCON 2006, IEEE Region 10 Conference.

Chan, L. L., Zhang, J. Z., Narayanan, M. R., Celler, B. G., & Lovell, N. H. (2008, February 13-15). *A Health Monitoring and Evaluation System for Assessing Care Needs of Residents in Aged-Care Facilities.* Paper presented at the IASTED Biomed. Eng., Innsbruck, Austria.

Chau, S., & Turner, P. (2006). Utilisation of mobile handheld devices for care management at an Australian aged care facility. *Electronic Commerce Research and Applications*, 5, 305–312. doi:10.1016/j.elerap.2006.04.005

Chazko, Z., & Ahmad, F. (2005). Wireless Sensor Network Based System for Fire Endangered Areas. In *Proceedings of the Third Intl. Conf. on Information Technology and Applications (ICITA'05) Volume 2* (pp. 203-207). Washington DC: IEEE Computer Society.

Cheek, P. (2005). Aging Well With Smart Technology. *Nursing Administration Quarterly*, 29(4), 329–338.

Cherukuri, S., Venkatasubramanian, K. K., & Gupta, S. K. S. (2003). BioSec: A biometric based approach for securing communication in wireless networks of biosensors implanted in the human body. In *Proceedings of the workshop on wireless security and privacy (wispr), international conference on parallel processing workshops* (pp. 432–439).

Chin, T. (2005, January, 17 2006). Untapped power: a physician's handheld. *AMNews*.

Chittleborough, C. R., Grant, J. F., Phillips, P. J., & Taylor, A. W. (2007). The increasing prevalence of diabetes in South Australia: the relationship with population ageing and obesity. *Public Health, 121*, 92–99. doi:10.1016/j.puhe.2006.09.017

Cho, H., Kang, M., Park, J., Park, B., & Kim, H. (2007). Performance analysis of location estimation algorithm in ZigBee networks using received signal strength. In *21st International Conference on Advanced Information Networking and Applications Workshops (AINAW'07), 21-23 May 2007* (pp. 302-306). Niagara Falls, Canada: IEEE Computer Society.

Choudhri. A., Kagal, L., Joshi, A., Finin, T. & Yesha, Y. (2003). PatientService: Electronic Patient Record Redaction and Delivery in Pervasive Environments. In *Fifth International Workshop on Enterprise Networking and Computing in Healthcare Industry.*

Choudhury, T. (2008). The Mobile Sensing Platform: An Embedded Activity Recognition System. *IEEE Pervasive Computing / IEEE Computer Society [and] IEEE Communications Society, 7*(2), 32–41.

Chu, Y., & Ganz, A. (2004). A Mobile Teletrauma System Using 3G Networks. *IEEE Transactions on Information Technology in Biomedicine, 8*(4), 456–462.

Clark, R. A., Inglis, S. C., McAlister, F. A., Cleland, J. G. F., & Steward, S. (2007). Telemonitoring or Structured Telephone Support Programmes for Patients with Chronic Heart Failure: Systematic Review and Meta-Analysis. *BMJ (Clinical Research Ed.), 334*, 942. doi:10.1136/bmj.39156.536968.55

*CMS Adds Searchable Database of Lowest-Quality Nursing Homes Nationwide to Web Site.* (2008). Kaiser Family Foundation.

Codd, E. F. (1970). A Relational Model of Data for Large Shared Data Banks. *Communications of the ACM, 13*(6), 377–387. doi:10.1145/362384.362685

Colagiuri, S., Colagiuri, R., & Ward, J. (1998). *National Diabetes Strategy and Implementation Plan.* Canberra, Australia: Diabetes Australia.

Collins, S. C., Bhatti, J. Z., Dexter, S. L., & Rabbitt, P. M. (1992). Elderly people in a new world: attitudes to advanced communications technologies. In Boumqa, H., & Graafmans, J. A. M. (Eds.), *Gerontechnology.* Amsterdam: IOS Press.

Consolvo, S., & Walker, M. (2003). Using the Experience Sampling Method to Evaluate Ubicomp Applications. *IEEE Pervasive Computing Magazine: The Human Experience, 2*(2), 24–31. doi:10.1109/MPRV.2003.1203750

Consolvo, S., Harrison, B., Smith, I., Chen, M. Y., Everitt, K., & Froehlich, J. (2007). Conducting In Situ Evaluations for and With Ubiquitous Computing Technologies. *International Journal of Human-Computer Interaction, 22*(1-2), 103–118. doi:10.1207/s15327590ijhc2201-02_6

Continuous Care (C-CARE). (2005). Retrieved December 15, 2008, from http://cordis.europa.eu/data/PROJ_FP5/ACTIONeqDndSESSIONeq112422005919ndDO-Ceq513ndTBLeqEN_PROJ.htm

Coronato, A., & Esposito, M. (2008). Towards an implementation of smart hospital: A localization system for mobile users and devices. In *Proceedings Sixth Annual IEEE International Conference on Pervasive Computing and Communications PERCOM 2008,* (pp. 715-719).

Corporation, W. (2005). Our products and services. About WebMD.com.

CosmoCom Showcases Telehealth at World Health Care Congress (2009). *Health &amp; Beauty Close-Up,* NA.

Crossbow Technology, Inc. (2008). *MICAz Datasheet.* Retrieved January 29, 2009, from http://www.xbow.com/Products/Product_pdf_files/Wireless_pdf/MICAz_Datasheet.pdf

Crossbow. (n.d.). *Home page.* Retrieved 13 Feb 2009 from http://www.xbow.com

Crowe, B. (1998). Cost-Effectiveness Analysis of Telemedicine. *Journal of Telemedicine and Telecare, 4*(Supplement), 1, 14–17. doi:10.1258/1357633981931867

Curtis, D. W., Pino, E. J., Bailey, J. M., Shih, E. I., Waterman, J., & Vinterbo, S. A. (2008). SMART - An Integrated Wireless System for Monitoring Unattended Patients. *Journal of the American Medical Informatics Association, 15*(1), 44–53. doi:10.1197/jamia.M2016

Czabke, A., D'Angelo, L. T., Niazmand, K., & Lüth, T. C. (2009). Ein kompaktes System zur Erfassung und Dokumentation von Bewegungsgewohnheiten. In *Proceedings of 2nd German AAL congress.*

Czarnecki, K., & Helsen, S. (2006). Feature-based survey of model transformation approaches. *IBM Systems Journal, 45*(3), 621–645.

D'Angelo, L., Weber, S., Honda, Y., Thiel, T., Narbonneau, F., & Lüth, T. C. (2008). A system for respiratory motion detection using optical fibers embedded into textiles. In *Engineering in Medicine and Biology Society, 2008. EMBS 2008. 30th Annual International Conference of the IEEE,* (pp. 3694-3697).

*Daily Activities.* (n.d.). Retrieved October 20, 2008, from http://seniors-site.com/nursingm/index.html

Dalal, S., Alwan, M., Seifrafi, R., Kell, S., & Brown, D. (2005). A Rule-Based Approach to the Analysis of Elders' Activity Data: Detection of Health and Possible Emergency Conditions. In *Proceedings of the AAAI 2005 Symposium, Workshop on Caring Machines: AI in Eldercare.*

Darkins, A., & Cary, M. (2000). *Telemedicine and Telehealth: Principles, Policies, Performance and Pitfalls.* New York: Springer Publishing Company.

Daumer, M., Thaler, K., Kruis, E., Feneberg, W., Staude, G., & Scholz, M. (2007). Steps towards a miniaturized, robust and autonomous measurement device for the long-term monitoring of patient activity: ActiBelt. *Biomedizinische Technik, 52,* 149–155. doi:10.1515/BMT.2007.028

David, P. (1994). *A revolution in seating - Nursing Home Technology.* Retrieved November 03, 2008.

Davies, S., Froggatt, K., & Meyer, J. (Eds.). (2009). *Understanding Home Care: A Research and Development Perspective.* London: Jessica Kingsley Publishers.

Davis, F. D. (1989). Perceived Usefulness, Perceived Ease Of Use, And User Acceptance Of Information Technology. *Management Information Systems Quarterly, 13*(3), 318–323. doi:10.2307/249008

Davis, F. D., & Venkatesh, V. (1995). *Measuring User Acceptance of Emerging Information Technologies: An Assessment of Possible Method Biases.* Paper presented at the 28th Hawaii Int'l Conf. System Sciences.

De Rossi, D., Carpi, F., Lorussi, F., Mazzoldi, A., Paradiso, R., Scilingo, E. P., & Tognetti, A. (2003). Electroactive fabrics and wearable biomonitoring devices. *AUTEX Research Journal, 3*(4), 180–185.

Debra, O., & Brain, H. (2006). A promising Technology to Reduce Social Isolation of Nursing Home Residents. *Journal of Nursing Care Quality, 21*(4), 302–306.

Del Vecchio, D., Hazlewood, V., & Humphrey, M. (2006, November). *Evaluating Grid portal security.* Paper presented at Supercomputing, Tampa, FL. DOC@HAND, 2006. Retrieved December 15, 2008, from http://services.txt.it/docathand/.

Demiris, G., Parker Oliver, D., Dickey, G., Skubic, M., & Rantz, M. (2008, April). Findings from a participatory evaluation of a smart home application for older adults. *Journal of Technology and Health Care, 16*(2), 111–118.

Demiris, G., Rantz, M. J., Aud, M. A., Marek, K. D., Tyrer, H. W., Skubic, M., & Hussam, A. A. (2004). Older adults' attitudes towards and perceptions of 'smart home' technologies: a pilot study. *Med. Inform. Taylor & Francis Healthsciences, 29*(2), 87–94. doi:10.1080/14639230410001684387

Demiris, G., Speedie, S. M., & Finkelstein, S. (2001). Change of patients' perceptions of TeleHomeCare. *Telemedicine Journal and e-Health, 7*(3), 241–249. doi:10.1089/153056201316970948

Dey, A. K., Salber, D., & Abowd, G. D. (2001). A Conceptual Framework and a Toolkit Supporting the Rapid Prototyping of Context-Aware Applications. *Human-Computer Interaction Journal, 16*(2-4), 97–166. doi:10.1207/S15327051HCI16234_02

DiabCostAustralia. (2002). *Assessing the Burden of Type 2 Diabetes in Australia.* Adelaide, Australia: DiabCost Australia.

Diabetes Australia. (2008). Diabetes in Australia. *Journal.* Retrieved from http://www.diabetesaustralia.com.au/Understanding-Diabetes/Diabetes-in-Australia/

Dishman, E. (2004). *Inventing Wellness Systems for Aging in Place.*

Dixon, T., & Webbie, K. (2006). *The National System for Monitoring Diabetes in Australia (AIHW Cat. No. CVD 32).* Canberra, Australia: Australian Institute of Health and Wealfare.

Doam, C. (2008). The Last Challenges and Barriers to the Development of Telemedicine Programs. *Studies in Health Technology and Informatics, 131*(1), 45–54.

Dorbritz, J., Ette, A., Gärtner, K., Grünheid, E., Mai, R., Micheel, F. et al. (2008). *Bevölkerung: Daten, Fakten, Trends zum demographischen Wandel in Deutschland.* Wiesbaden, Germany: Bundesinstitut für Bevölkerungsforschung und Statistisches Bundesamt.

Duda, R. O., Hart, P. E., & Stork, D. G. (2001). *Pattern Classification* (*Vol. 2*). New York: John Wiley & Sons, Inc.

Durable medical equipment: Scope and conditions. (2006). *CFR, 38,* 42.

Eley, R., Fallon, T., Soar, J., Buikstra, E., & Hegney, D. (2008). The status of training and education in information and computer technology of Australian nurses: a national survey. *Journal of Clinical Nursing, 17,* 2758–2767. doi:10.1111/j.1365-2702.2008.02285.x

Elite Care. (2008). *Elite Care.* Retrieved 2009, 2008, from http://www.elitecare.com/

Eljay, L. (2006). A Report on Shortfalls in Medicaid Funding for Nursing Home Care: American Health Care Association.

Emmerich, W., Butchart, B., Chen, L., Wassermann, B., & Price, S. L. (2006). Grid service orchestration using the Business Process Execution Language (BPEL). *Journal of Grid Computing, 3,* 283–304. doi:10.1007/s10723-005-9015-3

Endsley, M. R. (2000). Theoretical Underpinnings of Situation Awareness: A Critical Review. In M. R. Endsley, & D. J. Garland, Situation Awareness Analysis and Measurement (pp. 3-32). Mahwah, NJ: Lawrence Erlbaum Associates.

Eurosmart. (2008, April). *Smart USB Token.* White Paper. Retrieved February 17, 2009, from http://www.eurosmart.com/images/doc/WorkingGroups/NewFF/Papers/eurosmart_smart_usb_token_wp_april08.pdf

Eurostat/US Bureau of the Census. (2008, 03/09/2008). *People by age classes.* Retrieved 28/01/2009, from http://epp.eurostat.ec.europa.eu/portal/page?_pageid=1996,39140985&_dad=portal&_schema=PORTAL&screen=detailref&language=en&product=REF_TB_population&root=REF_TB_population/t_popula/t_pop/t_demo_pop/tps00010

Eyole-Monono, M., Harle, R., & Hopper, A. (2006). POISE: An inexpensive, low-power location sensor based on electrostatics. In *3rd Annual International Conference On Mobile and Ubiquitous Systems: Networks And Services (MobiQuitous 2006), 17–21 July 2006* (pp.1-3). San Jose, California: ICST.

Facts, N. (2006). *Today's Registered Nurse - Numbers and Demographics.* Washington, DC: A. N. Association.

Falck, T., Baldus, H., Espina, J., & Klabunde, K. (2007). Plug æn Play Simplicity for Wireless Medical Body Sensors. *Mobile Networks and Applications, 12,* 143–153. doi:10.1007/s11036-007-0016-2

Favela, J., Rodríguez, M. D., Preciado, A., & Gonzalez, V. M. (2004). Integrating Context-aware Public Displays into a Mobile Hospital Information System. *IEEE Trans. IT in BioMedicine, 8*(3), 279–286.

Fei, H., Meng, J., Wagner, M., & De-Cun, D. (2007). Privacy-Preserving Telecardiology Sensor Networks: Toward a Low-Cost Portable Wireless Hardware/Software Codesign. *IEEE Transactions on Information Technology in Biomedicine, 11*(6), 619–627.

Ferraiolo, D. F., Kuhn, R. D., & Chandramouli, R. (2003). *Role-Based Access Control*. Boston: Artech House Publishers.

Ferscha, A. (2007). Informative Art Display Metaphors. In *Proceedings of the 4th International Conference on Universal Access in Human-Computer Interaction (UAHCI 2007),* (pp. 82-92). Beijing, China: Springer LNCS.

Field, T., & Rochon, P. (2008). Costs associated with developing and implementing a computerized clinical decision support system for medication dosing for patients with renal insufficiency in the long-term care setting. *Journal of the American Medical Informatics Association, 15*(4), 466–472. doi:10.1197/jamia.M2589

Finch, C. (1999). Mobile computing in healthcare. *Health Management Technology, 20*(3), 63–64.

Finch, T. L., Mort, M., Mair, F. S., & May, C. R. (2008). Future Patients? Telehealthcare, Roles, and Responsibilities. *Health & Social Care in the Community, 16*(1), 86–95.

Finnema, E., de Lange, J., Droes, R. M., Ribbe, M., & Tilburg, W. (2001). The quality of nursing home care: do the opinions of family members change after implementation of emotion-oriented care? *Journal of Advanced Nursing, 35*(5), 728–732. doi:10.1046/j.1365-2648.2001.01905.x

Flores-Mangas, F., & Oliver, N. (2005). *Healthgear: A realtime wearable system for monitoring and analyzing physiological signals*. Technical Report MSR-TR-2005-182, Microsoft Research.

Fourty, N., Val, T., Fraisse, P., & Mercier, J.-J. (2005). Comparative analysis of new high data rate wireless communication technologies "from Wi-Fi to WiMAX". In. *Proceedings of the Joint International Conference on Autonomic and Autonomous Systems and International Conference on Networking and Services, ICAS-ICNS, 2005,* 66–71.

France, R., & Rumpe, B. (2007). Model-driven Development of Complex Software: A Research Roadmap. In *Proceedings of 29th Inernational Conference on Software Engineering*. Washington, DC: IEEE Computer Society.

Fraunholz, B., & Unnithan, C. (2007). Potential of Telemedicines of Preliminary Evaluation Through the Inovation Diffusion Lens. *International Journal of Healthcare Technology and Management, 8*(3/4), 315–332. doi:10.1504/IJHTM.2007.013166

*Frost and Sullivan Country Industry Forecast – European Union Healthcare Industry*. (2004, May 11). Retrieved from http://www.news-medical.net/print_article.asp?id=1405

Fulford-Jones, T. R. F., Wei, G. Y., & Welsh, M. (2004). A portable, low-power, wireless two-lead EKG system. *Engineering in Medicine and Biology Society, 2004. EMBC 2004.Conference Proceedings.26th Annual International Conference of the,* 1.

*Fun Times*. (n.d.). Retrieved October 20, 2008, from http://www.goldenlivingcenters.com/GGNSC

Gagnon, M. P., Légaré, F., Fortin, J. P., Lamothe, L., Labrecquel, M., & Duplantie, J. (2008). An Integrated Strategy of Knowledge Application for Optimal e-Health Implementation: A Multimethod Study Protocol. *BMC Medical Informatics and Decision Making, 8,* 17. doi:10.1186/1472-6947-8-17

Galarraga, M., Martínez, I., Serrano, L., de Toledo, P., Escayola, J., Fernández, J., et al. (2007a) Proposal of an ISO/IEEE11073 platform for healthcare telemonitoring: plug-and-play solution with new use cases. 29th Annual International Conference of the IEEE EMBS. Cité Internationale, Lyon, France, pp. 6711–6712.

Gao, T., Kim, M. I., White, D., & Alm, A. M. (2006). Iterative user-centered design of a next generation patient monitoring system for emergency medical response. In *AMIA Annual Symposium Proceedings*, (pp. 284-288).

Gao, T., Massey, T., Selavo, L., Crawford, D., Chen, B., & Lorincz, K. (2007, Sept.). The advanced health and disaster aid network: A light-weight wireless medical system for triage. *IEEE Transactions on Biomedical Circuits and Systems, 1*(3), 203–216. doi:10.1109/TB-CAS.2007.910901

Gao, T., Pesto, C., Selavo, L., Chen, Y., Ko, J. G., Lim, J. H., et al. (2008) Wireless Medical Sensor Networks in Emergency Response: Implementation and Pilot Results. In *Technologies for Homeland Security, 2008 IEEE Conference on,* (pp. 187-192).

Gasca, E., Favela, J., & Tentori, M. (2008). *Persuasive Virtual Communities to Promote a Healthy Lifestyle among Patients with Chronic Diseases.* Paper presented at the In Proc. of CRIWG, Omaha, Nebraska, September, 14-18.

Geisler, E., & Wickramasinghe, N. (2009). *The Role and Utilization of Wireless Technology in the Management and Monitoring of Chronic Diseases.* Washington, DC: IBM Center for the Business of Government.

General Accounting Office. (2004). *HS's efforts to promote health information technology and legal barriers to its adoption.* Washington, DC: Author.

Georgia Institute of Technology. (n.d.). *The Aware Home.* Retrieved from http://www.cc.gatech.edu/fce/ahri/projects/index.html

Geven, A., Tscheligi, M., Sorin, A., & Aronowitz, H. (2008). Presenting a speech-based mobile reminder system. In Proceedings of SiMPE 2008. Amsterdam, Netherlands.

Ghasemzadeh, H., Guenterberg, E., & Jafari, R. (2009). Energy-Efficient Information-Driven Coverage for Physical Movement Monitoring in Body Sensor Networks. *IEEE Journal on Selected Areas in Communications, 27*(1), 58–69.

Giani, A., Roosta, T., & Sastry, S. (2008, January). Integrity checker for wireless sensor networks in health care applications. In *Proceedings of the 2nd international conference on pervasive computing technologies for healthcare.*

Gill, TM, A. H., Han L. (2006). Bathing disability and the risk of long-term admission to a nursing home. *Journal of Gerontology, 61*(8), 821–825.

Gödde, F., Möller, S., Engelbrecht, K.-P., Kühnel, C., Schleicher, R., Naumann, A., & Wolters, M. (2008). Study of a Speech-based Smart Home System with Older Users. In *International Workshop on Intelligent User Interfaces for Ambient Assisted Living.*

Golant, S. M. (2008). The Future of Assisted Living Residences. In Golant, S. M., & Hyde, J. (Eds.), *The Assisted Living Residence* (pp. 3–45). Baltimore: The John Hopkins University Press.

Goldberg, S. a. (2002). *Building the Evidence for a standardized Mobile Internet (wireless) Environment in Ontario, Canada, January Update, Internal INET Documentation.* Ontario, Canada: INET.

Goldberg, S. a. (2002). *HTA Presentational Selection and Aggregation Component Summary. Internal INET Documentation.* Ontario, Canada: INET.

Goldberg, S. a. (2002). *Wireless POC Device Component Summary, Internal INET documentation.* Ontario, Canada: INET.

Goldberg, S. a. (2002). *HTA Presentation Rendering Component Summary, Internal INET documentation.* Ontario, Canada: INET.

Goldberg, S. a. (2002). *HTA Quality Assurance Component Summary, Internal INET documentation.* Ontario, Canada: INET.

Gopalsamy, C., Park, S., Rajamanickam, R., & Jayaraman, S. (1999). The Wearable Motherboard: The first generation of adaptive and responsive textile structures (ARTS) for medical applications. *Virtual Reality (Waltham Cross), 4,* 152–168. doi:10.1007/BF01418152

Gouaux, F., Simon-Chautemps, L., Adami, S., Arzi, M., Assanelli, D., Fayn, J., et al. (2003). Smart devices for the early detection and interpretation of cardiological syndromes. In *Proceedings 4th International IEEE EMBS Special Topic Conference on Information Technology Applications in Biomedicine*, (pp. 291-294).

Grabowski, P., Lewandowski, B., & Russell, M. (2004). *Access from J2ME-enabled mobile devices to Grid services* (White Paper). Poznan University of Technology, Poland.

Greenly, M., & Gugerty, B. (2002). How bar coding reduces medication errors. *Nursing, 32*(5), 70.

*Gridsphere Portal Framework*. (n.d.). Retrieved August 18, 2007, from http://www.gridsphere.org/gridsphere/gridsphere

Großschädl, J. (2006). TinySA: A security architecture for wireless sensor networks (extended abstract). In *Proceedings of the 2nd international conference on emerging networking experiments and technologies (conext 2006)*. New York: ACM Press.

Groth, D., & Skandier, T. (2005). *Network+ Study Guild*. Indianapolis: Wiley Publishing Inc.

Guang-Zhong, Y., Lo, B., Wang, L., Rans, M., Thiemjarus, S., Ng, J., et al. (2004). From Sensor Networks to Behavior Profiling: A Homecare Perspective of Intelligent Building. In *Proceedings of the IEE Seminar for Intelligent Buildings*.

Guilliani, V., Scopeletti, M., & Fornara, F. (2005). Elderly People at Home: Technological Help in Everyday Activities. In *IEEE, International Workshop on Robots and Human Interactive Communication*. Retrieved from http://www.dinf.ne.jp/doc/english/Us_Eu/conf/csun_99/session0260.html

Gura, N., Patel, A., Wander, A., Eberle, H., & Shantz, S. C. (2004). Comparing elliptic curve cryptography and RSA on 8-bit CPUs. In *Proceedings of the workshop on cryptography hardware and embedded systems (CHES 2004)*, (pp. 119–132).

Hailey, D., Ohinmaa, A., & Roine, R. (2004). Study Quality and Evidence of Benefit in Recent Assessments of Telemedicine. *Journal of Telemedicine and Telecare, 10*(6), 318–324. doi:10.1258/1357633042602053

Hall, E. S., Vawdrey, D. K., Knutson, C. D., & Archibald, J. K. (2003). Enabling remote access to personal electronic medical records. *IEEE Engineering in Medicine and Biology Magazine*, 133–139.

Halpern, J. Y., & Weissman, V. (2008). Using First-Order Logic to Reason about Policies. *ACM Transactions on Information and System Security, 11*, 1–41. doi:10.1145/1380564.1380569

Hamilton, B. (2006). *Evaluation design of the business case of health information technology in long-term care (Final report)*. Baltimore: Centers for Medicare and Medicaid Services.

Harris, Y., & Clauser, S. B. (2002). Achieving improvement through nursing home quality measurement. *Health Care Financing Review, 23*(4), 13.

Harrison, J. P., & Lee, A. (2006, Nov-Dec). The Role of e-Health in the Changing Healthcare Environment. *Nurs. Econ., 24*(6), 2388, 279.

Harrison, S. (2002). Telehealth skills hailed as answer to discharge delays: costs of high-tech monitoring systems compare favourably with long-term care. (news). *Nursing Standard, 17*(12), 7(1).

Hartung, C., Balasalle, J., & Han, R. (2005, January). *Node compromise in sensor networks: The need for secure systems* (Technical Report No. CU-CS-990-05). Department of Computer Science, University of Colorado.

Hayes, H. (2008). *Home Health Monitoring Saves the Government Big Bucks*. Retrieved from http://www.govhealthit.com/print/4_21/features/350570-1.html

Healy, M., Newe, T., & Lewis, E. (2007). Efficiently securing data on a wireless sensor network. *Journal of Physics: Conference Series, 76*.

Henkemans, O. A. B., Caine, K. E., Rogers, W. A., Fisk, A. D., Neerinx, M. A., & de Ruyter, B. (2007) Medical Monitoring for Independent Living: User-Centered Design of Smart Home Technologies for Older Adults. In *Proceedings of the 2007 Med-e-Tel conference for eHealth*.

Hetzel, L., & Smith, A. (2001). *The 65 and Over Population: 2000-Census 2000 Brief*. Washington, DC: U.S. CENSUS BUREAU.

Hightower, J., & Borriello, G. (2001). A survey and taxonomy of location systems for ubiquitous computing. *IEEE Computer, 34*(8), 57–66.

Hihnel, D., Burgard, W., Fox, D., Fishkin, K., & Philipose, M. (2004). Mapping and localization with RFID technology. In *IEEE International Conference on Robotics & Automation (ICRA '04), 26 April-1 May 2004*, (pp. 1015-1020). New Orleans, LA: IEEE Robotics and Automation Society.

Hii, P., & Zaslavsky, A. (2005). Improving location accuracy by combining WLAN positioning and sensor technology. In *Workshop on Real-World Wireless Sensor Networks (REALWSN'05), 20-21 June 2005*. Stockholm, Sweden: Swedish Institute of Computer Science.

Hill, J., Szewczyk, R., Woo, A., Hollar, S., Culler, D., & Pister, K. (2000). System architecture directions for networked sensors. *ACM SIGPLAN Notices, 35*(11), 93–104. doi:10.1145/356989.356998

Ho, L., Moh, M., Walker, Z., Hamada, T., & Su, C. F. (2005). *A prototype on RFID and sensor networks for elder healthcare: progress report* (pp. 70–75). Applications, Technologies, Architectures, and Protocols for Computer Communication.

Hoban, S. (2003). Activities plus at Montgomery Place: the "new" active senior wants to be entertained, enlightened, and engaged--and will let you know how. *Nursing Homes, 52*(6), 52–56.

Hogan, W. (2007). *The Organisation of Residential Aged Care for an Aging Population*. The Centre of Independent Studies Limitedo.

Holma, H., & Toskala, A. (Eds.). (2006). *HSDPA/HSUPA for UMTS*. New York: Wiley.

Holma, H., Toskala, A., Ranta-aho, K., & Pirskanen, J. (2007). High-Speed Packet Access Evolution in 3GPP Release 7. *IEEE Communications Magazine, 45*(2), 29–35.

Holmes, D. (2007). An evaluation of a monitoring system intervention: falls, injuries, and affect in nursing homes. *Clinical Nursing Research, 16*(4), 317–335. doi:10.1177/1054773807307870

*Home Care and Nursing Home Services*. (n.d.). Retrieved December 12, 2008, from http://dhs.dc.gov/dhs/cwp/view,a,3,Q,613301.asp

Hunt, D. (2007). *Urgent health system reform needed to tackle disease epidemic, says head of new University of Melbourne centre*. Retrieved 25 November, 2008, from http://uninews.unimelb.edu.au/view.php?articleID=4615

Hyde, J., Perez, R., & Reed, P. S. (2008). The Old Road Is Rapidly Aging. In Golant, S. M., & Hyde, J. (Eds.), *The Assisted Living Residence* (pp. 46–85). Baltimore: The Johns Hopkins University Press.

IBM Corporation. (2005). *IBM Websphere Workflow – Getting Started with Buildtime V. 3.6*.

ICIC. (2008). Improving Chronic Illness Care: The Chronic Care Model. *Journal*. Retrieved from http://www.improvingchroniccare.org/indix.php?p=The_Chronic_Care_Model&s=2

IEEE802. *15 TG3, IEEE 802.15 WPAN Task Group 3* (TG3). (n.d.). Retrieved from http://www.ieee802.org/15/pub/TG3.html

*IEEE802.15 TG4b*. (2001). IEEE802.15 TG4 Contributions, WPAN-LR Call For Proposals for Session #13/ Portland, Plenary, Bob Heile.

Inglesby, J., & Inglesby, T. (2005, September). Retrieved April 25, 2009, from http://www.psqh.com/sepoct05/barcodingrfid2.html

*Inspectors Often Overlook Serious Deficiencies at U.S. Nursing Homes* (GAO Report). (2008). Medical New Today.

Institute of Medicine. (1996). *Telemedicine: A Guide to Assessing Telecommunications for Health Care.* Washington, DC: National Academy Press.

Institute of Medicine. (2001). *Crossing the quality chasm: A new health system for 21st century.* Washington, DC: National Academy Press.

Intanagonwiwat, C., Govindan, R., & Estrin, D. (2000). Directed diffusion: A scalable and robust communication paradigm for sensor networks. In *Proceedings of 6th Annual Intl. Conf. on Mobile Computing and Networking.* Boston.

Integrating the Healthcare Enterprise (IHE). (2005). Retrieved December 15, 2008, from http://www.ihe.net/

International Classification of Functioning. Disability and Health (ICF). (2001) Geneva: World Health Organization (W.H.O.).

International Telecommunication Union. (2004). *Telecommunication Development Bureau, ITU-D Study Group 2. Question 14-1/2: Application of telecommunications in health care, technical information - A mobile medical image transmission system in Japan, PocketMI-MAS.* Rapporteurs Meeting Q14-1/2 Japan.

Internet Engineering Task Force. (2008). *The Transport Layer Security (TLS) Protocol Version 1.2.* Retrieved February 17, 2009, from http://tools.ietf.org/html/rfc5246

Intille, S. S. (2002). Designing a Home of the Future. *IEEE Pervasive Computing / IEEE Computer Society [and] IEEE Communications Society, 1*(2), 76–82. doi:10.1109/MPRV.2002.1012340

Intille, S. S., Larson, K., Beaudin, J. S., Nawyn, J., Tapia, E. M., & Kaushik, P. (2005). A living laboratory for the design and evaluation of ubiquitous computing technologies. In ACM New York (pp. 1941-1944)

Intille, S., Kukla, C., & Ma, X. (2002). *Eliciting user preferences using image-based experience sampling and reection.* Paper presented at the Extended Abstracts of the Conference on Human Factors in Computer Systems.

ISO/IEC. Integrated Circuit(s) Cards with Contacts – Part 7: Interindustry Commands for Structured Card Query Language (SCQL). (1999). *Standard ISO/IEC 7816-7.* International Standardization Organization.

ISTAT. (2006). Popolazione comunale per sesso, età e stato civile - Anni 2002-2005. *Informazioni, 29.*

Istepanian, R. S. H., & Chandran, S. (1999). Enhanced telemedicine applications with next generation of wireless systems. In *Proc. First Joint BMES/EMBS IEEE International Conference of Engineering in Medicine and Biology,* Atlanta.

Istepanian, R. S. H., & Lacal, J. C. (2003). *Emerging mobile communication technologies for health: some imperative notes on m-health.* Paper presented at the 25th Annual International Conference of the IEEE EMBS, New York.

Istepanian, R. S. H., Jovanov, E., & Zhang, Y. T. (2004). Guest Editorial Introduction to the Special Section on M-Health: Beyond Seamless Mobility and Global Wireless Health-Care Connectivity. *IEEE Transactions on Information Technology in Biomedicine, 8*(4), 405–414.

Jafari, R., Encarnacao, A., Zahoory, A., Brisk, P., Noshadi, H., & Sarrafzadeh, M. (2005) Wireless Sensor Networks For Health Monitoring. In *Second ACM/IEEE International Conference on Mobile and Ubiquitous Systems.*

Japan Statistics Bureau & Statistics Center. (2008, April 15). *Population by Age (Single Year), Sex and Sex ratio - Total population, Japanese population,* October 1, 2007. Retrieved 28/01/2009, from http://www.e-stat.go.jp/SG1/estat/ListE.do?lid=000001026128

Java Agent Development Framework. (n.d.). Retrieved May 15, 2008, from http://jade.tilab.com/

*Java Authentication and Authorization Service (JAAS) Reference Guide for the Java SE Development Kit 6.* (n.d.). Retrieved May 12, 2008, from http://java.sun.com/javase/6/docs/technotes/guides/security/jaas/JAASRefGuide.html

*Java CoG Kit.* (n.d.). Retrieved May 12, 2008, from http://www-unix.globus.org/cog/

Java Community Press. (n.d.). *JSR-168 Portlet Specification.* Retrieved August 18, 2007, from http://www.jcp.org/aboutJava/communityprocess/final/jsr168/

Jennett, P. A., Affleck Hall, L., Hailey, D., Ohinmaa, A., Andreson, C., & Thomas, R. (2003). The Socio-Economic Impact of Telehealth: A Systematic Review. *Telemed. Telecare, 9*(6), 311–320. doi:10.1258/135763303771005207

Jennett, P., & Watanabe, M. (2006). Healthcare and Telemedicine: Ongoing and Evolving Challenges. *Disease Management & Health Outcomes, 14*(1), 9–13. doi:10.2165/00115677-200614001-00004

Johnson, B., Wheeler, L., Dueser, J., & Sousa, K. (2000). Outcomes of the Kaiser Permanente Tele-Home Health Research Project. *Archives of Family Medicine, 9*(4), 40–45. doi:10.1001/archfami.9.1.40

Jones, V., Van Halteren, A., Widya, I., Dokovsky, N., Koprinkov, G., Bults, R., et al. (2005). Mobihealth: Mobile Services for Health Professionals, In R.S.H. Istepanian, C.S. Pattichis & S. Laxminarayan (Ed.), M-Health Emerging Mobile Health Systems, (pp. 237-246, Topics in Biomedical Engineering International Book Series). Berlin: Springer.

Jorgensen, J. B. (2002, August). *Coloured Petri Nets in UML-Based Software Development – Designing Middleware for Pervasive Healthcare.* Paper presented at the Fourth International Workshop on Practical Use of Coloured Petri Nets and the CPN Tools. Aarhus, Denmark.

Joshy, G., & Simmons, D. (2006). Diabetes information systems: a rapidly emerging support for diabetes surveillance and care. *Diabetes Technology & Therapeutics, 8*(5), 587–597. doi:10.1089/dia.2006.8.587

Jouault, F., & Kurtev, I. (2005). Transforming Models with ATL. In Proceedings of Model Transformations in Practice Workshop of MODELS'05.

Juels, A. (2006). RFID security and privacy: a research survey. *IEEE Journal on Selected Areas in Communications, 24*, 381–394. doi:10.1109/JSAC.2005.861395

Kannan, G., & Vijayakumar, S. (2008). Smart Home Testbed for Disabled People. *Mobile and Pervasive Computing, CoMPC.*

Kao, W. C., Chen, W. H., Yu, C. K., Hong, C. M., & Lin, S. Y. (2005). Portable Real-Time Homecare System Design with Digital Camera Platform. *IEEE Transactions on Consumer Electronics, 51*(4), 1035–1041.

Karantonis, D. M., Narayanan, M. R., Mathie, M., Lovell, N. H., & Celler, B. G. (2006). Implementation of a Real-Time Human Movement Classifier Using a Triaxial Accelerometer for Ambulatory Monitoring. *Information Technology in Biomedicine. IEEE Transactions on, 10*(1), 156–167.

Karjoth, G., Schunter, M., & Waidner, M. (2002). *Platform for Enterprise Privacy Practices: Privacy-Enabled Management of Customer Data* (pp. 69–84). Privacy Enhancing Technologies.

Karl, H., & Willig, A. (2005). *Protocols and Architectures for Wireless Sensor Networks.* New York: Wiley. doi:10.1002/0470095121

Karlof, C., Sastry, N., & Wagner, D. (2004, November). A link layer security architecture for wireless sensor networks. In Second ACM conference on embedded networked sensor systems (SenSys 2004) (pp. 162–175). TinySec.

Karp, B., & Kung, H. T. (2000). *GPSR: greedy perimeter stateless routing for wireless networks* (pp. 243–254). MOBICOM.

Kassim, M. R. M. (2007). Design, development and implementation of smart home systems using rf and power line communication. In *The 2nd National Intelligent Systems And Information Technology Symposium (ISITS'07),* Oct 30-31, 2007, ITMA -UPM, Malaysia.

Katz, S., Ford, A. B., Moskowitz, R. W., Jackson, B. A., & Jaffe, M. W. (1963). Studies of Illness in the aged. The Index of ADL: a Standardized Measure of Biological and Psychosocial Function. *Journal of the American Medical Association, 185,* 914–919.

Kavas, A. (2007). Comparative analysis of WLAN, WiMAX and UMTS Technologies. In *Progress In Electromagnetics Research Symposium 2007, Prague, Czech Republic,* (pp. 140-144).

Kemper, P., Komisar, H. L., & Alecixh, L. (2005). Long-Term Care Over What can Current Retirees Expect? *Inquiry, 42,* 15.

Khambati, A., Warren, J., Grundy, J., & Hosking, J. (2008). *A model driven approach to care planning systems for consumer engagement in chronic disease management.* Paper presented at the HIC 2008 Australia's Health Informatics Conference, Health Informatics Society of Australia Ltd (HISA).

Khatua, S., Dasgupta, S., & Mukherjee, N. (2006, June). *Pervasive access to the Data Grid.* Paper presented at the International Conference on Grid Computing and Applications, Las Vegas, NV.

Khoor, S., Nieberl, K., Fugedi, K., & Kail, E. (2001). Telemedicine ECG-telemetry with Bluetooth technology. In *2nd Annual Conference of Computers in Cardiology,* Rotterdam, Holland, (pp. 585–588).

Kidd, C. D., Orr, R., Abowd, G. D., Atkeson, C. G., Essa, I. A., MacIntyre, B., et al. (1999). *The Aware Home: A Living Laboratory for Ubiquitous Computing Research.* Paper presented at the Proceedings of the Second International Workshop on Cooperative Buildings, Integrating Information, Organization, and Architecture.

Kifor, T., Varga, L., Vazquez-Salceda, J., Alvarez, S., Miles, S., & Moreau, L. (2006). Provenance in Agent-Mediated Healthcare Systems. *IEEE Intelligent Systems, 21*(6), 38–46.

Killeen, J. P., Chan, T. C., Buono, C., Griswold, W. G., & Lenert, L. A. (2006). A wireless first responder handheld device for rapid triage, patient assessment and documentation during mass casualty incidents. In *AMIA Annual Symposium Proceedings,* (pp. 429-433).

King, W. R., & He, J. (2006). A meta-analysis of the technology acceptance model. *Information & Management, 43*(6), 740–755. doi:10.1016/j.im.2006.05.003

Kjeldskov, J., & Skov, M. (2004, June). *Supporting work activities in healthcare by mobile electronic patient records.* Paper presented at the 6th Asia-Pacific Conference on Human-Computer Interaction, Rotorua, New Zealand.

Klein, M., Schmidt, A., & Lauer, R. (2007). Ontology-Centred Design of an Ambient Middleware for Assisted Living: The Case of SOPRANO. In T. Kirste, B. König-Ries, & R. Salomon (Ed.), *Towards Ambient Intelligence: Methods for Cooperating Ensembles in Ubiquitous Environments (AIM-CU), Proceedings of the 30th Annual German Conference on Artificial Intelligence (KI 2007).* Osnabrück.

Kleinberger, T., Becker, M., Ras, E., Holzinger, A., & Muller, P. (2007). Ambient Intelligence in assisted living: Enable elderly people to handle future interfaces. *Lecture Notes in Computer Science, 4555,* 103–112. doi:10.1007/978-3-540-73281-5_11

Knuiman, M. W., Welborn, T. A., & Bartholomew, H. C. (1996). Self-reported health and use of health services: a comparison of diabetic and nondiabetic persons from a national sample. *Australian and New Zealand Journal of Public Health, 20*(3), 241–247. doi:10.1111/j.1467-842X.1996.tb01023.x

Koch, S. (2005). Home telehealth - Current state and future trends. *International Journal of Medical Informatics.*

Kohn, L. T., Corrigan, J. M., & Donaldson, M. S. (1999). *To err is human: Building a safer human system.* Washington, DC: National Academy Press.

Köngis, A. (2005). Model Transformation with Triple Graph Grammars. *In Proceedings of Model Transformations in Practice Workshop at MoDELS Conference.* Montego Bay, Jamaica.

Korhonen, I., & Bardram, J. E. (2004). Guest editorial introduction to the special section on pervasive healthcare. *IEEE Transactions on Information Technology in Biomedicine, 8*(3), 229–234. doi:10.1109/TITB.2004.835337

Koufi, V., & Vassilacopoulos, G. (2008, January). *HDG-Portal: A Grid Portal Application for Pervasive Access to Process-Based Healthcare Systems.* Paper presented at the 2nd International Conference in Pervasive Computing Technologies in Healthcare, Tampere, Finland.

Koufi, V., Papakonstantinou, D., & Vassilacopoulos, G. (2006, June). *Virtual patient record security on a Grid infrastructure.* Paper presented at the International Conference on Information Communication Technologies in Health (ICICTH'06), Samos, Greece.

Kramer, A., Bennett, R., Fish, R., Lin, C. T., Floersch, N., & Conway, K. (2004). *Case studies of electronic health records in post-acute and long-term care.* Washington, DC: U.S. Department of Health and Human Services.

Krizner, K. (2008). Digital Hospitals Aim to Document Better Outcomes. *Managed Healthcare Executive, 18*(4), 28–30.

Krontiris, I., Dimitriou, T., Soroush, H., & Salajegheh, M. (2008). In Lopez, J., & Zhou, J. (Eds.), *Wireless sensors networks security* (pp. 142–163). Amsterdam: IOS Press.

Krontiris, I., Giannetsos, Th., & Dimitriou, T. (2008). Launching a Sinkhole Attack in Wireless Sensor Networks; the Intruder Side. In *Proceeding of the first international workshop on security and privacy in wireless and mobile computing, networking and communications (SecPriWiMob 2008),* (pp. 526-531).

Krummenacher, R., & Strang, T. (2007). Ontology-Based Context Modeling. In *Proceedings of Context Awareness for Proactive Systems (CAPS 2007),* Guildford, UK.

Kühner, J. (2008). *Expert. NET Micro Framework.* New York: APRESS.

Kuhn, T., Gotzhein, R., & Webel, C. (2006). Model-Driven Development with SDL - Process, Tools, and Experiences. In O. Nierstrasz, J. Whittle, D. Harel, & G. Reggio (Ed.), *Proceedings of the 9th Intl. Conf. on Model Driven Engineering Languages and Systems.* (LNCS, pp. 83-97). Berlin: Springer Verlag.

Kulik, J., Heinzelman, W., & Balakrishnan, H. (2002). Negotiation-based protocols for disseminating information in wireless sensor networks. [New York: ACM.]. *Wireless Networks,* 169–185. doi:10.1023/A:1013715909417

Kulkarni, R., & Nathanson, L. A. (2005). *Medical Informatics in medicine.* E-Medicine at http://www.emedicine.com/emerg/topic879.htm

Kumar, S., & Krupinski, E. (Eds.). (2008). *Teleradiology.* New York: Springer Publishing Company. doi:10.1007/978-3-540-78871-3

Kurschl, W., Mitsch, S., & Schoenboeck, J. (2008, November). *Model-Driven Prototyping Support for Pervasive Health Care Applications.* Paper presented at the Software Engineering and Applications Conference, Orlando, Florida, USA.

Kurschl, W., Mitsch, S., Schönböck, J., & Beer, W. (2008). Modeling Wireless Sensor Networks based Context-Aware Emergency Coordination Systems. In *Proceedings of the 10th Intl. Conf. on Information Integration and Web-based Applications & Services (iiWAS2008)* (pp. 117-122). Linz, Austria: ACM Press.

Kutzik, D. M., Glascock, A. P., Lundberg, L., & York, J. (2008). Technological Tools of the Future. In Golant, S. M., & Hyde, J. (Eds.), *The Assisted Living Residence.* Baltimore: The Johns Hopkins University Press.

Kvedar, J., Wootton, R., & Dimnick, S. (Eds.). (2006). *Home Telehealth: Connecting Care Within the Community.* London: Royal Society of Medicine Press.

Kyriacou, E., Pavlopoulos, S., Berler, A., Neophytou, M., Bourka, A., & Georgoulas, A. (2003). Multi-purpose HealthCare Telemedicine Systems with mobile communication link support. *Biomedical Engineering Online, 2*(7).

Laakko, T., Leppänen, J., Lähteenmäki, J., & Nummiaho, A. (2008)... *Mobile Health and Wellness Application Framework Methods of Information in Medicine, 47*(3), 217–222.

Laberg, T. (2005). Smart Home Technology; Technology supporting independent living - does it have an impact on health? In E-health 05, Tromsø, Norway, 23 -24 May.

Labiod, H., Afifi, H., & De Santis, C. (2007). *Wi-Fi Bluetooth Zigbee and WiMax*. Dordrecht: Springer. doi:10.1007/978-1-4020-5397-9

Lacroix, A. (1999). International concerted action on collaboration in telemedicine: G8sub-project 4. *Studies in Health Technology and Informatics, 64*, 12–19.

Lahtela, A., Hassinen, M., & Jylha, V. (2008). RFID and NFC in healthcare: Safety of hospitals medication care. In *Second International Conference on Pervasive Computing Technologies for Healthcare*, (pp. 241-244).

Lange, C., & Ziese, T. (2006). *Gesundheit in Deutschland*. Berlin: Robert Koch-Institut.

Langheinrich, M. (2005). *Personal Privacy in Ubiquitous Computing*. Doctoral dissertation. ETH Zurich.

Lawton, M. P., & Brody, E. M. (1969). Assessment of Older People: Self-Mantaining and Instrumental Activities of Daily Living. *The Gerontologist, 9*(3), 179–186.

Le, X. H. B., Di Mascolo, M., Gouin, A., & Noury, N. (2007). Health Smart Home-Towards an assistant tool for automatic assessment of the dependence of elders. *Engineering in Medicine and Biology Society, 2007. EMBS 2007.29th Annual International Conference of the IEEE*, 3806-3809.

Leff, B. (2009). Defining and Disseminating the Hospital-at-Home Model. *Canadian Medical Association Journal, 180*(2). doi:10.1503/cmaj.081891

Lenert, L., Palmer, D., Chan, T., & Rao, R. (2005). An intelligent 802.11 triage tag for medical response to disasters. In *AMIA Annual Symposium Proceedings*, (pp. 440-444).

LeRouge, C., Garfield, M. J., & Hevner, A. R. (2002). Quality Attributes in Telemedicine Video Conferencing. In *Proceedings of the 35th Hawaii International Conference on System Sciences*, Hawaii.

Levis, P., Madden, S., Polastre, J., Szewczyk, R., Whitehouse, K., & Woo, A. (2005). TinyOS: An Operating System for Wireless Sensor Networks. In Weber, W., Rabaey, J., & Aarts, E. (Eds.), *Ambient Intelligence*. doi:10.1007/3-540-27139-2_7

Lewis, F. L. (2005). Wireless Sensor Networks. In Cook, D. J., & Das, S. K. (Eds.), *Smart Environments - Technology, Protocols, and Applications* (pp. 13–46). Mahwah, NJ: John Wiley & Sons.

Liebert, T. (2008, March). Ongoing concern over Pentagon network attack. *IT News Digest*. Retrieved February 17, 2009, from http://blogs.techrepublic.com.com/technews/?p=2098.

Lilley RC, L. P., Lambden P. (2006). *Medicines management for residential and nursing homes: a toolkit for best practice and accredited learning*. Seatle: Radcliffe.

Lin, C. C., Chiu, M. J., Hsiao, C. C., Lee, R. G., & Tsai, Y. S. (2006). Wireless health care service system for elderly with dementia. *IEEE Transactions on Information Technology in Biomedicine, 10*(4), 696–704. doi:10.1109/TITB.2006.874196

Lin, Y.-H., Jan, I.-C., Ko, P. C.-I., Chen, Y.-Y., Wong, J.-M., & Jan, G.-J. (2004). A wireless PDA-based physiological monitoring system for patient transport. *IEEE Transactions on Information Technology in Biomedicine, 8*(4), 439–447. doi:10.1109/TITB.2004.837829

Liu, A., & Ning, P. (2008). TinyECC: A configurable library for elliptic curve cryptography in wireless sensor networks. In *Proceedings of the International Conference on Information Processing in Sensor Networks (IPSN 2008), 0*, 245-256.

Lorincz, K., Malan, D. J., Fulford-Jones, T. R. F., Nawoj, A., Clavel, A., & Shnayder, V. (2004). Sensor networks for emergency response: Challenges and opportunities. *IEEE Pervasive Computing / IEEE Computer Society [and] IEEE Communications Society, 3*(4), 16–23. doi:10.1109/MPRV.2004.18

Losilla, F., Vicente-Chicote, C., Alvarez, B., Iborra, A., & Sanchez, P. (2007). Wireless Sensor Network Application Development: An Architecture Centric MDE Approach. In *Proceedings of the First European Conference on Software Architecture* (S. 179-194). Madrid, Spain: Springer.

Lovell, N. H., Celler, B. G., Basilakis, J., Magrabi, F., Huynh, K., & Mathie, M. (2002). *Managing chronic disease with home telecare: a system architecture and case study.* Paper presented at the Proceedings of the Second Joint EMBS/BMES Conference.\.

Lubrin, E., Lawrence, E., Navarro, K. F., & Zmijewska, A. (2006, July). Awareness of wireless sensor network potential in healthcare industry: A second UTAUT study. In *Proceedings of the IASTED international conference on wireless sensor networks,* Banff, Canada.

Lüder, M., Salomon, R., & Bieber, G. (2009). StairMaster: A New Online Fall Detection Device. *Proceedings of 2nd German AAL congress.*

MacLaughlin, E. J. (2005). Assessing medication adherence in the elderly: which tools to use in clinical practice? *Drugs & Aging, 22*(3), 55–231.

Madden, M., & Fox, S. (2006). Finding Answers Online in Sickness and in Health. *Pew Internet & American Life Project Report,* May 2.

Maglogiannis, I. (2004). Design and Implementation of a Calibrated Store and Forward Imaging System for Teledermatology. *Journal of Medical Systems, 28*(5), 455–467.

Maglogiannis, I., Apostolopoulos, N., & Tsoukias, P. (2004). Designing and Implementing an Electronic Health Record for Personal Digital Assistants (PDAs). *International Journal for Quality of Life Research, 2*(1), 63–67.

Maglogiannis, I., Delakouridis, K., & Kazatzopoulos, L. (2006). Enabling collaborative medical diagnosis over the Internet via peer to peer distribution of electronic health records. *J Medical Systems, Springer, 30*(2), 107–116.

Maglogiannis, I., Karpouzis, K., & Wallace, M. (2007). Image, Signal and Distributed Data Processing for Networked eHealth Applications. *IEEE Engineering in Medicine and Biology Magazine, 26*(5), 14–17.

Magnusson, L., Hanson, E., & Borg, M. (2004). *A literature review study of Information and Communication Technology as a support for frail older people living at home and their family carers.* Technology and Disability.

Maitland, J., Sherwood, S., Barkhuus, L., Anderson, I., Hall, M., Brown, B. et al. (2006). Increasing the Awareness of Daily Activity Levels with Pervasive Computing. *Proceedings of Pervasive Health,* 6.

Malamateniou, F., & Vassilacopoulos, G. (2003). Developing a virtual patient record using XML and web-based workflow technologies. *International Journal of Medical Informatics, 70*(2-3), 131–139. doi:10.1016/S1386-5056(03)00039-X

Malan, D. J., Welsh, M., & Smith, M. D. (2008). Implementing public-key infrastructure for sensor networks. *ACM Transactions on Sensor Networks, 4*(4), 1–23. doi:10.1145/1387663.1387668

Malan, D., Fulford-Jones, T., Welsh, M., & Moulton, S. (2004). Codeblue: An ad hoc sensor network infrastructure for emergency medical care. *International Workshop on Wearable and Implantable Body Sensor Networks.*

Malan, D., Jones, T. F., Welsh, M., & Moulton, S. (2004). CodeBlue: An Ad Hoc Sensor Network Infrastructure for Emergency Medical Care. *MobiSys, Workshop on Applications of Mobile Embedded Systems.*

Malan, D., Welsh, M., & Smith, M. (2004). A public-key infrastructure for key distribution in TinyOS based on elliptic curve cryptography. In *Proceedings of the first annual IEEE communications society conference on sensor and ad hoc communications and networks (SECON 2004)* (pp. 71-80).

Malasri, K., & Wang, L. (2008). Design and implementation of a secure wireless mote-based medical sensor network. In *Ubicomp '08: Proceedings of the 10th international conference on ubiquitous computing* (pp. 172–181). New York, NY, USA: ACM.

Mango, P., & Riefberg, V. (2008). Three Imperatives for Improving Health Care. *The McKinsey Quarterly*, (December): 2008.

Mankoff, J., Dey, A. K., Hsieh, G., Kientz, J., Lederer, S., & Ames, M. (2003). *Heuristic Evaluation of Ambient Displays*.

Manzo, M., Roosta, T., & Sastry, S. (2005). Time synchronization attacks in sensor networks. In *SASN '05: Proceedings of the 3rd ACM workshop on security of ad hoc and sensor networks* (pp. 107–116).

Marci Meingast, S. S. Tanya Roosta. (2006, August). Security and privacy issues with health care information technology. In *Embs '06: Proceedings of the 28th annual international conference of the IEEE engineering in medicine and biology society* (pp. 5453–5458).

Mareca Hatler, Darryl Gurganious, Charlie Chi. (2008, August). *WSN for healthcare* (Market Report). OnWorld.

Marsden, R. (1999). *What's new in Computer Access and Environmental Control Units (ECU's) at Madenta, Inc.*

Marsh, D. (2006). Capacitive touch sensors fulfill early promise. *EDN Europe*. Retrieved April 27, 2009, from http://www.edn.com/contents/images/6339808.pdf

Martinez, I., Escayola, J., Fernandez de Bobadilla, I., Martinez-Espronceda, M., Serrano, L., Trigo, J., et al. (2008). Optimization proposal of a standard-based patient monitoring platform for ubiquitous environments. In *30th Annual International Conference of the IEEE Engineering in Medicine and Biology Society, EMBC2008*, (pp. 1813 – 1816).

Martinez, L., & Gomez, C. (Eds.). (2008). *Telemedicine in the 21st Century*. Hauppauge, NY: Nova Science Publishers.

Masella, C., & Zanaboni, P. (2008). Assessment Models for Telemedicine Services in National Health Systems. *International Journal of Healthcare Technology and Management*, 9(5/6), 446–472. doi:10.1504/IJHTM.2008.020198

Massacci, F., & Zannone, N. (2004). *Privacy Is Linking Permission to Purpose* (pp. 179–191). Security Protocols Workshop.

Massachusetts Institute of Technology. (2003). *PlaceLab: A House_n + TIAX Initiative*. Cambridge, MA: Author. Retrieved from http://architecture.mit.edu/house_n/placelab.html

Massey, T., Gao, T., Welsh, M., Sharp, J. H., & Sarrafzadeh, M. (2006). The design of a decentralized electronic triage system. *AMIA Annual Symposium Proceedings*, (pp. 544-548).

MasterCard International. (2002). *MasterCard Open Data Storage Version 2.0*. Technical Specifications.

Mathie, M. J., Coster, A. C., Lovell, N. H., & Celler, B. G. (2004). Accelerometry: providing an integrated, practical method for long-term, ambulatory monitoring of human movement. *Physiological Measurement*, 25(2), R1–R20. doi:10.1088/0967-3334/25/2/R01

Mathie, M. J., Coster, A. C., Lovell, N. H., Celler, B. G., Lord, S. R., & Tiedemann, A. (2004). A pilot study of long-term monitoring of human movements in the home using accelerometry. *Journal of Telemedicine and Telecare*, 10(3), 144–151. doi:10.1258/135763304323070788

Matusitz, J., & Breen, G. M. (2007). Telemedicine: Its effects on health communication. *Health Communication*, 21(1), 10–21.

McCreadie, C., & Tinker, A. (2005). The Acceptabiliy of Assistive Technology to Older People. *Ageing and Society*, 25, 91–110. doi:10.1017/S0144686X0400248X

McElligott, L., Dillon, M., Leydon, K., Richardson, B., Fernström, M., & Paradiso, J. (2002). 'ForSe FIElds' - Force sensors for interactive environments. *Lecture Notes in Computer Science*, 2498, 321–328.

McGrath, S., Grigg, E., Wendelken, S., Blike, G., Rosa, M. D., Fiske, A., et al. (2003, November). *ARTEMIS: A vision for remote triage and emergency management information integration*. Dartmouth University.

McGraw, C. (2004). Multi-compartment medication devices and patient compliance. *British Journal of Community Nursing, 9*(7), 90–285.

McKinsey & Company. (2008). Why Americans Pay More for Health Care. *The McKinsey Quarterly*, (December): 2008.

McKnight's LTC News. (2005, July). 2005 software. *McKnight's Long-Term Care News, 43*.

Mendling, J., Strembeck, M., Stermsek, G., & Neumann, G. (2004, June). *An Approach to Extract RBAC Models for BPEL4WS Processes*. Paper presented at the 13th IEEE Int. Workshops on Enabling Technologies: Infrastructure for Collaborative Enterprises, Modena, Italy.

Messina, M., Lim, Y., Lawrence, E., Martin, D., & Kargl, F. (2008). Implementing and validating an environmental and health monitoring system. In *ITNG '08: Proceedings of the fifth international conference on information technology: New generations* (pp. 994–999).

Meyer, S., & Schulze, E. (2002). Smart Home and the Aging User. Trends and Analyses of Consumer Behaviour. In *Symposium "Domotics and Networking"*, *Miami*, 11/19-12.

Michael, S. J. C. (2000). Wireless clinical alerts for physiologic, laboratory and medication data. In *Proceedings / AMIA 2000 Annual Symposium*, (pp. 789-793).

Miller, J., & Mukerji, J. (2006, March). *MDA Guide Version 1.0.1*. Retrieved January 21, 2009, from http://www.omg.org/docs/omg/03-06-01.pdf

Mini, R. A., Loureiro, A., & Nath, B. (2005). A State-Based Energy Dissipation Model for Wireless Sensor Nodes. In *Proceedings of the 10th IEEE Conference on Emerging Technologies in Factory Automation*. Catania, Italy: IEEE Computer Society.

Mirza, F., Norris, T., & Stockdale, R. (2008). Mobile technologies and the holistic management of chronic diseases. *Health Informatics Journal, 14*(4), 309–321. doi:10.1177/1460458208096559

Mitchell, S., Spiteri, M. D., Bates, J., & Coulouris, G. (2000). *Context-Aware Multimedia Computing in the Intelligent Hospital*. Paper presented at the 9th European Workshop on ACM SIGOPS, New York.

Mitka, M. (2003). Approach could widen access for older patients. *Telemedicine eyes for mental health services, 290*(14), 22-25.

Mobile Devices For Healthcare Applications (MOBI-DEV). (2005). Retrieved December 15, 2008, from http://www.mobi-dev.arakne.it/

Moller, J., Renegar, Carrie. (2003). Bathing as a wellness experience. *Nursing Homes Long Term Care Management, 52*(10), 108.

Montgomery, K., Mundt, C., Thonier, G., Tellier, A., Udoh, U., Barker, V., et al. (2004) Lifeguard - A Personal Physiological Monitor For Extreme Environments. In Proceeding of 26th annual International of IEEE EMBS, (pp. 2192-2195).

Mor, V., Berg, K., Angelelli, J., Gifford, D., Morris, J., & Moore, T. (2003). The quality of quality measurement in U.S. nursing homes. *The Gerontologist, 43*(2), 37–46.

Mori, T., Noguchi, H., Takada, A., & Sato, T. (2004). Sensing Room: Distributed Sensor Environment for Measurement of Human Daily Behavior. In *First International Workshop on Networked Sensing Systems (INSS2004)*, (pp. 40-43).

Morrison, K., Szymkowiak, A., & Gregor, P. (2004). Memojog - an interactive memory aid incorporating mobile based technologies. In S. Brewster & M. Dunlop (Eds.), MobileHCI, September 13-16, Glasgow, UK, (LNCS 3160, pp. 481-485). Berlin: Springer-Verlag.

Mukamel, B. D., & Spector, D. W. (2000). Nursing home Costs and Risk-Adjusted Outcome Measures of Quality. *Medical Care, 38*(1), 32–35. doi:10.1097/00005650-200001000-00009

Mukhopadhyay, S., Paniyrahi, D., & Dey, S. (2004). Data aware, Low cost Error correction for Wireless Sensor Networks. In *IEEE Wireless Communications and Networking Conference*, Atlanta, (pp. 2492-2497).

Muller, M., Frankewitsch, T., Ganslandt, T., Burkle, T., & Prokosch, H. U. (2004). The Clinical Document Architecture (CDA) enables Electronic Medical Records to wireless mobile computing. [Amsterdam: IOS Press.]. *Medinfo, 107*, 1448-1452.

Munoz, M., Rodriguez, M. D., Favela, J., Martinez-Garcia, A. I., & Gonzalez, V. M. (2003). Context-Aware Mobile Communication in Hospitals. *IEEE Computer, 36*(9), 38-46.

Muras, J., Cahill, V., & Stokes, E. (2006). A taxonomy of pervasive healthcare systems. In *Pervasive Health Conference and Workshops*, (pp. 1-10).

Mynatt E.D., Rowan, J., Jacobs, A., & Craighill, S. (2001). Digital Family Portraits: Supporting Peace of Mind for Extended Family Members. *SIGCHI 2001 3*(1), 333-340.

Mynatt, E. D., Essa, I., & Rogers, W. (2000). Increasing the opportunities for aging in place. *Proceedings of the 2000 conference on Universal Usability*, 65-71.

National Institute of Standards and Technology (NIST). *Role Based Access Control (RBAC) and Role Based Security*. (n.d.). Retrieved October 16, 2007, from http://csrc.nist.gov/groups/SNS/rbac/

Neely, S., Stevenson, G., Kray, C., Mulder, I., Connelly, K., & Siek, K. A. (2008). Evaluating Pervasive and Ubiquitous Systems. *IEEE Pervasive Computing / IEEE Computer Society [and] IEEE Communications Society, 7*(3), 85-88. doi:10.1109/MPRV.2008.47

Nehmer, J., Becker, M., Karshmer, A. I., & Lamm, R. (2006). Living Assistance Systems - An Ambient Intelligence Approach. In *Proceedings of the 28th Intl. Conf. on Software Engineering* (pp. 43-50). Shanghai, China: ACM Press.

Nesbit, T. (2006). Rural Outreach in Home Telehealth: Assessing Challenges and Reviewing Successes. *Telemedicine Journal and e-Health, 12*(2), 107–113. doi:10.1089/tmj.2006.12.107

Netics. (2008). *Le ICT nelle Regioni e Province Autonome. Rapporto 2008*.

Neville, G., Greene, A., McLeod, J., & Tracy, A. (2002). Mobile phone text messaging can help young people with asthma. *British Medical Journal, 325*, 600. doi:10.1136/bmj.325.7364.600/a

Ng, H. S., Sim, M. L., & Tan, C. M. (2006). Security issues of wireless sensor networks in healthcare applications. *BT Technology Journal, 24*(2), 138–144. doi:10.1007/s10550-006-0051-8

Ni Scanaill, C., Carew, S., Barralon, P., Noury, N., Lyons, D., & Lyons, G. M. (2006). A Review of Approaches to Mobility Telemonitoring of the Elderly in Their Living Environment. Annals of Biomedical Engineering. *The Journal of the Biomedical Engineering Society, 34*(4).

Ni, Q., Trombetta, A., Bertino, E., & Lobo, J. (2007). Privacy-aware role based access. In *Proceedings of the 12th ACM symposium on Access control models and technologie*, (pp. 41-50).

Nick, M., & Becker, M. (2007). A Hybrid Approach to Intelligent Living Assistance. In *Proceedings of the 7th Intl. Conf. on Hybrid Intelligent Systems* (pp. 283-289). Washington, DC: IEEE Computer Society.

Nielsen, J. (1994). Heuristic evaluation. In *Usability Inspection Methods*. New York: John Wiley & Sons.

Norris, A. C. (2002). *Essentials of Telemedicine and Telecare*. Chichester, UK: Wiley.

Noury, N., Fleury, A., Rumeau, P., Bourke, A. K., Laighin, G. Ó., Rialle, V., et al. (2007). Fall detection –principles and methods. In *Proceedings of the 29th Annual International Conference of the IEEE EMBS, 23-26 August 2007* (pp. 1663-1666). Lyon, France: IEEE-EMBS.

Nursing Home Data Compendium. (2007). In CMS (Ed.): HS.gov.

NURSING HOMES. (2008). Federal Monitoring Surveys Demonstrate Continued Understatement of Serious Care Problems and CMS Oversight Weaknesses. In Office, S. G. A. (Ed.), *U* (*Vol. 517*). GAO.

O'Connor, J. (2005). Feds provide info on LTC tech products on market.(Technology)(Long Term Care)(Brief Article). *McKnight's Long-Term Care News, 14*(11).

O'Connor, J. (2008). Nursing homes up on technology. (NEWS). *McKnight's Long-Term Care News, 29*(12), 3(1).

O'Connor, M. C. (2006). Testing Ultrasound to Track, Monitor Patients. *RFID Journal, 1*(31), 2.

Ohta, S., Nakamoto, H., Shinagawa, Y., & Tanikawa, T. (2002). A health monitoring system for elderly people living alone. *Journal of Telemedicine and Telecare, 8*(3), 151–156. doi:10.1258/135763302320118997

Open Grid Services Architecture - Data Access and Integration (OGSA-DAI). (n.d.). Retrieved October 12, 2007, from http://www.ogsadai.org.uk/

Opie, A. (1998). Nobody's asked me for my view: users' empowerment by multidisciplinary health teams. *Qualitative Health Research, 18*, 188–206. doi:10.1177/104973239800800204

Organization for the Advancement of Structured Information Standards (OASIS). *Core and Hierarchical Role Based Access Control (RBAC) Profile of XACML v2.0.* (n.d.). Retrieved May 12, 2008, from http://docs.oasis-open.org/xacml/2.0/access_control-xacml-2.0-rbac-profile1-spec-os.pdf

Orwat, C., Graefe, A., & Faulwasser, T. (2008). Towards pervasive computing in health care - a literature review. *BMC Medical Informatics and Decision Making, 8*, 26. doi:10.1186/1472-6947-8-26

Otis, P. (1997). Don't worry, The Carpet is Keep Watching. *BusinessWeek,*1.

Overview Medicaid Program. (2006). *General Information* (In, C. M. S., Ed.).

Oviatt, S. L., & Cohen, P. R. (2000). Multimodal interfaces that process what comes naturally. *Communications of the ACM, 43*(3), 45–53. doi:10.1145/330534.330538

Paksuniemi, M., Sorvoja, H., Alasaarela, E., & Myllyla, R. (2006). Wireless sensor and data transmission needs and technologies for patient monitoring in the operating room and intensive care unit. In 27th Annual Int. Conf IEEE EMBS05, (pp. 5182-5185).

Palen, L., & Dourish, P. (2003). *Unpacking 'privacy' for a networked world.* Paper presented at the Conference on Human factors in computing systems.

Palokari, S. (2007, November 5). *Turvana hälyttävä matto.* Helsingin Sanomat, p. D4. (In Finnish)

Paradiso, R., Loriga, G., & Taccini, N. (2005). A Wearable Health Care System Based on Knitted Integrated Sensors. *IEEE Transactions on Information Technology in Biomedicine, 9*(3), 337–344.

Park, A. (2008). America's Health Check-up. *Time Magazine, 172*(22), 41–49.

Parker, O. D., Demiris, G., Day, M., Courtney, K. L., & Porock, D. (2006). Tele-hospice support for elder caregivers of hospice patients: two case studies. *Journal of Palliative Medicine, 9*(2), 54–59.

Pasley, J. (2005). How BPEL and SOA are changing web services development. *IEEE Internet Computing, 9*(3), 60–67. doi:10.1109/MIC.2005.56

Patient Placement Systems Unveils Referral Automation Vision Center. (2009). *PRWeb*, NA.

Pattichis, C. S., Kyriacou, E., Voskarides, S., Pattichis, M. S., Istepanian, R., & Schizas, C. N. (2002). Wireless Telemedicine Systems: An Overview. *IEEE Antennas and Propagation Magazine, 44*(2), 143–153.

Pear, R. (2008). Serious Deficiencies in Nursing Homes Are Often Missed. *New York Times.*

Pear, R. (2008). Violations Reported at 94% of Nursing Homes. *New York Times.*

Pearlman, L., Welch, V., Foster, I., Kesselman, C., & Tuecke, S. (2002, June). *A Community Authorization Service for Group Collaboration.* Paper presented at the 3rd IEEE International Workshop on Policies for Distributed Systems and Networks, Monterey, California, USA.

Pentland, A. (2004). Healthwear: Medical technology becomes wearable. *Computer, 37*(5), 42–49. doi:10.1109/MC.2004.1297238

Pereira, A. L., Muppavarapu, V., & Chung, S. M. (2006). Role-Based Access Control for Grid database services using the community authorization service. *IEEE Transactions on Dependable and Secure Computing, 3*(2), 156–166. doi:10.1109/TDSC.2006.26

Perry, M., Dowdall, A., Lines, L., & Hone, K. (2004). Multimodal and ubiquitous computing systems: supporting independent-living older users. *IEEE Transactions on Information Technology in Biomedicine, 8*(3), 258–270. doi:10.1109/TITB.2004.835533

Peter, D. (2001). *The Nurse Shortage: Perspectives from Current Direct Care Nurses and Former Direct Care Nurses* (Report).

Philipose, M., Fishkin, K. P., Perkowitz, M., Patterson, D. J., Fox, D., & Kautz, H. (2004). Inferring activities from interactions with objects. *Pervasive Computing, IEEE, 3*(4), 50–57. doi:10.1109/MPRV.2004.7

Pino, E., Ohno-Machado, L., Wiechmann, E., & Curtis, D. (2005). Real-Time ECG Algorithms for Ambulatory Patient Monitoring. In *AMIA Annual Symposium Proceedings,* (pp. 604-608).

Polit, F. D., & Beck, T. C. (2004). *Nursing Research: Principles and Methods.* Wickford, RI: Lippincott-Raven Publishers.

Pollack, M. (2005). Intelligent technology for an aging population: The Use of AI to Assist Elders with Cognitive Impairment. *AI Magazine, 26*(2), 9–24.

Pollack, M. E., Brown, L., Colbry, D., McCarthy Colleen, E., Orosz, C., & Peintner, B. (2003). *Autominder: An Intelligent Cognitive Orthotic System for People with Memory Impairment.* Robotics and Autonomous Systems.

Pomberger, G., & Weinreich, R. (1994). The role of prototyping in software development. In *Proceedings of the 13th Intl. Conf. on Technology of Object-Oriented Languages and Systems.* Versailles, France: Prentice Hall.

Poon, E. G., Jha, A. K., Christino, M., Honour, M. M., Fernandopulle, R., & Middleton, B. (2006). Assessing the level of healthcare information technology adoption in the United States: A snapshot. *BMC Medical Informatics and Decision Making, 6*, 1. doi:10.1186/1472-6947-6-1

*Popular Mechanics.* (2004, 06). Robots Help Japan Care For Its Elderly. Retrieved 30/01/2009, 2009, from http://www.popularmechanics.com/science/technology_watch/1288241.html

Porter, M., & Tiesberg, E. (2006). *Re-defining health care delivery.* Boston: Harvard Business Press.

Poulton, B. C. (1999). User involvement in identifying health needs and shaping and evaluating services: is it being raised? *Journal of Advanced Nursing, 30*(6), 1289–1296. doi:10.1046/j.1365-2648.1999.01224.x

Poulymenopoulou, M., Malamateniou, F., & Vassilacopoulos, G. (2005). Emergency Healthcare Process Automation using Workflow Technology and Web Services. *International Journal of Medical Informatics, 28*(3), 195–207.

Pucheral, P., & Yin, S. (2007). System and Method of Managing Indexation of Flash Memory. *European Patent by Gemalto and INRIA,* N° 07290567.2.

Pucheral, P., Bouganim, L., Valduriez, P., & Bobineau, C. (2001). PicoDBMS: Scaling down database techniques for the smartcard. [VLDBJ]. *Very Large Data Bases Journal, 10*(2-3), 120–132.

Quigley, G., & Tweed, C. (1999). *Costs benefits analysis for assistive technologies. Research report on EPSRC GR/M05171.* Belfast, UK: Queen's University of Belfast.

Rabaey, J. M., Ammer, M. J., da Silva, J. Jr, Patel, D., & Roundy, S. (2000). PicoRadio Supports Ad Hoc Ultra-Low Power Wireless Networking. *Computer, 33*(7), 42–48.

Rachlis, M. (2006). *Key to sustainable healthcare system.* Available http://www.improveinchroniccare.org

Radermacher, W. (2007). *Demografischer Wandel in Deutschland.* Wiesbaden: Statistisches Bundesamt.

Radin, P. (2006). To me, it's my life: medical communication, trust, and activism in cyberspace. *Social Science & Medicine, 6,* 591–601. doi:10.1016/j.socscimed.2005.06.022

Raju, M. (2007). *Heart-Rate and EKG Monitor Using the MSP430FG439* [Electronic Version].

Ramachandran, R., Ramanna, L., Ghasemzadeh, H., Pradhan, G., Jafari, R., & Prabhakaran, B. (2008). Body Sensor Networks to Evaluate Standing Balance: Interpreting Muscular Activities Based on Inertial Sensors. In *The 2nd International Workshop on Systems and Networking Support for Healthcare and Assisted Living Environments (HealthNet),* Breckenridge.

Ranganathan, A., & McFaddin, S. (2004, June). *Using processes to coordinate web services in pervasive computing environments.* Paper presented at the IEEE International Conference on Web Services (ICWS'04), San Diego, CA.

Rantanen, J., Impio, J., Karinsalo, T., Malmivaara, M., Reho, A., Tasanen, M., & Vanhala, J. (2002). *Smart clothing prototype for the arctic environment. Personal and Ubiquitous Computing.* Berlin: Springer.

Rantz, M. J., Marek, K. D., Aud, M., Tyrer, H. W., Skubic, M., & Demiris, G. (2005). A Technology and Nursing Collaboration to Help Older Adults Age in Place. *Nursing Outlook, 53*(1), 40–45. doi:10.1016/j.outlook.2004.05.004

Rantz, M. J., Skubic, M., Miller, S. J., & Krampe, J. (2008). Using Technology to Enhance Aging in Place. In *Proceedings of the International Conference on Smart Home and Health Telematics* (pp. 169-176). Berlin: Springer-Verlag.

Rao, S., & Troshani, I. (2007). A MC-ER Initial Selection of Content, Markets, and Distribution Channels for the Australian Mobile Content – Export Research Initiative. Adelaide, Australia: m.Net Corporation Ltd.

Rasmussen, B., Wellard, S., & Nankervis, A. (2001). Consumer issues in navigating health care services for type I diabetes. *Journal of Clinical Nursing, 10,* 628–634. doi:10.1046/j.1365-2702.2001.00550.x

Ratnasamy, S., Karp, B., Yin, L., Yu, F., Estrin, D., Govindan, R., et al. (2002). GHT: A geographic Hash Table for Data-Centric Storage. In *Proceedings of the First ACM Intl. Workshop on Wireless Sensor Networks and Applications* (pp. 78-87). Atlanta, GA: ACM.

Reach, G., Zerrouki, D., Leclercq, D., & d'Ivernois, J. F. (2005). Adjusting insulin doses: from knowledge to decision. *Patient Education and Counseling, 56*(1), 98–103. doi:10.1016/j.pec.2004.01.001

Redfern, S., Hannan, S., Norman, I., & Martin, F. (2002). Work satisfaction, stress, quality of care and morale of older people in a nursing home. *Health & Social Care in the Community, 10*(6), 17–35. doi:10.1046/j.1365-2524.2002.00396.x

Redmond, S. J., Lovell, N. H., Basilakis, J., & Celler, B. G. (2008). *ECG quality measures in telecare monitoring.* Paper presented at the Proc. 30th Annual Int. Conf IEEE EMBC08, 20th-24th Aug, Vancouver Canada.

Reilly, J., & Bischoff, J. (2008). Remote Monitoring Tested. *Technology and Health Care, 34*(9), 12–14.

Reiter, T. (2008). *T.R.O.P.I.C.: Transformations On Petri Nets In Color.* PhD Thesis, Johannes Kepler University, Faculty of Bioinformatics, Linz.

Rialle, V., Lamy, J. B., Noury, N., & Bajolle, L. (2003). Telemonitoring of patients at home: a software agent approach. *Computer Methods and Programs in Biomedicine, 72*(3), 257–268.

Rimminen, H., & Sepponen, R. (2009). Biosignals with a floor sensor. In *Second International Conference on Biomedical Electronics and Devices (BIODEVICES 2009), 14-17 January 2009* (pp. 125-130). Porto, Portugal: INSTICC.

Rimminen, H., Lindström, J., & Sepponen, R. (2009). Positioning accuracy and multi-target separation with a human tracking system using near field imaging. *International Journal on Smart Sensing and Intelligent Systems, 2*. Retrieved April 27, 2009, from http://www.s2is.org/Issues/v2/n1/papers/paper9.pdf

Rimminen, H., Linnavuo, M., & Sepponen, R. (2008). Human tracking using near field imaging. In *Second International Conference on Pervasive Computing Technologies for Healthcare (PervasiveHealth 2008), 30 January -1 February 2008* (pp.148-151).Tampere, Finland: ICST.

Robinson, K. (2003). Technology can't replace compassion in health care. *Critical Care Choices, 34*(1), 1.

Robots may be next solution to nursing shortage. (2003). *Managed Care Weekly*, 102.

Rogers, Y., Connelly, K., Tedesco, T., Hazlewood, W., Kurtz, A., Hall, R. E., et al. (2004). *Why It's Worth the Hassle: The Value of In-Situ Studies When Designing Ubicomp.* Paper presented at the Mobile Human-Computer Interaction – MobileHCI 2004.

Römer, K. (2005). *Time Synchronization and Localization in Sensor Networks.* Phd Thesis, Swiss Federal Institute of Technology Zürich (ETH Zürich), Zürich, Schweiz.

Ropponen, A., Linnavuo, M., & Sepponen, R. (2009). LF indoor location and identification system. *International Journal on Smart Sensing and Intelligent Systems, 2.* Retrieved April 27, 2009, from http://www.s2is.org/Issues/v2/n1/papers/paper6.pdf

Røstad, L., & Nytrø, O. (2008). Personalized access control for a personally controlled health record. In *Proceedings of the 2nd ACM workshop on Computer security architectures* (pp. 9-16).

Rowland, D. (2003). An ageing population: emergence of a new stage of life? In Khoo, S., & McDonald, P. (Eds.), *The Transformation of Australia's Population: 1970-2030* (pp. 239–265). Sydney: UNSW Press.

Rudi, R., & Celler, B. G. (2006). *Design and implementation of expert-telemedicine system for diabetes management at home.* Paper presented at the International Conference on Biomedical and Pharmaceutical Engineering 2006 (ICBPE2006), IEEE, 11-14 December 2006, Singapore.

Russell, L. B., Churl Suh, D., & Safford, M. M. (2005). Time requirements for diabetes management: too much for many? *The Journal of Family Practice, 54*(1), 52–56.

Salvador, C. H. (2005). Airmed-Cardio: A GSM and Internet Services-Based System for Out-of-Hospital Follow-Up of Cardiac Patients. *IEEE Transactions on Information Technology in Biomedicine, 9*(1), 73–85.

Samarati, P., & di Vimercati, S. D. C. (2000). Policies, Models, and Mechanisms. In *Foundations of Security Analysis and Design on Foundations of Security Analysis and Design 2000* (pp. 137–196). Access Control.

Sanchez, D., Tentori, M., & Favela, J. (2008, March-April). Activity recognition for the smart hospital. *IEEE Intelligent Systems, 23*(2), 50–57. doi:10.1109/MIS.2008.18

Sanchez, J., Calcaterra, G., & Tran, Q. Q. (2005). Automation in the Home: The Development of an Appropriate System representation and its effects on reliance. In *Proceedings of the Human Factors and Ergonomics Society 49th Annual Meeting (HFES'05).* Santa Monica, CA: Human Factors and Ergonomics Society.

Sanders, J., & Bashshur, R. (1995). Challenges to the Implementation of Telemedicine. *Telemedicine Journal, 3*, 115–123.

Sandhu, J. S., Agogino, A. M., & Agogino, A. K. (2004). *Wireless Sensor Networks for Commercial Lighting Control: Decision Making with Multi-agent Systems.*

Santana, P. C., Castro, L. A., Preciado, A., Gonzalez, V. M., Rodriguez, M. D., & Favela, J. (2005). *Preliminary Evaluation of Ubicomp in Real Working Scenarios.* Paper presented at the 2nd Workshop on Multi-User and Ubiquitous User Interfaces MU3I, January 9, 2005, San Diego, USA.

Saranummi, N., & Wactlar, H. (2008). Editorial: Pervasive Healthcare. Selected papers from the pervasive healthcare 2008 conference, Tampere, Finland. *Methods of Information in Medicine, 47*(3), 175–177.

Schäfer, G., Baryn, M., Fritz, M., Augier, A. J., & Wieland, U. (2008). *Europe in Figures - Eurostat yearbook 2008.* Statistical Office of the European Communities.

Schanze, T., Hesse, L., Lau, C., Greve, N., Haberer, W., & Kammer, S. (2007). An Optically Powered Single-Channel Stimulation Implant as Test System for Chronic Biocompatibility and Biostability of Miniaturized Retinal Vision Prostheses. *Biomedical Engineering. IEEE Transactions on, 54,* 983–992.

Schauerhuber, A., Schwinger, W., Retschitzegger, W., Wimmer, M., & Kappl, G. (2007). *A Survey on Web Modeling Approaches for Ubiquitous Web Applications.* Vienna: Vienna University of Technology.

Schepers, J., & Wetzels, M. (2007). A meta-analysis of the technology acceptance model: Investigating subjective norm and moderation effects. *Information & Management, 44*(1), 90–103. doi:10.1016/j.im.2006.10.007

Schiffer, S. (1998). *Visuelle Programmierung.* Phd Thesis, Johannes Kepler University, Linz.

Schmitt, L., Falck, T., Wartena, F., & Simons, D. *(2007a). Towards plug-and-play interoperability for wireless personal telehealth systems. In* IFMBE Proceedings of the 4th Interim Workshop on Wearable and Implantable Body Sensor Networks, *(pp. 257–263).*

Schmitt, L., Falck, T., Wartena, F., & Simons, D. (2007b) Novel ISO/IEEE 11073 standards for personal telehealth systems interoperability. In *2007 Joint Workshop on High Confidence Medical Devices, Software, and Systems and Medical Device Plug-and-Play Interoperability,* (pp. 146–148).

Schwinger, W., Grün, C., Pröll, B., & Retschitzegger, W. (2008). Context-Awareness in Mobile Tourism Guides. In Khalil-Ibrahim, I. (Ed.), *Handbook of Research in Mobile Multimedia.* Hershey, PA: IGI Global.

Selwyn, N. (2004). The Information Aged: A Qualitative Study of Older Adults' Use of Information and Communications Technology. *Journal of Aging Studies, 18,* 369–384. doi:10.1016/j.jaging.2004.06.008

Shah, P. J., Aroul, P., Hande, A., & Bhatia, D. (2007). Remote Cardiac Activity Monitoring Using Multi-Hop Wireless Sensor Networks. *Engineering in Medicine and Biology Workshop, 2007 IEEE Dallas,* 142-145.

Sharma, S. K., Xu, H., Wickramasinghe, N., & Ahmed, N. (2006). Electronic Healthcare: Issues and Challenges. *International Journal of Electronic Healthcare, 2*(1), 50–65. doi:10.1504/IJEH.2006.008693

Shields, S. (2005, March 23). Culture Change in Nursing homes. *The Commonwealth Fund.*

Shimizu, K. (1999). Telemedicine by Mobile Communication. *IEEE Engineering in Medicine and Biology Magazine, 18*(4), 32–44.

Shnayder, V., Chen, B., Lorincz, K., Fulford-Jones, T. R. F., & Welsh, M. (2005). Sensor Networks for Medical Care. In *Proceedings of the 3rd international conference on Embedded networked sensor systems,* (pp. 314-314).

Sidorov, J. (2006). It Ain't Necessarily So: The Electronic Health Record and the Unlikely Prospect of Reducing Healthcare Costs. *Health Affairs, 25*(4), 1079–1085. doi:10.1377/hlthaff.25.4.1079

Silva, J., Zamarripa, S., Strayer, P., Favela, J., & González, V. (2006). *Empirical Evaluation of a Mobile Application for Assisting Physicians in Creating Medical Notes.* Paper presented at the Proceedings of the 12th Americas Conference on Information Systems (AMCIS 2006), Acapulco, Mexico, August 4-6, 2006.

Sisko, A., Truffer, C., & Smith, S. (2009). Health Spending Projections Through 2018: Recession Effects Add Uncertainty to Outlook. *Health Affairs, 24*(February), 346–357. doi:10.1377/hlthaff.28.2.w346

Skulimowski, A. M. (2006). *The Challenges to the Medical Decision Making System posed by mHealth.* Kraków, Poland: Centre for Decision Sciences and Forecasting, Progress & Business Foundation, Institute for Prospective Technological Studies (IPTS). Available http://ipts.jrc.ec.europa.eu/home/report/english/articles/vol81/ICT1E816.htm

Sloan, F., & Shayne, M. (1993). Long-Term Care, Medicaid, and the Impoverishment of the Elderly. *The Milbank Quarterly, 70*(4), 19.

Sloane, E. B. (2006). The emerging health care IT infrastructure.(Tech Talk). *24x7, 11*(12), 42(43).

Sloane, E. B. (2009). Regulatory overview (Networking). *24x7, 14*(4), 24(22).

SOPRANO Consortium. (2007). *Review state-of-the-art and market analysis.* Deliverable D1.1.2.

Spiekermann, S. (2008). *User Control in Ubiquitous Computing: Design Alternatives and User Acceptance.* Aachen, Germany: Shaker Verlag.

Srovnal, V., & Penhaker, M. (2007). *Health Maintenance Embedded Systems in Home Care Applications.* Paper presented at the Systems, ICONS '07, Second International Conference on.

St. Joseph Convent retirement and nursing home. (2007). *McKnight's Long-Term Care News,* 1.

Stahl, T., Völter, M., Efftinge, S., & Haase, A. (2007). Modellgetriebene Softwareentwicklung (Vol. 2). Heidelberg, Germany: dpunkt.verlag.

Stanford, V. (2002). Using Pervasive Computing to Deliver Elder Care. *IEEE Pervasive Computing / IEEE Computer Society [and] IEEE Communications Society,* 10–13. doi:10.1109/MPRV.2002.993139

Stanford, V. (2003). Beam Me Up, Doctor McCoy. *IEEE Pervasive Computing / IEEE Computer Society [and] IEEE Communications Society, 2*(3), 13–18. doi:10.1109/MPRV.2003.1228522

Stankovic, J. A., Lee, I., Mok, A., & Rajkumar, R. (2005, November). Opportunities and Obligations for Physical Computing Systems. *IEEE Computer, 38*(11), 23–31.

Stieglitz, T., Schuetter, M., & Koch, K. P. (2005). Implantable biomedical microsystems for neural prostheses. *Engineering in Medicine and Biology Magazine, IEEE, 24,* 58–65. doi:10.1109/MEMB.2005.1511501

Stoa, S., Balasingham, I., & Ramstad, T. A. (2007). Data throughput optimization in the IEEE 802.15.4 medical sensor networks. In IEEE international symposium on circuits and systems (pp. 1361-1364).

Strang, T., & Linnhoff-Popien, C. (2004). A Context Modeling Survey. *Proceedings of the 1st Intl. Workshop on Advanced Context Modelling, Reasoning And Management at UbiComp.* Nottingham, England.

Stroetmann, K. A., Jones, T., Dobrev, A., & Stroetmann, V. N. (2006). eHealth is Worth It—The Economic Benefits of Implemented eHealth Solutions at Ten European Sites. *European Communities.*

Stroetmann, V. N., Cleland, J. G., Stroetmann, K. A. & Westerteicher, Ch. (2000). Evaluation Telehealth Homecare Services—The TEN-HMS Project: Medical, Quality of Life and Economic Efficiency Aspects. *Gesellschaft für Biomedizinische Technologien in Ulm e.V.*

Sunny, C., Katherine, E., Ian, S., & James, A. L. (2006). Design requirements for technologies that encourage physical activity, *Proceedings of the SIGCHI conference on Human Factors in computing systems.* Montreal, Quebec, Canada: ACM.

Suzuki, R., Ogawa, M., Otake, S., Izutsu, T., Tobimatsu, Y., & Izumi, S. (2004). Analysis of activities of daily living in elderly people living alone: single-subject feasibility study. *Telemedicine Journal and e-Health, 10*(2), 260–276. doi:10.1089/tmj.2004.10.260

Szczechowiak, P., Oliveira, L. B., Scott, M., Collier, M., & Dahab, R. (2008). NanoECC: Testing the limits of elliptic curve cryptography in sensor networks. In *Proceedings of the 5th European conference on wireless sensor networks (EWSN),* (Vol. 4913, p. 305-320). Berlin: Springer.

Tachakra, S., Wang, X. H., Istepanian, R. S. H., & Song, Y. H. (2003). Mobile e-Health: The Unwired Evolution of Telemedicine. *Telemedicine Journal and e-Health, 9*(3), 247–257.

Taentzer, G. (2004). *AGG: A Graph Transformation Environment for Modeling and Validation of Software in Application of Graph Transformations with Industrial Relevance. In 2nd Intl. Workshop of AGTIVE.* Charlottesville, NC: Springer.

Takizawa, M. S. (2001). Telemedicine System Using Computed Tomography Van of High-Speed Telecommunication Vehicle. *IEEE Transactions on Information Technology in Biomedicine, 5*(1), 2–9.

Tamura, T., Kawarada, A., Nambu, M., Tsukada, A., Sasaki, K., & Yamakoshi, K. (2007). E-Healthcare at an experimental welfare techno house in Japan. *The Open Medical Informatics Journal, 1,* 1–7. doi:10.2174/1874431100701010001

Tamura, T., Togawa, T., Ogawa, M., & Yoda, M. (1998). Fully automated health monitoring system in the home. *Medical Engineering & Physics, 20,* 573–579. doi:10.1016/S1350-4533(98)00064-2

Tan, C., Wang, H., Zhong, S., & Li, Q. (2008). Body sensor network security: an identity-based cryptography approach. In *WiSec '08: Proceedings of the first ACM conference on wireless network security* (pp. 148–153). New York, NY, USA: ACM.

Tan, J. (Ed.). (2008). *Healthcare Information Systems and Informatics: Research and Pratices.* Hershey, PA: IGI Global Publishers.

Tapia, E., Intille, S. S., & Larson, K. (2004). Activity Recognition in the Home Using Simple and Ubiquitous Sensors. In Pervasive Computing (pp. 158-175).

Tarricone, R., & Tsouros, A. D. (2008). *Home Care in Europe.* World Health Organisation.

Tashiro, S., & Murakami, T. (2008). Step Passage Control of a Power-Assisted Wheelchair for a Caregiver. *Industrial Electronics. IEEE Transactions on, 55,* 1715–1721.

Telehealth can improve quality of life. (2009). *Nursing Standard, 23*(24), 21(21).

Telemonitoring, S. I. C. An Updated Review of the Applicability of ISO/IEEE 11073 Standards for Interoperability in Telemonitoring. In *29th Annual International Conference of the IEEE Engineering in Medicine and Biology Society, 2007. EMBC 2007,* (pp. 6161 – 6165).

Tentori, M., & Favela, J. (2008, April-June). Activity-aware computing for healthcare. *IEEE Pervasive Computing / IEEE Computer Society [and] IEEE Communications Society, 7*(2), 51–57. doi:10.1109/MPRV.2008.24

Tentori, M., Favela, J., & Gonzalez, V. (2006). Quality of Privacy (QoP) for the Design of Ubiquitous Healthcare Applications. *Journal of Universal Computer Science, 12*(3), 252–269.

Tentori, M., Favela, J., & Rodriguez, M. (2006). Privacy-aware Autonomous Agents for Pervasive Healthcare. *IEEE Intelligent Systems, 21*(6), 55–62. doi:10.1109/MIS.2006.118

The Globus Alliance. (n.d.). *The Globus Toolkit.* Retrieved December 12, 2008, from http://www.globus.org/

Thomas, M. P., Burruss, J., Cinquini, L., Fox, G., Gannon, D., & Gilbert, L. (2005). Grid portal architectures for scientific applications. *Journal of Physics: Conference Series, 16,* 596–600. doi:10.1088/1742-6596/16/1/083

Thompson, L. T., Dorsey, M. A., Miller, I. K., & Parrott, R. (Eds.). (2003). Telemedicine: Expanding healthcare into virtual environments. Mahwah, NJ: Handbook of health communication.

Tong, B., & Stevenson, C. (2007). *Comorbidity of cardiovascular disease, diabetes and chronic kidney disease in Australia, AIHW cat. no. CVD 37.* Canberra, Australia: AIHW.

Triantafyllidis, A., Koutkias, V., Chouvarda, I., & Maglaveras, N. (2008). An open and reconfigurable wireless sensor network for pervasive health monitoring. In *Proceedings Second International Conference on Pervasive Computing Technologies for Healthcare PervasiveHealth 2008*, (pp. 112-115).

Troshani, I., & Rao, S. (2007a). The diffusion of mobile services in Australia: an evaluation using stakeholder and transaction cost economics theories. *IADIS International Journal of WWW/Internet, 5*(2), 40-57.

Tsipouras, M. G., Fotiadis, D. I., & Sideris, D. (2005). An arrhythmia classification system based on the RR-interval signal. *Artificial Intelligence in Medicine, 33*(3), 237–250. doi:10.1016/j.artmed.2004.03.007

Tyrer, H. W., Alwan, M., Demiris, G., He, Z., Keller, J., Skubic, M., et al. (2006). Technology for Successful Aging. In *Proceedings of the 28th Intl. Conf. of the IEEE Engineering in Medicine and Biology Society (EMBS)*, (pp. 3290-3293). New York: IEEE Computer Society.

Tyrer, H. W., Aud, M. A., Alexander, G., Skubic, M., & Rantz, M. (2007). Early Detection of Health Changes in Older Adults. In *Proceedings of the 29th Intl. Conf. of the IEEE EMBS* (pp. 4045-4048). Lyon, France: IEEE Computer Society.

*Ubiquitous, Permanent and Intelligent Access to Patients' Medical Files (DOCMEM)*. (2003). Retrieved December 15, 2008, from http://cordis.europa.eu/data/PROJ_FP5/ACTIONeqDndSESSIONeq112422005919ndDOCeq2361ndTBLeqEN_PROJ.htm

Uhsadel, L., Poschmann, A., & Paar, C. (2007). Enabling Full-Size Public-Key Algorithms on 8-bit Sensor Nodes. In *Proceedings of european workshop on security in adhoc and sensor networks (ESAS 2007)* (Vol. 4572, pp.73–86). Berlin: Springer-Verlag.

US Census Bureau. (2008, 13/08/2008). *Projected Population by Single Year of Age, Sex, Race, and Hispanic Origin for the United States: July 1, 2000 to July 1, 2050*. Retrieved 27/01/2009, from http://www.census.gov/population/www/projections/downloadablefiles.html

Van Eyk, H., & Baum, F. (2002). Learning about inter-agency collaboration: Trialling collaborative projects between hospitals and community health services. *Health & Social Care in the Community, 10*(4), 262–269. doi:10.1046/j.1365-2524.2002.00369.x

Vandewalle, J.-J (2004). Smart Card Research Perspectives. *LNCS Construction and Analysis of Safe, Secure and Interoperable Smart devices*.

Vanjara, P. (2006). Application of mobile technologies in healthcare diagnostics and administration. In Lazakidou, A. (Ed.), *Handbook of Research on Informatics in Healthcare and Medicine* (pp. 113–130). Hershey, PA: Idea Group.

Varginadis, Y., Gouvas, P., Bouras, T., & Mentzas, G. (2008). Conceptual Modeling of Service-Oriented Programmable Smart Assistive Environments. In F. Makedon, & L. Baillie (Ed.), *Proceedings of the 1st ACM Intl. Conf. on Pervasive Technologies Related to Assistive Environments, PETRA*, Athens, Greece.

Varshney, U. (2003, Dec.). Pervasive healthcare. *Computer, 36*(12), 138–140. doi:10.1109/MC.2003.1250897

Varshney, U. (2006). Using wireless technologies in healthcare. *International Journal of Mobile Communications, 4*(3), 354–368.

Venkatasubramanian, K., & Gupta, S. (2007). Security in distributed, grid, mobile, and pervasive computing. In Y. Xiao (Ed.), (p. 443-464). Auerbach Publications, CRC Press. Jih, W., Cheng, S., Hsu, J. Y., & Tsai, T. (2005). Context-aware access control in pervasive healthcare. In EEE '05 workshop: Mobility, agents, and mobile services.

Victorian Government. (2007). *Diabetes Prevention and Management: A Strategic Framework for Victoria 1007-2010*. Melbourne, Australia: Victorian Government, Department of Human Services.

Villalba, E., Ottaviano, M., Arredondo, M. T., Martinez, A., & Guillen, S. (2006). Wearable Monitoring System for Heart Failure Assessment in Mobile Environment. *Computers in Cardiology, 33*, 237–240.

Vincent, C., Drouin, G., & Routhier, F. (2002). Examination of new environmental control applications. *Assistive Technology, 14*(2), 98–111.

Virone, G., Alwan, M., Dalal, S., Kell, S. W., Turner, B., & Stankovic, J. A. (2008). Behavioral Patterns of Older Adults in Assisted Living. *IEEE Transactions on Information Technology in Biomedicine, 12*(3), 12. doi:10.1109/TITB.2007.904157

Virone, G., Wood, A., Selavo, L., Cao, Q., Fang, L., Doan, T., et al. (2006). An Assisted Living Oriented Information System Based on a Residential Wireless Sensor Network. In *Proceedings of the 1st Transdisciplinary Conf. on Distributed Diagnosis and Home Healthcare,* (pp. 95-100). Arlington, VA: IEEE Computer Society.

VivoMetrics. (2009). *VivoMetrics LifeShirt System Technology.* Retrieved from http://www.vivometrics.com

Völter, M., Haase, A., Efftinge, S., & Kolb, B. (2006). Graphical Modeling Framework. *iX, 12,* 17.

Voon, R., Celler, B. G., & Lovell, N. H. (2008). *The use of an energy monitor in the management of diabetes: a pilot study.* Diabetes Technology and Therapeutics.

Wade, E., & Asada, H. (2007, Jan.-March). Conductive fabric garment for a cable-free body area network. *IEEE Pervasive Computing / IEEE Computer Society [and] IEEE Communications Society, 6*(1), 52–58. doi:10.1109/MPRV.2007.8

Wald, H., & Shojania, K. G. (2001). Incident reporting. In Shojania, K. G., Ducan, B. W., McDonald, K. M., & Wachter, R. M. (Eds.), *Making health care safer: A critical analysis of patient safety practices* (pp. 41–47). Rockville, MD: Agency for Healthcare Research and Quality.

Wang, X. H., Gu, T., Zhang, D. Q., & Pung, H. K. (2004). Ontology Based Context Modeling and Reasoning using OWL. In *Proceedings of the Intl. Conf. on Pervasive Computing and Communication* (pp. 18-22). Washington, DC: IEEE Computer Society.

Ward, J. A., Lukowicz, P., Troster, G., & Starner, T. E. (2006). Activity Recognition of Assembly Tasks Using Body-Worn Microphones and Accelerometers. *IEEE Transactions on Pattern Analysis and Machine Intelligence, 28*(10), 1553–1567.

Warren, S., Lebak, J., Yao, J., Creekmore, J., Milenkovic, A., & Jovanov, E. (2005). Interoperability and security in wireless body area network infrastructures. In *Proceedings of the 27th annual international conference of the IEEE engineering in medicine and biology society,* (pp. 3837–3840).

Warren, S., Yao, J., & Barnes, G. E. (2002). Wearable sensors and component-based design for home health care. *Annual International Conference of the IEEE Engineering in Medicine and Biology - Proceedings, 3,* 1871-1872.

Washington, DC, USA: IEEE Computer Society. Orwat, C., Graefe, A., & Faulwasser, T. (2008, June). Towards pervasive computing in health care - a literature review. *BMC Medical Informatics and Decision Making, 8,* 26–44. doi:10.1186/1472-6947-8-26

Waterman, J., Curtis, D., Goraczko, M., Shih, E., Sarin, P., Pino, E., et al. (2005). Demonstration of SMART (Scalable Medical Alert Response Technology). *AMIA 2005 Annual Symposium.*

Webb, A. (2001). *The Impact of the Cost of Long-Term Care on the Saving of the Elderly.* New York: International Longevity Center.

Weber, J. S., Clippingdale, B., & Pollack, M. E. (2007). The Michigan Autonomous Guidance System. In *Proceedings of the 2nd International Conference on Technology and Aging.*

Weber, W., Rabaey, J. M., & Aarts, E. H. L. (2005). *Ambient Intelligence.* Berlin: Springer. doi:10.1007/b138670

Weiser, M. (1991). The Computer for the 21st Century. *Scientific American, 265*(3), 94–104.

Weiser, M. (1998). The future of ubiquitous computing on campus. *Communications of the ACM, 41*(1), 41–42. doi:10.1145/268092.268108

Wellard, S. J., Rennie, S., & King, R. (2008). Perceptions of people with type 2 diabetes about self-management and the efficiency of community based services. *Contemporary Nurse, 29*(2), 218–226.

Whitten, P., Doolittle, G., & Heilmich, S. (2001). Telehospice: using telecommunication technology for terminally ill patients. *Comput-Mediat Commun, 6*(4), 43–47.

WHO. (2006). *Building FOUNDATIONS eHealth.*

WHO. (2008). *Home Care in Europe.*

Wickramasinghe, N., & Geisler, E. (Eds.). (2008). *Encyclopedia of Healthcare Information Systems.* Hershey, PA: IGI Global Publishers.

Wickramasinghe, N., & Goldberg, S. (2003). *The wireless panacea for healthcare.* Paper presented at the 36th Hawaii International Conference on System Sciences, Hawaii, 6-10 January, IEEE.

Wickramasinghe, N., & Goldberg, S. (2004). How M=EC2 in healthcare. *International Journal of Mobile Communications, 2*(2), 140–156. doi:10.1504/IJMC.2004.004664

Wickramasinghe, N., & Misra, S. (2004). A wireless trust model for healthcare. *International Journal of e-Health, 1*, 60-77.

Wickramasinghe, N., & Schaffer, J. (2006). Creating knowledge driven healthcare processes with the intelligence continuum. *International Journal of Electronic Healthcare, 2*(2), 164–174.

Wickramasinghe, N., Goldberg, S., & Bali, R. (2007). Enabling Superior M-health Project Success: A tri-Country Validation. *Intl. J. Services and Standards, 4*(1), 97–117. doi:10.1504/IJSS.2008.016087

Wickramasinghe, N., Schaffer, J., & Geisler, E. (2005). Assessing e-health. In Spil, T., & Schuring, R. (Eds.), *E-Health Systems Diffusion and Use: The Innovation, The User, and The User IT Model.* Hershey, PA: Idea Group.

Wild, S., Roglic, G., Green, A., Sicree, R., & King, H. (2004). Global prevalence of diabetes: estimates for the year 2000 and projections for 2030. *Diabetes Care, 27*, 1047–1053. doi:10.2337/diacare.27.5.1047

Wilken, O., Huelsmann, N., & Hein, A. (2009). Bestimmung von Verhaltensmustern basierend auf der Nutzung elektrischer Geräte. *Proceedings of 2nd German AAL congress.*

Williams, G., Doughty, K., & Bradley, D. A. (1998). A systems approach to achieving CarerNet-an integrated and intelligent telecare system. *Information Technology in Biomedicine. IEEE Transactions on, 2*(1), 1–9.

Williams, L. (2003). Medication-Monitoring Lawsuit: Case Study and Lessons Learned. *Nursing Homes/Long Term Care Management, 3.*

Wilson, L. S., Ho, P., Bengston, K. J., Dadd, M. J., Chen, C. F., Huynh, C., et al. (2001). *The CSIRO hospital without walls home telecare system.* Paper presented at the Intelligent Information Systems Conference, The Seventh Australian and New Zealand 2001.

*WiMedia Alliance.* (n.d.). Retrieved from http://www.wimedia.org.

Wiser, M. (1991). The Computer of the twenty-first century. *Scientific American*, 94–110.

Wixon, D., Jones, S., Tse, L., & Casaday, G. (1994). Inspections and design reviews: Framework, history, and reflection. In *Usability Inspection Methods.* New York: John Wiley & Sons.

Wolf, A. (2003). *Behind Closed Doors.* NFPA Journal.

Wolf, D. A., & Jenkins, C. (2008). Family Care and Assisted Living. In Golant, S. M., & Hyde, J. (Eds.), *The Assisted Living Residence.* Baltimore: The Johns Hopkins University Press.

Wolf, P., Schmidt, A., & Klein, M. (2008). SOPRANO - An extensible, open AAL platform for elderly people based on semantical contracts. In *Proceedings of the 3rd Workshop on Artificial Intelligence Techniques for Ambient Intelligence*, Patras, Greece.

Wolfstadt, J. (2008). The effect of computerized physician order entry with clinical decision support on the rates of adverse drug events: a systematic review. *Journal of General Internal Medicine, 23*(4), 451–458. doi:10.1007/s11606-008-0504-5

Wood, A., Virone, G., Doan, T., Cao, Q., Selavo, L., & Wu, Y. (2006). *ALARM-NET: Wireless Sensor Networks for Assisted-Living and Residential Monitoring.* USA: University of Virginia, Department of Computer Science.

Wood, A., Virone, G., Doan, T., Cao, Q., Selavo, L., Wu, Y., et al. (2006). *ALARM-NET: Wireless sensor networks for assisted-living and residential monitoring* (Tech. Rep. No. CS-2006-1). Department of Computer Science, University of Virginia.

Wootton, R. (2001). Telemedicine. *British Medical Journal, 323*, 4.

Wozak, F., Ammenwerth, E., Hoerbst, A., Soegner, P., Mair, R., & Schabetsberger, T. (2008, May). *IHE Based Interoperability – Benefits and Challenges.* Paper presented at the 21st International Congress of the European Federation for Medical Informatics (MIE), Göteborg, Sweden.

Wu, C. W., & Tay, Y. C. (1999). A Multicast Protocol for Ad hoc Wireless Networks. In *IEEE MILCOM'99.* AMRIS.

Wunderlich, G. S., & Kohler, P. O. (2001). *Improving the quality of long-term care: 4. Information systems for monitoring Quality.* Washington, DC: National Academy Press.

Wylde, M. A. (2008). The Future of Assisted Living: Residents' Perspectives 2006-2026. In Golant, S. M., & Hyde, J. (Eds.), *The Assisted Living Residence.* Baltimore: The Johns Hopkins University Press.

Yamaguchi, A., Ogawa, M., Tamura, T., & Togawa, T. (1998). *Monitoring behavior in the home using positioning sensors.* Paper presented at the Engineering in Medicine and Biology Society, 1998. Proceedings of the 20th Annual International Conference of the IEEE.

Yamazaki, T. (2006). Beyond the Smart Home. *Proceedings of the 2006 International Conference on Hybrid Information Technology-Volume 02*, 350-355.

Yang, A.Y., Jafari, R., Sastry, S.S., & Bajcsy, R. (2009). Distributed Recognition of Human Actions Using Wearable Motion Sensor Networks. *Journal of Ambient Intelligence and Smart Environments.*

Yang, N., Barringer, H., & Zhang, N. (2007). A Purpose-Based Access Control Model. In *Symposium in Information Assurance and Security,* (pp. 143-148).

Yao, J., & Warren, S. (2005). Applying the ISO/IEEE 11073 standards to wearable home health monitoring systems. *Journal of Clinical Monitoring and Computing, 19*(6), 427–436. doi:10.1007/s10877-005-2033-7

Yao, J., Shmitz, R., & Warren, S. (2005). A wearable point-of-care system for home use that incorporates plug-and-play and wireless standards. *IEEE Transactions on Information Technology in Biomedicine, 9*(3), 363–371. doi:10.1109/TITB.2005.854507

Yin, S., Pucheral, P., & Meng, X. (2009). A Sequential Indexing Scheme for Flash-Based Embedded Systems. In *International Conference on Extending Database Technology (EDBT).*

Yu, P., Li, H., & Gagnon, M.-P. (2008). Health IT acceptance factors in long-term care facilities: a cross-sectional survey. *International Journal of Health Informatics.* doi:10.1016/j.ijmedinf.2008.07.006

Zaad, L., & Allouch, S. B. (2008). *The Influence of Control on the Acceptance of Ambient Intelligence by Elderly People: An Explorative Study.* Paper presented at the Proceedings of the European Conference on Ambient Intelligence, Nuremberg, Germany.

Zamarripa, M. S., Gonzalez, V. M., & Favela, J. (2007). *The Augmented Patient Chart: Seamless Integration of Physical and Digital Artifacts for Hospital Work.* Paper presented at the HCI.

Zhang, D., Gu, T., & Wang, X. (2005). Enabling context-aware Smart Home with Semantic Web Technologies. *International Journal of Human-friendly Welfare Robotic Systems, 4*(6).

Zhang, X., Parisi-Presicce, F., Sandhu, R., & Park, J. (2005). Formal model and policy specification of usage control. *ACM Transactions on Information and System Security, 8,* 351–387. doi:10.1145/1108906.1108908

Zhao, F., & Guibas, L. (2004). *Wireless Sensor Networks - An Information Processing Approach.* San Francisco: Morgan Kaufmann.

Zigbor, J. C., & Songer, T. J. (2001). External barriers to diabetes care: addressing personal and health systems issues. *Diabetes Spectrum, 14,* 23–28. doi:10.2337/diaspect.14.1.23

Zimmerman, T., Smith, J., Paradiso, J., Allport, D., & Gershenfeld, N. (1995). Applying electric field sensing to human computer interfaces. In SIGCHI conference on Human factors in computing systems, May 7-11 1995 (pp. 280–287). Denver, CO: ACM Press.

# About the Contributors

**Antonio Coronato** received the degree in information engineering at the University "Federico II" of Naples in the 1998. He is a researcher at the Institute for High Performance Computing and Networking (ICAR) of the italian National Research Council (CNR). He is grant professor of Software Engineering at the University "Federico II" of Naples and Object Oriented Programming at the Second University of Naples. He is an associate editor for the *Journal of Security and Communication Networks*, a member of the international editorial board for the *Journal of Smart Home*, the *Journal of Multimedia and Ubiquitous Engineering* and the *Journal of Software Architecture*. He is also involved in the organization of several international conferences on pervasive computing. His research interests are in the field of pervasive computing, middleware and component-based architectures and dependable computing.

**Giuseppe De Pietro** received the degree in electronic engineering at the University "Federico II" of Naples in the 1988. He is a senior researcher at the Institute for High Performance Computing and Networking (ICAR) of the Italian National Research Council (CNR). He is grant professor of Information Systems at the Second University of Naples. He is a member of the international editorial board for the *Journal of Smart Home* and the *Journal of Multimedia and Ubiquitous Engineering*. He is also involved in the organization of several international conferences on pervasive computing. His research interests are in the field of pervasive computing, graphics and virtual reality environments, middleware and component-based architectures, software engineering. He is a member of the IEEE.

\* \* \*

**Tristan Allard** is a Ph.D. Student at University of Versailles, France. He received his engineering degree from the ESILV, France, in 2006 and his M. S. degree with highest honours from the University of Versailles in 2007. His research interests encompass privacy and data distribution.

**Nicolas Anciaux** is a Researcher at INRIA, France. He received his Ph.D. in Computer Science from the University of Versailles in 2004. After one year at University of Twente, Netherlands, he joined the SMIS (Secured and Mobile Information Systems) at INRIA Rocquencourt. His main research area is embedded data management and privacy, in particular in the context of ambient intelligence. He has co-authored more than fifteen journal and conference papers.

**Luc Bouganim** is a Director of Research at INRIA Rocquencourt. He obtained a PhD and the Habilitation à Diriger des Recherches, both from the University of Versailles in 1996 and 2006, respectively.

He worked as an assistant professor from 1997 to 2002 when he joined INRIA. Luc co-authored more than 60 conference and journal papers, an international patent and was the recipient of 4 international awards. Since 2000, Luc is strongly engaged in research activities on ubiquitous data management and data confidentiality. He is currently the vice-head of the SMIS (Secured and Mobile Information Systems) research team.

**Leroy Lai Yu Chan** received the B.E. (Hons) degree in electrical engineering and the M.Biomed.E degree in biomedical engineering from the University of New South Wales (UNSW), Sydney, Australia, in 2001. Currently, he is pursuing the Ph.D. degree at the School of Electrical and Telecommunications Engineering at UNSW. His research focuses on smart wireless sensor networks for residential aged care management and care level classification.

**Branko George Celler** received the B.Sc. degree in computer science and physics, the B.E. (Hons) degree in electrical engineering, and the Ph.D. degree in biomedical engineering from the University of New South Wales (UNSW), Sydney, Australia, in 1969, 1972, and 1978, respectively. From 1977 to 1980, he was a Postdoctoral Fellow working at the Johns Hopkins School of Medicine in Baltimore, MD. He returned to UNSW in 1981 as a Lecturer, where he was appointed an Associate Professor in 1991 and a Professor in January 1997. Prof. Celler is a Foundation Member of the Australian College of Medical Informatics and was the Foundation Co-Director of the Centre for Health Informatics at UNSW.

**Hsiao-Hwa Chen** is currently a full Professor in Department of Engineering Science, National Cheng Kung University, Taiwan, and he was the founding Director of the Institute of Communications Engineering of the National Sun Yat-Sen University, Taiwan. He received BSc and MSc degrees from Zhejiang University, China, and PhD degree from University of Oulu, Finland, in 1982, 1985 and 1990, respectively, all in Electrical Engineering. He has authored or co-authored over 200 technical papers in major international journals and conferences, five books and several book chapters in the areas of communications, including the books titled "Next Generation Wireless Systems and Networks" (512 pages) and "The Next Generation CDMA Technologies" (468 pages), both published by John Wiley and Sons in 2005 and 2007, respectively. He has been an active volunteer for IEEE various technical activities for over 20 years. Currently, he is serving as the Chair of IEEE ComSoc Radio Communications Committee, and the Vice Chair of IEEE ComSoc Communications \& Information Security Technical Committee. He served or is serving as symposium chair/co-chair of many major IEEE conferences, including VTC, ICC, Globecom and WCNC, etc. He served or is serving as Associate Editor or/and Guest Editor of numerous important technical journals in communications. He is serving as the Chief Editor (Asia and Pacific) for Wiley's Wireless Communications and Mobile Computing (WCMC) Journal and Wiley's International Journal of Communication Systems, etc. He is the Editor-in-Chief of Wiley' Security and Communication Networks journal (www.interscience.wiley.com/journal/security). He is also an adjunct Professor of Zhejiang University, China, and Shanghai Jiao Tung University, China.

**Dorothy Curtis** is a Research Scientist at the Computer Science and Artificial Intelligence Laboratory (CSAIL) at the Massachusetts Institute of Technology in Cambridge, Massachusetts, USA. Her work focuses on physiological monitoring and indoor location systems. She has built other real-time systems, in the fields of computer networking and shipboard collision detection and avoidance and navigation. Other computer science interests include natural language processing, compilers, and object-oriented databases. She holds degrees from the Massachusetts Institute of Technology, Boston University, and Simmons College.

**Axel Czabke** was born in Munich, Germany, on April 17th 1981. He studied mechanical engineering with focus on mechatronics and systematical product development. In 2008 he received his Dipl.-Ing. degree (M.S.) from the Technical University of Munich, Germany. He is currently working toward the Doctorate degree at the Department of Micro Technology and Medical Device Technology of the Technical University of Munich. His research interests include the development of mobile assistant devices for elderly people and analysis of activity patterns.

**Lorenzo T. D'Angelo** was born in La Spezia, Italy, on January 6th 1983. He studied mechanical engineering with focus on mechatronics at the Technical University of Karlsruhe, Germany. He received the Dipl.-Ing. degree (M.S.) in 2006. He is currently working toward the Doctorate degree at the Department of Micro Technology and Medical Device Technology of the Technical University of Munich. His research interests include the development of intelligent textiles, mobile assistant devices for elderly people and activity logging.

**Arianna D'Ulizia** received her degree in Computer Science Engineering at the University of Rome 'La Sapienza' in 2005 and her doctoral degree in Computer Science and Automation at the 'Roma Tre' University in 2009. She is actually researcher at the Institute of Research on Population and Social Policies of the National Research Council of Italy. She is the author of more than 30 papers on books and conferences. She is mainly interested in Human Computer Interaction, Multimodal Interaction, Visual Languages, Visual Interfaces and Geographical Query Languages.

**Jesus Favela** is a professor of computer science at CICESE, where he leads the Mobile and Ubiquitous Healthcare Laboratory. His research interests include ambient computing, medical informatics, and human computer-interaction. Since 2001 much of his efforts have focused on the design and evaluation of ubiquitous computing environments for healthcare. In collaboration with public and private Mexican hospitals his research team has conducted fieldwork studies to gain a better understanding of current work practices and design and evaluate pervasive computing technology for such complex environments. He holds a Bs from the Universidad Nacional Autónoma de México (UNAM) and received a MSc and PhD from the Massachusetts Institute of Technology (MIT). He's a member of the ACM and former president of the Sociedad Mexicana de Ciencia de la Computación (SMCC).

**Fernando Ferri** received the degree in Electronics Engineering and the PhD in Medical Informatics. He is actually senior researcher at the National Research Council of Italy. From 1993 to 2000 he was professor of "Sistemi di Elaborazione" at the University of Macerata. He is the author of more than 100 papers in international journals, books and conferences. His main methodological areas of interest are: Human-Computer Interaction, Visual Languages, Visual Interfaces, Sketch-based Interfaces, Multimodal Interfaces, Data and knowledge bases, Geographic Information Systems and Virtual Communities. He has been responsible of several national and international research projects.

**Eliezer (Elie) Geisler** is the IIT Distinguished Professor at the Stuart School of Business, Illinois Institute of Technology and Director of the IIT Center for the Management of Medical Technology.

He holds a doctorate from the Kellogg School at Northwestern University. Dr. Geisler authored over 100 papers in the areas of technology and innovation management, the evaluation of R&D, science and technology, knowledge management, and the management of healthcare and medical technology. He authored and edited twelve books. He consulted for major corporations and for many U.S. federal departments. Dr. Geisler is the co-founder of the annual conferences on the Hospital of the Future, and the Health Care Technology Management Association. His current research interests include the metrics of technological innovation and knowledge, and knowledge management in complex systems.

**Steve Goldberg** started his 24-year information technology career at Systemhouse Ltd. At Crowntek, he developed a $30 million IT services business. During his tenure at Cybermation, he transformed the organization from mainframe to client/server solution delivery. Prior to INET, at Compugen he successfully built and managed teams to deliver enterprise e-business solutions. Mr. Goldberg has a B.A. (Economics & Computer Science) from the University of Western Ontario. He is on the Editorial Board of the International Journal of Networking and Virtual Organizations, and has many papers accepted under peer review at international conferences and published in international journals.

**Victor M. Gonzalez** is a Lecturer (Assistant Professor) in Human-Computer Interaction at the Manchester Business School of the University of Manchester, United Kingdom. He is an applied computer science researcher, focusing on studying and designing for the 'praxis' of work, personal and social spheres of human activity. Dr. Gonzalez is a Senior Research Fellow of CRITO (Centre for Research on Information Technology and Organizations) at the University of California at Irvine. He received a Ph.D. and Master degrees in Information and Computer Science from the University of California at Irvine and a Master degree in Telecommunications and Information Systems from the University of Essex, United Kingdom. He is a member of BCS HCI, IEEE, ACM SIGCHI and vice-president of SIG-CHI Mexican Chapter.

**Patrizia Grifoni** received the degree in Electronics Engineering. He is actually researcher at the National Research Council of Italy. From 1994 to 2000 she was professor of "Elaborazione digitale delle immagini" at the University of Macerata. She is the author of more than 80 papers in international journals, books and conferences. Her scientific interests have evolved from Query Languages for statistical and Geographic Databases to the focal topics related to Human-Computer Interaction, Multimodal Interaction, Visual Languages, Visual Interfaces, Sketch-based Interfaces, Accessing Web Information and Virtual Communities. She was responsible of several research projects.

**Tiziana Guzzo**: she received the degree in Sociology and the PhD in Theory and Social Research at the University of Rome "La Sapienza". She is actually researcher at the Institute of Research on Population and Social Policies of the National Research Council of Italy. From 2005 to 2008 she was professor of Sociology at the University of Catanzaro. Her main areas of interest are: Social Science, Information Communication Technologies, Communication Science, Social Networks and Risk Governance.

**Yutaka Kimura** received MD from Kansai Medical School in 1981. Since 1981, he has been a post-doctoral fellow at University of Connecticut University and University of Toronto, Canada. Since 2006 he joined Kansai Medical School, Health centre as a Director. He is currently a Professor and Director, Kansai Medical School, Health Science Centre. His interests include prevention of metabolic syndrome, home health care, and sport medicine.

**Werner Kurschl** is a professor in the Department Software Engineering at the Upper Austria University of Applied Sciences, School of Informatics, Communication, and Media. He holds a PhD and MS from the Johannes Kepler University Linz. He is the head of the Smart environments and mobile enterprise (SMART) research group, which is working on wireless sensor networks for eldercare and industrial appliances, ambient-assisted living, position and tracking technologies, speech processing applications, and cloud computing. He teaches wireless sensor networks, component-based software development and software architectures, web architectures and frameworks, and mobile computing at the university.

**Vassiliki Koufi** was born in Athens, Greece. She received a B.Sc. in Informatics from the University of Piraeus (2001) and an M.Sc. in Data Communication Systems from Brunel University, UK (2003). Since 2003 she is a Ph.D candidate in the Department of Digital Systems at the University of Piraeus while she works as a network engineer in the Network Management Center at the University of Piraeus. She has been actively involved in several projects concerning the development of healthcare information systems and other web-based applications as well as the development and management of telecommunication services and applications. Her research interests include ubiquitous and pervasive healthcare, context-aware healthcare information systems, process-oriented web-based and grid-based healthcare information systems and healthcare information systems security.

**Ioannis Krontiris** is a researcher at Computer Science in the School of Mathematics and Computer Science at University of Mannheim, Germany. He holds a Master degree from Carnegie Mellon University, Pennsylvania, USA and a PhD degree from Mannheim University, Germany. Dr. Krontiris has been working for several years in the area of embedded distributed systems and especially security in wireless sensor networks. His main technical interests lie in the areas of pervasive healthcare, and reliability and privacy of distributed systems.

**Tim Christian Lueth**, full professor, was born in Hamburg, Germany, on November 30th 1965. In combination of functions, he is director (chair) of the Institute for Micro Technology and Medical Device Technology (MIMED) of the Technical University of Munich, Germany and also co-director of the Central Institute of Medical Engineering (IMETUM) of the Technical University of Munich. He is member of the Mechanical Engineering Faculty and the Medical Faculty (Klinikum rechts der Isar, MRI). End of 2006, Dr. Lueth recieved an appointment as full professor (status only) at the University of Toronto, Canada, the Department of Medical Imaging. Prof. Dr. Lueth received a Dipl.-Ing. degree (M.S.) in electrical engineering of the Technical University Darmstadt in 1989, his Ph.D. in robotics of the University Karlsruhe, 1993, and the state doctorate (Habilitation, Priv. Doz.) for computer science of the University Karlsruhe in 1997. He received several fellowships and awards for his work.

**Matti Tapio Linnavuo** was born in Porvoo, Finland, in 1954. He received his M.Sc. degree in 1978 and Lic. (Tech) degree in 1982 in electrical engineering from Helsinki University of Technology, Espoo, Finland. He has worked as Acting Professor in hardware technologies at Helsinki University of Technology, and as a project manager at Instrumentarium Oy, Finland. His present position is Laboratory Manager at the Department of Electronics, Helsinki University of Technology, Espoo, Finland. His main interests are medical electronics and health care instrumentation. Mr. Linnavuo is a member of the Finnish Society of Electronics Engineers and the Finnish Association of Graduate Engineers.

**Nigel Hamilton Lovell** received the B.E. (Hons.) and Ph.D. degrees from the University of New South Wales (UNSW), Sydney, Australia. He is currently a Professor of Biomedical Engineering at the Graduate School of Biomedical Engineering, UNSW, and an Adjunct Professor in the School of Electrical Engineering and Telecommunications, UNSW. He is the author or coauthor of more than 300 refereed journals, conference proceedings, book chapters and patents. His current research interests include cardiac modeling, home telecare technologies, biological signal processing and visual prosthesis design. He has served in numerous roles on the Administrative Committee of the IEEE Engineering in Medicine and Biology Society, including Vice President for Member and Student Activities and Vice President for Conferences.

**Lucila Ohno-Machado**, MD, PhD, Professor and Chief of the Division of Biomedical Informatics at UCSD, holds a medical degree from the University of São Paulo in Brazil and a PhD in Medical Information Sciences and Computer Science from Stanford University where she was a research fellow in medicine from 1991 to 1996. She served as an instructor, assistant professor, and associate professor in the Department of Radiology and the Division of Health Sciences and Technology at Harvard-MIT, where she developed and taught new graduate courses in the computer science department. She is an elected fellow of the American College of Medical Informatics and of the American Institute for Medical and Biological Engineering. Besides her UCSD responsibilities, she is associate editor of the Journal of the American Medical Informatics Association, and will also serve as associate editor of the Journal of Biomedical Informatics starting 2010. She chairs the scientific program committee for the 2009 American Medical Informatics Association Annual Symposium.

**Ilias Maglogiannis** (imaglo@ucg.gr) received a Diploma in Electrical & Computer Engineering and a Ph.D. in Biomedical Engineering and Medical Informatics from the National Technical University of Athens (NTUA) Greece in 1996 and 2000 respectively. From 1996 until 2000 he worked as a Researcher in the Biomedical Engineering Laboratory in NTUA. Since 2001 he was a Lecturer in the Dept of Information and Communication Systems Engineering in University of the Aegean. Since 2008 he serves as Assistant Professor in the Dept of Computer Science and Biomedical Informatics in the University of Central Greece. He has been principal investigator in many European and National Research programs in Biomedical Engineering and Informatics. He has served on program committees of national and international conferences and he is a reviewer for several scientific journals. His scientific activities include biomedical engineering, image processing, computer vision and multimedia communications. He is the author of over one hundred (100) publications in the above areas. He is a member of the IEEE, the SPIE, and the Hellenic Association of Biomedical Engineering.

**Flora Malamateniou** was born in Athens, Greece. She received the B.Sc degree in Statistics from the University of Piraeus in 1993 and the M.Sc and the Ph.D degree in Health Informatics from the University of Athens in 1995 and 1999, respectively. She has worked as a senior researcher at Research Academic Computer Technology Institute, Greece during 2000-2004 and at Informatics and Telematics Institute Centre for Research and Technology, Greece during 2004-2008. She has been actively involved in many national and EU-funded R&TD projects and in the European IST programmes, E2R I/II, TENCompetence, iCLASS, C-CARE and LIMBER. Currently, she is an Assistant Professor at the Department of Digital Systems of the University of Piraeus. Her current research interests include process-oriented, web-based healthcare information systems, pervasive healthcare, virtual healthcare records, information security and workflow systems.

**Stefan Mitsch** studied Software Engineering at the Upper Austria University of Applied Sciences in Hagenberg from 2000 to 2004. After his diploma thesis on performance profiling of mobile Java applications at the Siemens Corporate Technology Research Department in Munich, Stefan Mitsch joined the R&D department of the Upper Austria University of Applied Sciences, School of Informatics, Communications, and Media (Hagenberg Campus) as a researcher, working from 2004 to 2009 in several projects situated in the area of Ubiquitous Industrial Environments and Wireless Sensor Networks. Since 2009 Stefan Mitsch is affiliated with the Department of Bioinformatics at the Johannes Kepler University Linz as project assistant and PhD student in the BeAware! project focusing on situation awareness.

**Isao Mizukura\*** received BS and MS form Faculty of Engineering, Keio University in 1974,1976 respectively. Sine 1976 he joined at Mitsubishi Electric Co. Ltd. He is currently a manager of health promotion section Nagoya Engineering office at Mitsubishi Electric Engineering Co.Ltd. He is also a Ph.D candidate of Graduate school of Engineering. Chiba University. He developed several medical and care devices such as servo-controlled Exercise therapy devices. From 2003 to 2006 he has been a member of the national project of Home-healthcare in Japan with 12 companies, which he involves an analysis, and synthesis of telecare data processing.

**Esteban Pino,** ScD, is an assistant professor at the Electrical Engineering Department at the Universidad de Concepción in Concepción, Chile. He graduated as an electronics engineer and then obtained a MSc degree from the same institution. After a short period in the industry, he pursued doctoral studies while actively involved in the Biomedical Engineering program planning and creation in 2005. He was a research fellow at the Brigham and Women's Hospital in Boston, Massachusetts, working on ambulatory patient monitoring from 2004 to 2006. His research interests include distributed monitoring systems and biomedical signal processing.

**Philippe Pucheral** is Professor at the University of Versailles, currently in secondment at INRIA Rocquencourt where he is heading the SMIS (Secured and Mobile Information Systems) research team. He obtained a PhD in Computer Science from the University Paris 6 in 1991 and the Habilitation à Diriger des Recherches from the University of Versailles in 1999. He (co-) authored more than 60 conference and journal papers, 4 international patents, 4 books and was the recipient of 4 international awards (EDBT'92, VLDB'2000, e-gate'2004, SIMagine'2005). His domain of interest covers database systems, mobile and embedded databases and database security.

**Henry Jouni Alex Rimminen** was born in Helsinki, Finland, in 1981. He received his M.Sc. degree in electrical engineering from Helsinki University of Technology, Espoo, Finland, in 2006. He joined the Department of Electrical and Communications Engineering, Helsinki University of Technology, as a student in 2001. He is a corporal in the Finnish army reserve, and is currently working as a research scientist at the Applied Electronics research group, Department of Electronics, Helsinki University of Technology, Espoo. His main interests are embedded systems and capacitive sensors. Mr. Rimminen is a member of the Finnish Society of Electronics Engineers and the Finnish Association of Graduate Engineers.

**Johannes Schönböck** studied Software Engineering for Business and Finance at the Upper Austrian University of Applied Science in Hagenberg from 2001 to 2005. During his study, he did his internship as well as my diploma thesis at the Siemens Corporate Technology Research Department in Munich focusing on Model-Driven Software Development (MDSD). From 2005 to 2009 Johannes Schönböck worked at the R&D department of the Upper Austria University of Applied Sciences, School of Informatics, Communication, and Media (Campus Hagenberg) in the area of Wireless Sensor Networks and MDSD . Since March 2009 he is working at the Business Informatics Group at the Technical University of Vienna as project assistant and PhD student in the TROPIC project focusing on model transformations.

**Thomas Stair** graduated from Harvard Medical School, completed residency training in emergency medicine at Georgetown University, and served on the faculty at Georgetown for twenty years, where he was director of clinical informatics, assistant dean for continuing medical education, residency director and chair of emergency medicine. Ten years ago he returned to teach at Harvard and also sees patients in the Emergency Department of Brigham and Women's Hospital. He has edited and co-authored textbooks of emergency medicine, published articles on technology assessment, volunteered with the National Disaster Medical System and served as the President of the Society for Academic Emergency Medicine.

**Toshiyo Tamura** received his BS and MS degrees from Keio University, Japan, in 1971 and 73, respectively and Ph.D. from Tokyo Medical and Dental University in 1980. He is currently a Professor, Department of Medical System Engineering, Graduate School of Engineering, Chiba University, Japan. He also holds several adjunct positions in universities in Japan. His research interests include biomedical instrumentation, biosignal processing, telemedicine telecare and home care technology. His research has resulted in over 100 reviewed articles. He has served as a chair of IEEE/EMBS Tokyo Chapter in 1996-2000, and the Asian Pacific representative for the EMBS from 2000 to 2004. He is currently a board member of Japanese society of Medical electronics and Biological Engineering Also he serves as the Editor-in-chief of the Japanese Journal of Medical electronics and Biological Engineering in 2008-2010.

**Haruyuki Tatsumi** received MD from Yamagata University School of Medicine in 1982. From 1984 to 1998, he has been working at Department Anatomy, Osaki University, Since 1999, he joined at Department of Anatomy, Sapporo Medical School as an Associated Professor. He is currently a Professor in Department Biological informatics and Anatomy,, Sapporo Medical University. His interests include anatomy, bioinformatics and internet application on home health care.

**Monica Tentori** is a lecturer in computer science at UABC, Ensenada, México. Much of her research is an intersection of computer science, behavioral sciences, design and several other fields of study with the aim at understanding the interactions between people, technology and the environment to develop ubiquitous environments to effectively enhance humans interactions with their world and particularly to improve the lifestyle of people with cognitive disabilities and their caregivers. Her past work has involved the design of ubiquitous applications in support of hospital work. Her research interests include ubiquitous computing, HCI, Medical Informatics, Mobile Computing and CSCW. She holds a Bs from the Universidad Autónoma de Baja California (UABC) and received a MSc and PhD from the Centro Investigación Científica y de Educación Superior de Ensenada (CICESE).

**Romuald Thion** received his Ph.D. in computer science from the University of Lyon (Institut National des Sciences Appliquées de Lyon - INSA) in 2008. His main research interests are databases, logic, access control, privacy and formal management of obligations. He is currently a postdoctoral research fellow in the LICIT (Legal Issues in Communication and Information Technologies) team at INRIA Grenoble.

**Indrit Troshani**, PhD MSc is a senior lecturer in Information Systems at the University of Adelaide Business School. Malaysia. His research interests include adoption and diffusion of network innovations in Business-to-Business (B2B) settings and mobile services. Dr Troshani has contributed to the body of knowledge in electronic commerce and information systems by co-authoring refereed journal and international conference publications. His work has appeared in European Journal of Innovation Management, Electronic Markets, International Journal of E-Business Research, Journal of Theoretical and Applied Electronic Commerce Research, International Journal of Mobile Communications and others.

**Giuseppe Turchetti** holds a Laurea Degree in economics from the University of Pisa and a PhD in economics and management from the Scuola Superiore Sant'Anna (SSSA) in Pisa, where he is Associate Professor of Economics and Management. He is cofounder of two Research Centers of SSSA on Technologies and Services for the Support of Longevity and on Management and Innovation, and Director of the Research Centre on European Transplantation Management (ETXMAN Centre) of SSSA. Dr. Turchetti's main research interests are in the fields of organization, financing and evaluation of healthcare services and technologies, and in the area of the economic issues of litigation and pain and suffering. He is author/coauthor of seven books and of over eighty scholarly papers/book chapters.

**George Vassilacopoulos** was born in Athens, Greece, received his Ph.D. degree from the University of London, U.K. and he is currently a Professor at the Department of Digital Systems of the University of Piraeus. He has been an advisor of health informatics to the Greek Minister of Health, a member of the board of two major Athens hospitals and an advisor of informatics to the National Ambulance Service of Greece. He has actively participated in several research and development projects at both National and European levels. His research interests include healthcare information systems, workflow systems, healthcare systems security, web-based healthcare information systems and electronic patient records. He has authored numerous publications in these areas in international journals and refereed conferences. He is a member of BCS and IEEE.

**Demosthenes Vouyioukas** received the Diploma in Electrical and Computer Engineering from the National Technical University of Athens, Greece, in 1996 and the Ph.D. degree in Wireless Communications from the School of Electrical and Computer Engineering in National Technical University of Athens, in July 2003. He also received a Joint Engineering-Economics M.Sc. from the National Technical University of Athens. Since 2004 he was an adjunct lecturer and researcher of the Department of Information and Communication Systems Engineering at the University of the Aegean located at Samos Island, Greece. Now, he serves as Assistant Professor at the same Department. The areas of expertise are wireless communications systems, analog and digital communication systems, Wireless Sensors and Broadband Networks, Digital Video Broadcasting (DVB), Satellite Systems, DVB-RCS, UMTS and HSPA systems and applications and MIMO systems. Within these topics he has published more than 50 journals, book chapters and international conferences and he is also reviewer in several scientific journals. He is a member of IEEE since 1997, a member of the Communication Society of the Greek Section of IEEE and also a member of the Technical Chamber of Greece since 1997.

**Nilmini Wickramasinghe**, PhD MBA researches and teaches within Information Systems. She is well published having written several books, over 100 refereed scholarly papers and co-edited an encyclopedia. Currently, she is the associate director of the Center for Management Medical Technology (CMMT) at Illinois Institute of Technology, USA and holds a professor position at RMIT University, Australia. In addition, she is the editor-in-chief of the international journal of networking and virtual orgnaisations (IJNVO) and the inaugural editor-in-chief of the international journal of biomedical engineering and technology (IJBET) both published by InderScience.

**Yang Xiao** worked in industry as a MAC (Medium Access Control) architect involving the IEEE 802.11 standard enhancement work before he joined Department of Computer Science at The University of Memphis in 2002. He is currently with Department of Computer Science (with tenure) at The University of Alabama. He was a voting member of IEEE 802.11 Working Group from 2001 to 2004. He is an IEEE Senior Member. He is a member of American Telemedicine Association. He currently serves as Editor-in-Chief for International Journal of Security and Networks (IJSN), International Journal of Sensor Networks (IJSNet), and International Journal of Telemedicine and Applications (IJTA). He serves as a referee/reviewer for many funding agencies, as well as a panelist for NSF and a member of Canada Foundation for Innovation (CFI)'s Telecommunications expert committee. He serves on TPC for more than 100 conferences such as INFOCOM, ICDCS, MOBIHOC, ICC, GLOBECOM, WCNC, etc. He serves as an associate editor for several journals, e.g., IEEE Transactions on Vehicular Technology. His research areas are security, telemedicine, robot, sensor networks, and wireless networks. He has published more than 300 papers in major journals, refereed conference proceedings, book chapters related to these research areas. Dr. Xiao's research has been supported by the US National Science Foundation (NSF), U.S. Army Research, Fleet & Industrial Supply Center San Diego (FISCSD), and The University of Alabama's Research Grants Committee. Dr. Xiao is a Guest Professor of Jilin University, and an Adjunct Professor of Zhejiang University. Email: yangxiao@ieee.org

**Shuyan Xie** studies at University of Alabama within the Health Care Management undergraduate program, and she is a candidate of the manager assistant at Veteran Affair Medical Center after graduation. Since 2008, she has worked for Professor Yang Xiao where her jobs have included writing papers on various healthcare topics, assisting in health-care organization surveys, and visiting nursing homes and different health-care providers. During her past four years, Shuyan had experience in teaching aerobic classes as a group leader--- planning, coordinating, and directing operation of the patient information system as an administrative assistant at National Maternity Hospital in Dublin, Ireland. These duties combine with her special interest in healthcare development of healthcare management in varieties. In her spare time, she likes to travel, do yoga, reading etc. Shuyan can be reached at rainnyxie@gmail.com.

**James Zhaonan Zhang** received the B.E. (Hons) degree in telecommunications engineering and the M.Biomed.E degree in biomedical engineering from the University of New South Wales (UNSW), Sydney, Australia, in 2006. Currently, he is pursuing the Ph.D. degree at the School of Electrical and Telecommunications Engineering at UNSW. His research focuses on knowledge management, data fusion and decision support based on wireless sensor network technology.

# Index